Practical Allergy

Practical Allergy

Etan C. Milgrom, MD
Acute Care Staff Physician
University Park Health Center
Clinical Associate Professor of Family
    Medicine
Keck School of Medicine
University of Southern California
Los Angeles, California

Richard P. Usatine, MD
Professor and Vice Chair for Education
Director of Medical Student Education
Department of Family and Community
    Medicine
University of Texas Health Science Center
San Antonio, Texas

Ricardo Antonio Tan, MD
Practicing Allergist
California Allergy and Asthma Medical Group,
    Inc.
Los Angeles, California

Sheldon L. Spector, MD
Clinical Professor of Medicine
Division of Allergy and Clinical Immunology
Department of Medicine
UCLA School of Medicine
Director
California Allergy and Asthma Medical Group,
    Inc.
Los Angeles, California

2004

Mosby
An Affiliate of Elsevier

Mosby

An Affiliate of Elsevier

The Curtis Center
Independence Square West
Philadelphia, Pennsylvania 19106

PRACTICAL ALLERGY   ISBN 0-32301236-1

NOTICE

Allergy/Immunology is an ever-changing field. Standard safety precautions must be followed, but as new research and clinical experience broaden our knowledge, changes in treatment and drug therapy may become necessary or appropriate. Readers are advised to check the most current product information provided by the manufacturer of each drug to be administered to verify the recommended dose, the method and duration of administration, and contraindications. It is the responsibility of the licensed prescriber, relying on experience and knowledge of the patient, to determine dosages and the best treatment for each individual patient. Neither the publisher nor the author assumes any liability for any injury and/or damage to persons or property arising from this publication.

Library of Congress Cataloging-in-Publication Data
Practical allergy / [edited by] Etan C. Milgrom ... [et al.]—1st ed.
      p. ; cm.
    Includes bibliographical references and index.
    ISBN 0-323-01236-1
    1. Allergy. I. Milgrom, Etan C.
  [DNLM: 1. Hypersensitivity—diagnosis. 2. Hypersensitivity—therapy. 3. Patient Education. 4. Primary Health Care—methods. WD 300 P8948 2004]
  RC584.P685 2004
  616.97—dc22   2003059692

Acquisitions Editor: Thomas H. Moore
Developmental Editor: Marla Sussman

Printed in China.

Last digit is the print number: 9   8   7   6   5   4   3   2   1

"... endow me with the strength to equally serve humankind,
to simply see in each individual, a fellow human being in pain ..."
"THE PHYSICIAN'S PRAYER," MAIMONIDES

To my wife Debby and children Jonathan, Sarah, and Hannah
for their boundless love and devotion

my parents Jo and Jacob Milgrom who gave me passion for learning
Beverly and Lou Barak who taught me dedication.

To my lovely wife Janna and my wonderful children Rebecca and Jeremy
for all their love and support through the many life changes over the past year

my sister Karen, I wish her many years of health and happiness.

To Patricio and Leticia Tan, for all their love, sacrifices,
and support through the years.

To my wife, Judith Spector and three wonderful children:
Daniel, Tahlia, and Ilana.

PREFACE

Practical Allergy is a hands-on guide created to facilitate the diagnosis and treatment of allergic disorders with a focus on patient needs and concerns. Written with primary care clinicians in mind, this practical guide provides essential knowledge for experienced physicians, midlevel practitioners, residents, and medical students. Readers will find valuable learning opportunities throughout, specifically geared toward diagnosing and treating the most common allergic conditions seen in the offices of primary care, allergy, and ENT clinicians.

One of the unique features of this book is its editorial team, consisting of a highly experienced family physician, two veteran allergists, and led by a skilled family physician who completed an allergy and immunology fellowship. The result is a book that organically blends the varied expertise of the writers and translates into an eminently useful approach to the learning and utilization of cutting-edge techniques in the diagnosis and treatment of allergy and immunology that are immediately applicable in the day-to-day primary care setting.

The text is divided into three sections. The first section covers common, clinically relevant topics in the field of allergy and immunology. The second section focuses on hands-on clinical allergy skills that can be learned and applied in primary care offices. Each technique discussed is intended to help fine-tune our readers' diagnostic and management skills. The final section, the appendix, contains a compilation of relevant reference material frequently used in busy allergy practices.

Full-color photographs and illustrations are presented frequently throughout the book in an effort to enhance learning the diagnoses and treatments of allergic disorders. Far from being merely a "how-to" guide, our book provides the necessary foundation and supporting literature to help readers practice evidence-based allergy. Where appropriate, we also provide rationales for deciding when to refer difficult cases. All chapters are edited in an outline fashion to make the text especially user friendly and to allow for easy access to important and pertinent information. Where appropriate, practice guidelines, internet resources, ICD–9 codes, and diagnosis and management algorithms are readily available.

Practical Allergy also comes with a CD-ROM devoted to patient education. Information on this CD-ROM was gathered and developed over many years of clinical practice and with direct feedback from hundreds of patients. It has been formatted to provide readily accessible, easy-to-understand handouts for adult and pediatric patients. These handouts can be easily modified to fit specific practice requirements. Additional patient education material can also be found at the end of most chapters. The CD-ROM also contains a short video segment of rhinolaryngoscopy for clinicians who are interested in exploring this technique further.

The CD-ROM and other resources in this book will enhance your ability to communicate with your patients about their allergic disorders. It is our strongly held belief that promotion of patient-clinician communication heightens patient compliance and ultimately leads to improved therapeutic responses. Indeed, by trying to see disease through the eyes of our patients, we render care that is more sensitive to their feelings, needs, and concerns, which, ultimately, can only better the care that we provide.

Special thanks are due to all the contributors to this book for their time and dedication. We are especially grateful to Marla Sussman, Developmental Editor at Elsevier Science, for her unfailing perseverance and the considerable expertise that helped to create this book. We would also like to acknowledge Dr. Thomas Zuber, Dr. Daniel Stulberg, and Hollister-Stier Laboratories LLC, for generously sharing their photographs.

CONTRIBUTORS

Joe Belleau, MD
Fellow
Department of Allergy and Immunology
University of Tennessee, Memphis
Memphis, TN

George W. Bensch, MD
Chief
Allergy, Immunology & Asthma Resident Training
    Program
San Joaquin Hospital
Acampo, CA

Joanne Blessing-Moore, MD
Clinical Assistant Professor
Department of Immunology
Stanford University Hospital
Palo Alto, CA

Adrian M. Casillas, MD
Assistant Professor of Medicine
Department of Medicine, Division of Clinical
    Immunology and Allergy
David Geffen School of Medicine at University of
    California, Los Angeles
Los Angeles, CA

Mark S. Dykewicz, MD
Professor of Internal Medicine
Director, Training Program in Allergy and Immunology
Division of Allergy and Immunology, Department of
    Internal Medicine
St. Louis University School of Medicine
Attending Staff Physician
Department of Internal Medicine
St. Louis University Hospital
St. Louis, MO

Brian H. Halstater, MD
Assistant Clinical Professor
Assistant Residency Director
Department of Family Medicine
David Geffen School of Medicine at University of
    California, Los Angeles
Los Angeles, CA

Phillip L. Lieberman, MD
Clinical Professor
Department of Medicine and Pediatrics
University of Tennessee College of Medicine
Memphis, TN

Guillermo R. Mendoza, MD
Chief
Department of Allergy
Kaiser Napa Solano
The Permanente Medical Group
Vacaville, CA

Etan C. Milgrom, MD
Acute Care Staff Physician
University Park Health Center
Clinical Associate Professor of Family Medicine
Keck School of Medicine
University of Southern California
Los Angeles, CA

John E. Moffitt, MD
Associate Dean for Graduate Medical Education
Professor
Department of Pediatrics, Division of Allergy and
    Immunology
University of Mississippi Medical Center
Jackson, MS

Marc A. Riedl, MD
Fellow
Department of Medicine, Division of Clinical
    Immunology and Allergy
David Geffen School of Medicine at University of
    California, Los Angeles
Los Angeles, CA

Sheldon L. Spector, MD
Clinical Professor of Medicine
Division of Allergy and Clinical Immunology
Department of Medicine
UCLA School of Medicine
Director
California Allergy and Asthma Medical Group, Inc.
Los Angeles, CA

William W. Storms, MD
Clinical Professor
University of Colorado Health Sciences Center
Practicing Allergist
Asthma and Allergy Associates
Colorado Springs, CO

Ricardo Antonio Tan, MD
Practicing Allergist
California Allergy and Asthma Medical Group, Inc.
Los Angeles, CA

Abba I. Terr, MD
Clinical Professor
Attending Physician
Department of Medicine
University of California, San Francisco
Attending Physician
Department of Medicine
California Pacific Medical Center
San Francisco, CA

Richard P. Usatine, MD
Professor and Vice Chair for Education
Director of Medical Student Education
Department of Family and Community Medicine
University of Texas Health Science Center
San Antonio, TX

Anne B. Yates, MD
Associate Professor of Pediatrics
Director, Division of Pediatric Allergy–Immunology
Department of Pediatrics
University of Mississippi Medical Center
Jackson, MS

CONTENTS

Plants of Allergenic Importance (Listed alphabetically and depicted on opening page of each chapter or appendix)

Practical Allergy

SECTION I
Core Topics

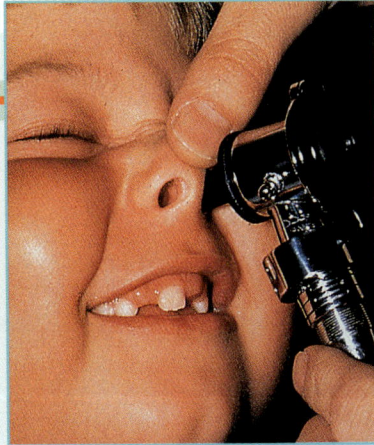

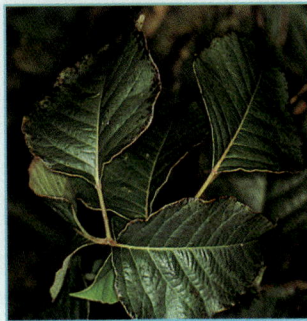

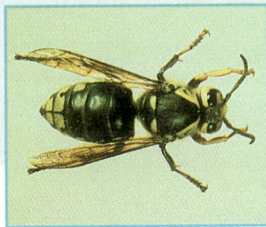

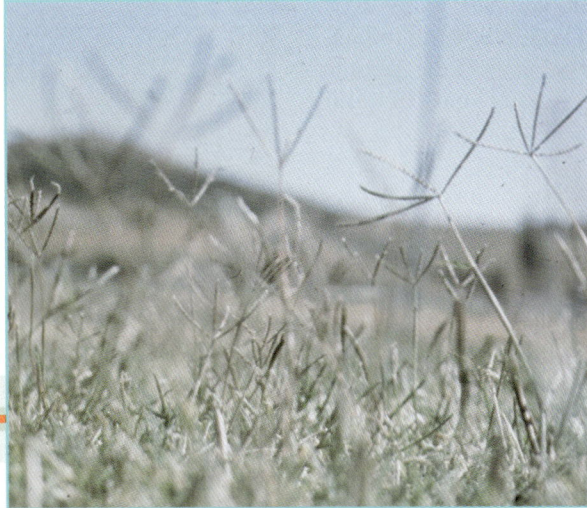

CHAPTER 1
Rhinitis

Mark S. Dykewicz

I. Introduction

Rhinitis is an inflammation of the membranes lining the nose. Symptoms are variable but may include nasal congestion, rhinorrhea, sneezing, itching of the nose, and postnasal drainage. Although sometimes mistakenly viewed as trivial conditions, symptoms of allergic and nonallergic rhinitis may significantly impact the patient's quality of life by causing fatigue, headache, cognitive impairment, decreased work and school performance, and impairment of other activities of daily living.[1] Appropriate management of rhinitis may be an important component in effective management of coexisting or complicating respiratory conditions, such as asthma, sinusitis, or chronic otitis media.[1] Rhinitis may be caused by allergic, nonallergic, infectious, hormonal, occupational, and other factors. The etiology and clinical manifestations of each of these forms of rhinitis will be reviewed separately, followed by discussion of a diagnostic approach to rhinitis and treatment approaches for rhinitis generally.

II. Epidemiology

A. Estimates of the prevalence of rhinitis vary widely, in part because of different definitions of disease in different epidemiologic studies. Seasonal allergic rhinitis (hay fever) occurs in at least 10%–20% of the population, and one study reported a prevalence of physician-diagnosed allergic rhinitis in 42% of 6-year-old children.[1,2]

B. Overall, allergic rhinitis affects 20–40 million individuals in the United States annually.[1]

1. In 80% of cases, allergic rhinitis develops before age 20. A child has a greater chance of developing allergic rhinitis if both parents have a history of allergic disorders than if only one parent has such a history.

2. Children in families with a bilateral family history of allergy generally develop symptoms before puberty; those with a unilateral family history tend to develop symptoms later in life or not at all.

3. There is an increased prevalence of allergic rhinitis in higher socioeconomic classes, in nonwhites, and in some polluted urban areas. For reasons that are unclear, allergic rhinitis apparently is becoming more common.

III. Etiology and Clinical Manifestations

A. Allergic Rhinitis

1. **Etiology**

   Allergic rhinitis results from IgE antibody-mediated responses to allergen that cause release of inflammatory mediators (e.g., histamine and leukotrienes) and cytokines, and mucosal inflammation driven by interaction between resident and infiltrating inflammatory cells. Sensory nerve activation, plasma leakage, and congestion of venous sinusoids also contribute.

2. **Clinical Manifestations**
   a. **Symptoms.** Common symptoms include sneezing, nasal congestion, rhinorrhea, and postnasal drainage. Congestion results from nasal mucosal edema, impairing normal airflow (Fig. 1-1).
   b. **Related symptoms.** Allergic rhinitis often coexists with allergic conjunctivitis and its symptoms of itchy, watery eyes and increased lacrimation.
   c. **Relation to allergen exposure.** Early-phase responses cause symptoms within an hour of acute allergen exposure. Late-phase responses cause symptoms 4 or more hours after allergen exposure and lead to chronic symptoms, especially nasal congestion.
   d. **Seasonal/perennial patterns.** Allergic rhinitis may occur:
      1) Only during specific seasons
      2) Perennially with seasonal exacerbations
      3) Perennially without seasonal exacerbations
      4) Sporadically after specific exposures
         a) *Seasonal allergic rhinitis* is caused by IgE-mediated reaction to seasonal aeroallergens such as pollens, grasses (Fig. 1-2), trees (Fig. 1-3), weeds (Fig. 1-4) (the pollen count of ragweed peaks in

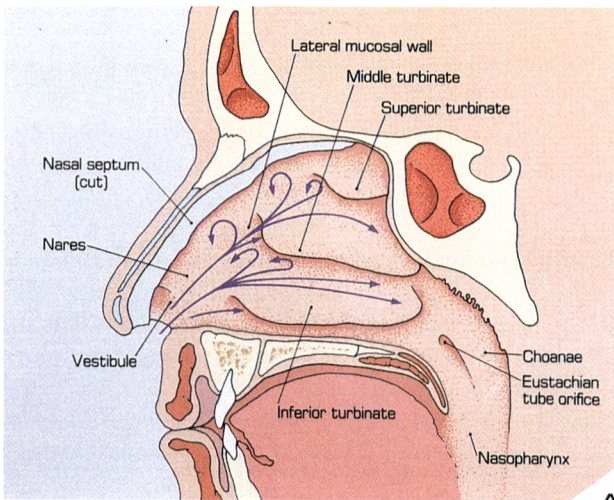

Figure 1-2 Bermuda grass, a common grass antigen that typically pollinates in the springtime. (Courtesy of Hollister-Stier Laboratories.)

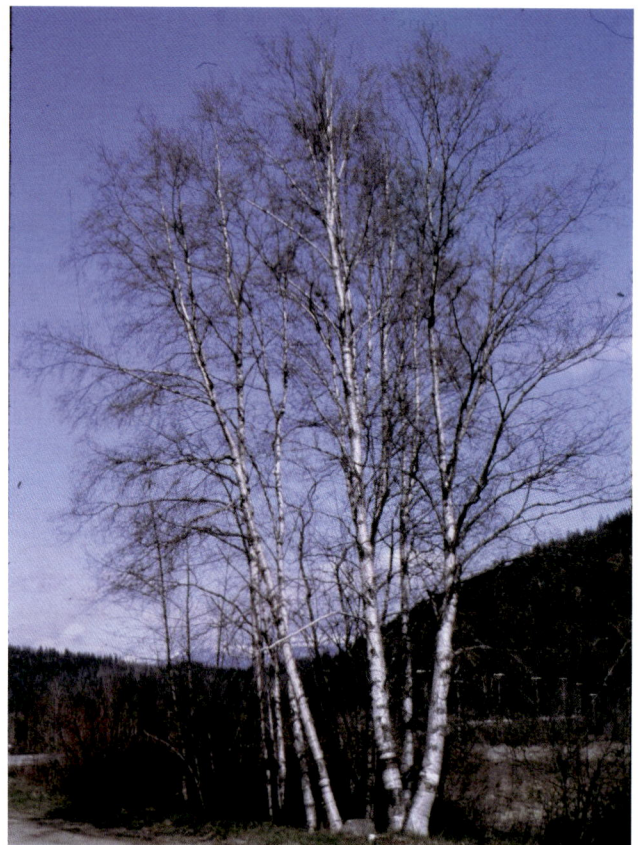

Figure 1-1 Schematic representation of the inside of the nose, illustrating how inspired air, after entering the nose, circulates over, under, and around the inferior, middle, and superior nasal turbinates. Mucosal edema in rhinitis impairs airflow, causing nasal congestion. (Reproduced with permission from Fireman P, Slavin RG: Atlas of Allergies, 2nd ed. London: Mosby-Wolfe, 1996.)

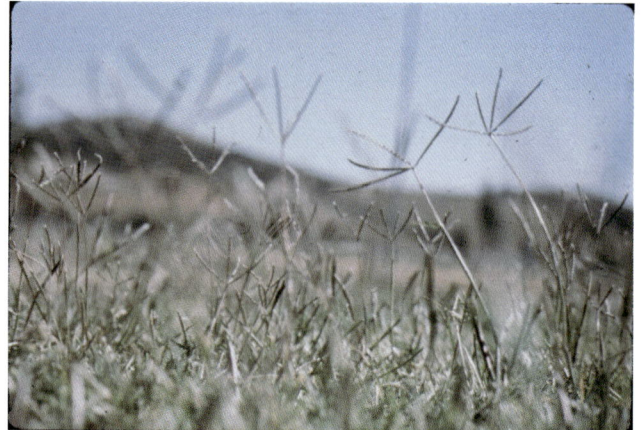

Figure 1-3 Paper birch, a common tree antigen that typically pollinates in the summertime. (Courtesy of Hollister-Stier Laboratories.)

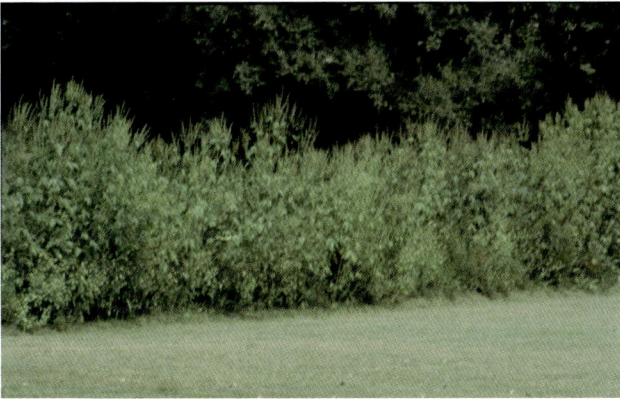

Figure 1-4 Giant ragweed, a common weed, especially in the northeastern United States. (Courtesy of Hollister-Stier Laboratories.)

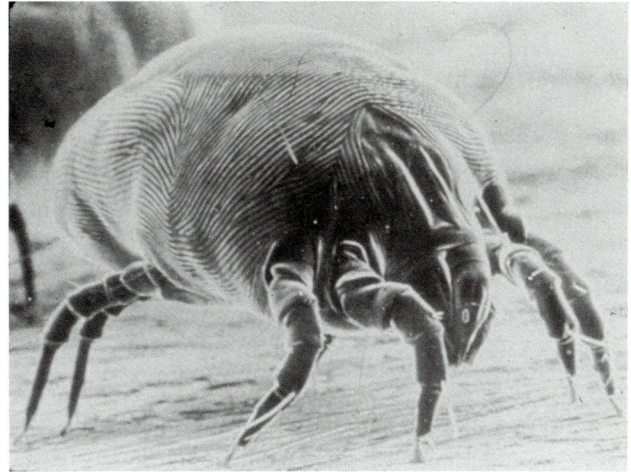

Figure 1-6 House dust mite, *Dermatophagoides farinae*. Its fecal particles are the sensitizing allergic trigger. (Courtesy of Hollister-Stier Laboratories.)

September, often forcing individuals who are allergic to it to vacation during that month far away from where it pollinates), and sometimes molds (Fig. 1-5).

b) *Perennial allergic rhinitis* is caused by IgE-mediated reaction to perennial environmental aeroallergens such as dust mites (Fig. 1-6), molds, animal allergens, cockroaches, some occupational allergens, and in some climates perennial pollens.

B. Nonallergic Rhinitis Syndromes

Nonallergic rhinitis is actually a group of disorders characterized by sporadic or persistent perennial symptoms of rhinitis that do not result from IgE antibody-mediated mechanisms. Examples of nonallergic rhinitis are infectious rhinitis, nonallergic rhinitis without eosinophils (vasomotor rhinitis), nonallergic rhinitis with eosinophilia

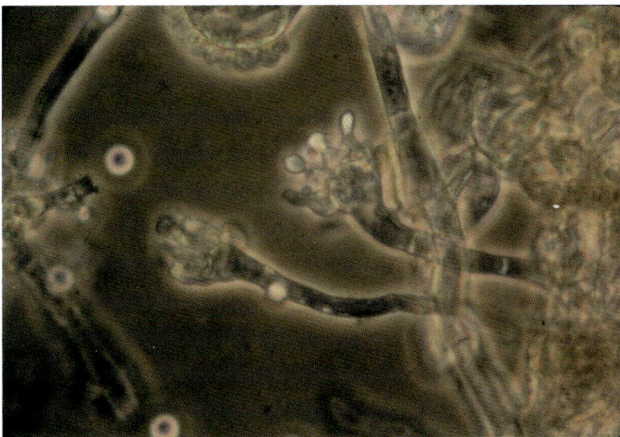

Figure 1-5 Aspergillus spores. Microscopic view of a mold that causes bronchopulmonary aspergillosis. (Courtesy of Hollister-Stier Laboratories.)

syndrome (NARES), hormonal rhinitis, certain types of occupational rhinitis, and gustatory and drug-induced rhinitis.

C. Infectious Rhinitis

1. *Etiology*
   a. Infectious rhinitis may be acute or chronic. Acute infectious rhinitis is usually caused by one of a large number of viruses, but the viral infection commonly precipitates a secondary bacterial infection with sinus involvement.
   b. Chronic infectious rhinitis is almost always due to bacterial infection of the nose that is associated with bacterial sinusitis, collectively referred to as rhinosinusitis.
2. *Clinical Manifestations*
   a. Manifestations may include nasal congestion, rhinorrhea, sneezing, and fever. Infectious rhinitis is sometimes confused with allergic rhinitis. Patients with infectious rhinitis may complain of a constant cold with variable symptoms, including postnasal drainage with cough, mucopurulent nasal discharge, facial pain and pressure, and a decrease in olfaction.
   b. The presence of purulent-appearing secretions may also occur from noninfectious rhinitis.

D. Nonallergic, Noninfectious Rhinitis Without Eosinophilia

1. *Etiology*
   a. Nonallergic, noninfectious rhinitis without eosinophilia refers to chronic nasal symptoms that are not driven by immunologic or infectious mechanisms and are usually not associated with nasal eosinophilia. It is likely that this diagnosis

actually refers to a heterogeneous group of disorders with different mechanisms that are not yet defined.

  b. The term *vasomotor rhinitis* is often used as an interchangeable term, although it has the additional connotation of abnormal vascular responses that probably are not present in many patients identified with this diagnosis.

  2. *Clinical Manifestations*
     a. Most patients develop an acute increase in rhinitis symptoms in response to environmental conditions such as cold air, temperature changes, strong odors, and inhaled irritants.
     b. In addition, ingestion of alcohol can aggravate symptoms through vasodilation of the nasal mucosa. The symptoms of this form of nonallergic rhinitis may be indistinguishable from those of perennial allergic rhinitis, although sneezing and conjunctival symptoms tend to be more prominent in allergic rhinitis.

E. Nonallergic Rhinitis with Eosinophilia Syndrome

  1. *Etiology*
     NARES (nonallergic rhinitis with eosinophilia syndrome) is characterized by nasal eosinophils in the absence of allergic disease defined by clinically significant, positive immediate skin tests or specific IgE antibodies in the serum.
  2. *Clinical Manifestations*
     Patients have perennial symptoms of sneezing, profuse rhinorrhea, nasal pruritus, and occasionally loss of sense of smell. These symptoms may be indistinguishable from those of perennial allergic rhinitis or nonallergic rhinitis without nasal eosinophils.

F. Occupational Rhinitis

Occupational rhinitis is defined as rhinitis in response to airborne substances in the workplace, whether mediated by allergic (IgE antibody) or nonallergic mechanisms (e.g., laboratory animal antigen, wood dusts, grains, chemicals). It often coexists with occupational asthma and may precede the development of occupational asthma.

G. Hormonal Rhinitis

  1. *Etiology*
     Pregnancy and hypothyroidism are causes of hormonal rhinitis. However, during pregnancy, other causes of rhinitis, such as allergic rhinitis, infectious rhinitis, and rhinitis medicamentosa (see Drug-Induced Rhinitis, following), are more often responsible for rhinitis symptoms.
  2. *Clinical Manifestations*
     In pregnancy, symptoms—prominently nasal congestion—are typically present from the second month

to term, but they usually disappear soon after delivery if there is no history of preexisting rhinitis.

H. Drug-Induced Rhinitis

Drug-induced rhinitis may be caused by a number of systemic medications, including angiotensin-converting enzyme (ACE) inhibitors, β-blockers, reserpine, guanethidine, phentolamine, methyldopa, chlorpromazine, aspirin and other nonsteroidal anti-inflammatory drugs (NSAIDs), and oral contraceptives.[1] Rhinitis medicamentosa commonly refers to the overuse of nasally inhaled vasoconstrictor (decongestant) agents such as the OTC products oxymetazoline or phenylephrine. Repeated use of cocaine may also produce rhinitis.

I. Gustatory and Food-Related Rhinitis

  1. *Etiology*
     Rhinitis that occurs after the ingestion of foods or alcoholic products may be due to vagally mediated mechanisms, nasal vasodilation, food allergy, or other undefined mechanisms.
  2. *Clinical Manifestations*
     Food allergy is a rare cause of rhinitis without associated gastrointestinal, dermatologic, or systemic manifestations. Copious watery rhinorrhea occurring immediately after ingestion of foods, particularly hot and spicy foods, is termed gustatory rhinitis and is vagally mediated. It appears to become more prevalent with aging.

IV. Differential Diagnosis

Symptoms resembling those of rhinitis may arise from structural/mechanical factors or inflammatory/immunologic factors.

A. Structural/Mechanical Factors

  1. Deviated septum/septal wall anomalies
  2. Hypertrophic turbinates
  3. Adenoidal hypertrophy
  4. Foreign bodies
  5. Nasal tumors
     a. Benign
     b. Malignant
  6. Choanal atresia

B. Inflammatory/Immunologic Factors

  1. Nasal polyps
     a. The presence of nasal polyps is suggested by unvarying nasal congestion.
     b. Nasal polyps may occur in conjunction with chronic rhinitis or sinusitis and may contribute significantly to the patient's symptoms.
     c. In adults, nasal polyps may be associated with sensitivity to aspirin and other NSAIDs, and with asthma ("aspirin triad").

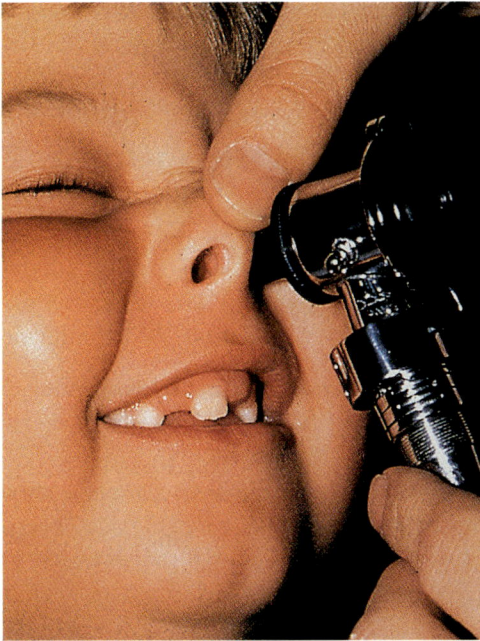

Figure 1-7 Inspection of nasal mucosa with speculum. Insertion of an illuminated nasal speculum permits magnified visualization of the anterior nose. (Reproduced with permission from Zitelli BJ, Davis HW: Pediatric Physical Diagnosis. St. Louis: Mosby, 1987.)

    d. Nasal polyps in children should raise concern about cystic fibrosis.

2. Sarcoidosis
3. Midline granuloma
4. Wegener's granulomatosis
5. Systemic lupus erythematosis
6. Sjögren's syndrome
7. Cerebrospinal fluid rhinorrhea

V. History

A. Symptoms (e.g., rhinorrhea, nasal congestion): Duration and Severity

1. Are the symptoms unilateral (suggesting an anatomic basis)?
2. Assessing the symptoms can aid in the diagnosis and in selecting medication.

B. Do the Symptoms Suggest an Allergic Basis?

1. Is there a seasonal pattern in this and previous years consistent with the allergen season?
2. If symptoms are perennial, it may be impossible to distinguish allergic from nonallergic rhinitis on the basis of the history. An allergic basis is somewhat more likely if associated conjunctival symptoms are present.
3. Sensitivity to house dust mites is suggested if symptoms increase with dusting or vacuuming.
4. A mold sensitivity is suggested if symptoms increase with cutting grass or raking leaves.

5. A pet allergy is suggested if acute symptoms occur with pet exposure or if symptoms improve during extended periods away from pets.

C. A temporal relation to food suggests gustatory rhinitis or, rarely, a true food allergy.

D. Medications used for symptoms, their effectiveness, and side effects

E. Coexisting medical conditions (e.g., otitis media, sinusitis, asthma)

F. Medications being taken for other conditions (could these cause rhinitis?)

VI. Physical Examination

A. Nasal Examination

Assess appearance of nasal mucous membranes and nasal septum, patency of nasal passages, other causes of nasal obstruction (e.g., nasal polyps, septal deviation), quality and quantity of nasal discharge (a purulent discharge suggests infection) (Figs. 1-7 to 1-9).

B. Other Examinations

1. Eyes (conjunctivitis?)
2. Ears (signs of otitis?)
3. Pharynx (postnasal drainage present, character?)
4. Lungs (signs of asthma?)

VII. Diagnostic Testing

A. Sensitivity to Specific Allergens

1. Testing for sensitivity to specific allergens can help determine whether there is an allergic basis to the

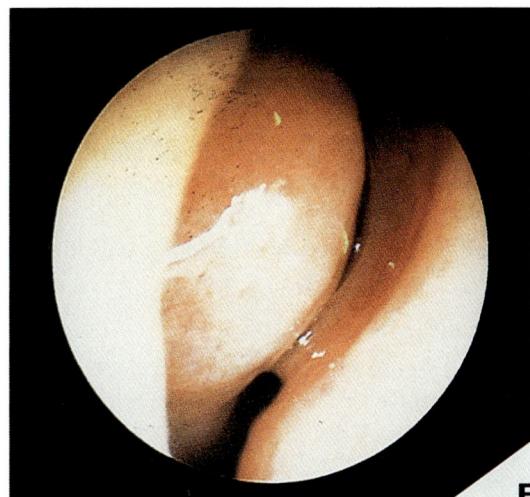

Figure 1-8 Nasal obstruction from engorged nasal mucosa including inferior turbinate. (Reproduced with permission from Fireman P, Slavin RG: Atlas of Allergies, 2nd ed. London: Mosby-Wolfe, 1996.)

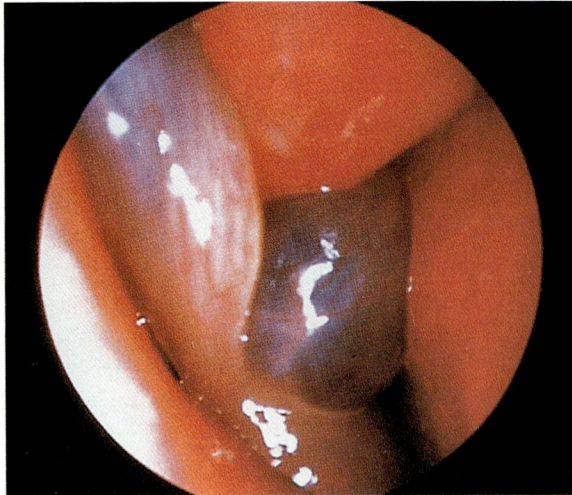

Figure 1-9 Appearance of nasal polyps on rhinoscopy. Polyps are more gray-blue than surrounding nasal mucosa, and have a translucent appearance. (Courtesy of Dr. Sylvan Stool, Department of Otolaryngology, University of Pittsburgh School of Medicine.)

rhinitis, thereby helping to direct allergen avoidance measures, choice of medication, and, in selected cases, whether allergen immunotherapy is a consideration for long-term management. Such testing is probably not required if the patient has rhinitis limited to a single season and responds well to simple empirical therapy. Chapter 12 covers this topic in greater detail.

2. Although current in vitro tests for specific IgE are approaching skin tests in sensitivity, skin testing still is generally more cost-effective, particularly when multiple allergens are relevant to disease.[1] Chapter 13 covers this topic in greater detail.

3. Even if tests for immediate hypersensitivity are positive for allergen sensitivity, poor correlation between allergen exposure and symptoms suggests that those allergens are not the cause of symptoms.

4. Negative skin tests rule out allergic rhinitis in nearly all cases.

5. Oral antihistamines, phenothiazines, and tricyclic antidepressants can inhibit allergen skin tests, whereas corticosteroids do not. (Corticosteroids do inhibit delayed hypersensitivity skin testing, e.g., PPD, patch testing, and anergy skin testing.)

B. Serum IgE

Neither total serum IgE levels nor peripheral eosinophil levels are sensitive or specific for identifying an allergic basis to rhinitis.

C. Nasal Cytology

Nasal cytology may aid in differentiating allergic rhinitis and NARES from other forms of rhinitis, such as vasomotor or infectious rhinitis. However, there is lack of expert consensus about whether nasal cytology should be routinely used in the diagnosis of rhinitis.[1] Chapter 19 covers this topic in greater detail.

VIII. Therapy and Management

A stepwise approach is recommended, with individualization of treatment based on the specific symptoms present and their severity, the likely basis for the rhinitis, the cost-effectiveness and side effects of the treatment, and the patient's preference and compliance.[1,3,4]

A. Avoidance of Known Rhinitis Triggers (e.g., allergens, irritants) (see Appendix 7 and patient education CD)

1. Patients allergic to outdoor allergens should be counseled to minimize time outside, keep doors and windows closed, and, if practical, use air conditioning.

2. For patients allergic to house dust mites, the most effective approach to reduce mite exposure is to encase pillows and mattresses with covers impermeable to house dust mites.[5] Polyester "hypoallergenic" pillows are actually no better than feather down pillows.

3. If patients are allergic to pets, advising patients to keep pets out of the bedroom is reasonable, but only complete removal of pets from the home is reliably effective.

B. Pharmacotherapy

1. The choice of medication should take into account the type of rhinitis most likely present.
   a. Oral antihistamines are generally not effective in nonallergic rhinitis.[1,4]
   b. Nasal corticosteroids and nasal antihistamines are of value in both allergic and nonallergic rhinitis.[1,4]
   c. Intranasal anticholinergic agents are of particular value in gustatory and vasomotor rhinitis.[1,4]

2. Specific pharmacologic considerations for episodic (E) or persistent (P) rhinitis symptoms
   a. Second-generation oral antihistamines (Table 1-1)
      1) Reduce allergic rhinitis and conjunctivitis symptoms (E or P).
      2) Second-generation antihistamines should usually be considered before first-generation (sedating) antihistamines because the patient may not perceive impairments to driving or thinking caused by the latter.[1,4]
   b. Nasally inhaled corticosteroids (Table 1-2)
      1) Generally the most effective agents to control symptoms (P) of allergic and nonallergic rhinitis.[1]

TABLE 1-1

Oral Antihistamines

H₁ Receptor Antagonist	Formulation	Recommended Dose	
		Adult	*Child*
First-generation (sedating)			
Chlorpheniramine (Chlor-Trimeton)	4, 8, 12 mg tablets 2.5 mg/5 mL syrup	8–12 mg bid	0.35 mg/kg/d 2–5 yr: 1 mg dose 6–11 yr: 2 mg dose (both given every 4–6h)
Diphenhydramine (Benadryl)	25 mg tablets 12.5 mg/5 mL liquid	25–50 mg q4–6h	5 mg/kg/d given every 4–6h 2–6 yr: 6.25 mg/dose, max. 37.5 mg/d 6–12 yr: 12.5–25 mg/dose, max. 150 mg/d
Hydroxyzine (Atarax, Vistaril)	10, 25, 50, 100 mg tablets 10 mg/5 mL syrup	25 mg tid–qid	2 mg/kg/d <6 yr: 50 mg/d ≥6 yr: 50–100 mg/d (both divided into 3–4 doses)
Cyproheptadine (Periactin)	4 mg scored tablet	4 mg tid	2–6 yr: 2 mg bid–tid 7–14 yr: 4 mg bid–tid
Second-generation (nonsedating)			
Fexofenadine (Allegra)	30, 60, 180 mg tablets	60 mg bid 180 mg bid	6–11 yr: 30 mg 2×/d
Cetirizine (Zyrtec)	5, 10 mg 1 mg/1 mL syrup	5–10 mg/d	2–5 yr: 2.5 mg/d ≥6 yr: 5–10 mg/d
Desloratadine (Clarinex)	5 mg tablets	5 mg/d	≥12 yr: 5 mg/d
Loratadine (Claritin)	10 mg tablets 10 mg dissolving tablets (Reditabs) 5 mg/5 mL syrup	10 mg/d 2 tsp/d	2–5 yr: 5 mg/d ≥6 yr: 10 mg/d

2) May also reduce symptoms of allergic conjunctivitis.
3) Optimally used with regular dosing, but can benefit allergic rhinitis with PRN dosing.[6]
4) Patients should be instructed to direct the spray away from the nasal septum to prevent septal perforation.
5) If prolonged use (e.g., >4–6 weeks), periodic examination of the nasal septum is recommended to detect mucosal erosions that may precede perforation.
6) Newer agents generally have an excellent safety profile in adults
7) For use of nasal corticosteroids in children, see Special Considerations in Children, discussed later.
8) Nasal dexamethasone may cause adrenal suppression in recommended doses.
   c. Oral decongestants
   1) Reduce nasal congestion (E or P).
   2) Principal side effects: nervousness, insomnia, tachycardia.

3) Pseudoephedrine is probably less likely to cause hypertension than phenylephrine.
   d. Decongestant nasal sprays (e.g., oxymetazoline, phenylephrine)
   1) Limit to 3–5 days of use to avoid rebound congestion.
   2) If the initial nasal examination shows mucosal edema so severe that delivery of other topical nasal sprays to superior regions of the nose would be impaired, the use of decongestant nose sprays 15–20 minutes prior to the use of other sprays should be considered (for 3–5 days only).
   e. Intranasal antihistamines (e.g., azelastine) (Table 1-3)
   1) For allergic (E or P) or nonallergic rhinitis symptoms. For allergic rhinitis, intranasal antihistamines are equally as effective as or more effective than oral antihistamines, but less effective than nasal corticosteroids.[7,8]
   2) To avoid a bitter taste, the patient should be instructed to spray with the head tilted forward and the nose ponting to the ground.

TABLE 1-2

Nasal Corticosteroid Sprays

Agent	Trade Name(s)	Dose per Inhalation	Adult Dosage	Pediatric Dosage
Beclomethasone dipropionate	Beconase AQ Vancenase Pockethaler	42 μg	1–2 sprays per nostril bid	≥12 yr: same as adults 6–12 yr: 1–2 sprays per nostril 2×/d
	Vancenase AQ Double Strength	84 μg	1–2 sprays per nostril 1×/d	≥6 yr: same as adults
Budesonide	Rhinocort Aqua	32 μg	1–4 sprays per nostril 1×/d	6–12 yr: 1–2 sprays per nostril 1×/d
Flunisolide	Nasarel	25 μg	2 sprays per nostril bid	≥14 yr: same as adults
	Nasalide			6–14 yr: 1 spray per nostril 3×/d or 2 sprays per nostril 2×/d
Fluticasone propionate	Flonase	50 μg	2 sprays per nostril 1×/d or 1 spray per nostril bid	≥6 yr: same as adults; start with 1 spray per nostril 1×/d
Mometasone	Nasonex (AQ)	50 μg	2 sprays per nostril 1×/d	≥12 yr: same as adults 3–12 yr: 1 spray per nostril 1×/d 6–11 yr: 2 sprays per nostril 1×/d
Triamcinolone acetonide	Nasacort	55 μg	1–2 sprays per nostril 1×/d	≥12 yr: same as adults
	Nasacort AQ	55 μg	1–2 sprays per nostril 1×/d	6–11 yr: 2 sprays per nostril 1×/d ≥12 yr: same as adults
	Tri Nasal	50 μg	2–4 sprays per nostril 1×/d or 2 sprays per nostril 2×/d	≥12 yr: same as adults
Dexamethasone sodium phosphate	Dexacort	84 μg	2 sprays per nostril bid–tid	6–12 yr: 1–2 sprays per nostril bid, depending on age

f. Intranasal ipratropium (see Table 1-3): Effective for rhinorrhea (E or P), but not other rhinitis symptoms.[9]

g. Intranasal cromolyn (see Table 1-3)
   1) May reduce allergic symptoms (P) in some patients (optimally dosed 4–6 times a day), or to prevent symptoms (E) when used 20–30 minutes prior to acute allergen exposure.
   2) Less effective than oral antihistamines, intranasal antihistamines, or cortico-steroids.[4,10]
   3) Excellent safety profile.

h. Systemic corticosteroids
   1) A short course (e.g., 5–7 days, 30 mg/day of prednisone or equivalent in adults) of oral corticosteroids is of benefit and may be needed for intractable nasal symptoms.[11]
   2) For oral agents (e.g., prednisone) once- or twice-daily administration is preferred.
   3) The use of injectable, prolonged-acting cor-ticosteroids is discouraged because of greater potential risks.[1]

i. Oral antileukotriene agents: Some but not all data suggest their effect is additive to that of oral anti-histamines, but their place in therapy needs further definition.[1,12]

C. Allergen Immunotherapy (Vaccines)

1. High-dose immunotherapy is highly effective in con-trolling symptoms of allergic rhinitis in appropriately selected patients.[1,4]

TABLE 1-3

Noncorticosteroid Nasal Sprays*

Class/Agent	Trade Name(s)	Adult Dosage	Pediatric Dosage
Intranasal antihistamines			
Azelastine hydrochloride	Astelin Nasal	2 sprays (137 µg/ spray) per nostril 2×/d	5–12 yr: 1 spray per nostril 2×/d ≥12 yr: same as adults
Intranasal mast cell stabilizers			
Cromolyn	Nasalcrom	1 spray (5.2 mg/spray) per nostril 3–4×/d (q4–6h); may increase up to 6×/d	≥6 yr: same as adults
Intranasal anticholinergics			
Ipratropium bromide	Atrovent Nasal 0.03% 0.06%	2 sprays (21 µg/spray) per nostril 2–3×/d 2 sprays (42 µg/spray) per nostril 3–4×/d	≥6 yr: same as adults ≥12 yr: same as adults

*In addition, a variety of nasal decongestant sprays are available for over-the-counter use. Use should be limited to 3–5 days.

2. Patients with allergic rhinitis should be considered candidates for immunotherapy based on the duration of their symptoms during the year (e.g., if long allergen season or perennial symptoms), symptom severity, failure or unacceptability of other treatment modalities, and possibly as a means of preventing worsening of rhinitis or the development or worsening of comorbid conditions (e.g., asthma, sinusitis, middle ear disease).

3. Selection of the immunotherapy extract should be based on correlation between the presence of specific IgE antibodies (demonstrated by allergy skin tests or in vitro tests) and the patient's history. Chapter 11 and Appendix 1 cover this topic in greater detail.

More severe rhinitis may require multiple therapeutic interventions, including the use of multiple medications, evaluation for possible complications and allergic factors, and instruction in or modification of the immunotherapy and medication program.

IX. Special Considerations in Patient Subsets

A. Children

1. *Diagnosis*
   a. Viral-induced rhinitis averages 6 episodes per year at ages 2–6 years.
   b. In addition to rhinitis, nasal obstruction may occur from structural defects, adenoidal hypertrophy, or a foreign body in the nose.
   c. Nasal polyps (rare in childhood) may be associated with cystic fibrosis, ciliary dyskinesia, or chronic infection.

2. *Treatment*
   a. Oral second-generation antihistamines and nasal cromolyn are first-line treatments for allergic rhinitis.
   b. Nasal corticosteroids are the most effective treatment for allergic rhinitis, but they should be used at the lowest effective dose, and the child's height must be monitored.[1,3,4]
   c. If nasal corticosteroids are used, they should be used in conjunction with other medications and avoidance measures and, if appropriate, immunotherapy to reduce the corticosteroid dose.[1]

B. Elderly Patients

1. *Diagnosis*
   a. Allergic rhinitis is less common than cholinergic hyperreactivity, medication-induced rhinitis, or sinusitis in patients over age 65.[13]
   b. Antihypertensive medications should be considered as a possible cause of nasal congestion in this age group.

2. *Treatment*
   Rhinorrhea associated with cholinergic hyperreactivity (e.g., gustatory rhinitis) may respond to intranasal ipratropium.

C. Pregnant Patients

1. Chlorpheniramine and tripelennamine have been the preferred antihistamines for use in pregnant patients.[1] Of the second-generation antihistamines, loratadine and cetirizine have FDA category B ratings.

2. Nasal cromolyn has reassuring safety data and may be considered first for allergic rhinitis.

3. Intranasal corticosteroids may be used for intractable symptoms or as an alternative to oral therapy. Of the intranasal corticosteroids, budesonide has an FDA category B rating.
4. Oral decongestants are best avoided in the first trimester because of risk of gastroschisis.[1,13]
5. Allergen immunotherapy may be continued in patients during pregnancy, although doses should not be increased.[1,13]

X. When to Obtain Consultation

Referral for an allergy or immunology evaluation should be considered when:

A. Allergic/environmental triggers must be identified.

B. Rhinitis is inadequately controlled, such as:

1. The patient needs additional education in allergen avoidance measures.

TABLE 1-4

Stepwise Approach to Pharmacotherapy for Seasonal Allergic Rhinitis

Avoidance of allergic factors and irritants is the first step in the management of the patient with allergic rhinitis.

Severity	Daily Medication	Quick-Relief Medication
Intermittent symptoms	None	
Persistent mild-to-moderate disease Consider referral to an allergy/ immunology specialist or otolaryngologic allergy specialist for consultation or comanagement.	Oral nonsedating H_1-antihistamine (with or without a decongestant combination). **or** Topical nasal corticosteroid (preferably start therapy 1–2 weeks before season and continue through season). **consider** Topical nasal antihistamine; nasal cromolyn sodium for children. If there are prominent eye symptoms: topical ocular antihistamine with or without vasoconstrictor, topical ocular mast cell stabilizer, and/or topical ocular NSAID.	Rapid onset, oral, nonsedating H_1-antihistamine. **or** Topical nasal antihistamine. **consider** Nasal cromolyn sodium as a preventive measure before anticipated allergen exposures.
Severe disease Referral to an allergy/immunology specialist or otolaryngologic allergy specialist for consultation or comanagement is recommended.	Topical nasal corticosteroid (preferably start therapy 1–2 weeks before season and continue through season). **and** Oral nonsedating H_1-antihistamine (with or without a decongestant combination). **consider** Topical nasal antihistamine; nasal cromolyn sodium for children. **and** (if needed) A short course (3–10 days) of oral corticosteroids. If there are prominent eye symptoms: topical ocular antihistamine with or without vasoconstrictor, topical ocular mast cell stabilizers, and/or topical ocular NSAIDS.	

From Nelson HS, Rachelevsky GS, Bernick J, et al: Rhinitis. In The Allergy Report, Vol 2. Diseases of the Atopic Diathesis, pp 1–172. Milwaukee: American Academy of Allergy, Asthma and Immunology, 2000. Reproduced with permission.

TABLE 1-5

Stepwise Approach to Pharmacotherapy for Perennial Allergic Rhinitis

Avoidance of allergic factors and irritants is the first step in the management of the patient with allergic rhinitis.

Severity	*Daily Medication*	*Quick-Relief Medication*
Intermittent symptoms	None	
Persistent mild-to-moderate disease Consider referral to an allergy/immunology specialist or otolaryngologic allergy specialist for consultation or comanagement.	Oral nonsedating H_1-antihistamine (with or without a decongestant combination). **and/or** Topical nasal corticosteroid. **consider** Topical nasal antihistamine. Children should start with oral nonsedating H_1-antihistamine or nasal cromolyn sodium.	Rapid onset, oral, nonsedating H_1-antihistamine. **or** Topical nasal antihistamine. **consider** Nasal cromolyn sodium as a preventive measure before anticipated allergen exposures.
Severe disease Referral to an allergy/immunology specialist or otolaryngologic allergy specialist for consultation or comanagement is recommended.	Topical nasal corticosteroid. **and** Oral nonsedating H_1-antihistamine (with or without a decongestant combination). **and** (if needed) A short course (3–10-days) of oral corticosteroid.	

From Nelson HS, Rachelevsky GS, Bernick J, et al: Rhinitis. In The Allergy Report, Vol 2. Diseases of the Atopic Diathesis, pp 1–172. Milwaukee: American Academy of Allergy, Asthma and Immunology, 2000. Reproduced with permission.

---

2. Medication side effects or rhinitis symptoms impair patient performance (e.g., school, work, driving).

C. Rhinitis is prolonged or associated with complications or comorbid conditions (e.g., otitis media, sinusitis, nasal polyps, asthma).

D. The patient has required oral corticosteroids, more than two courses per year, to manage symptoms of rhinitis.

E. Multiple medications are necessary over a prolonged period of time.

F. Allergen immunotherapy is a consideration.

XI. Practice Guidelines

General stepwise medical treatment of allergic rhinitis can be found in Tables 1-4 and 1-5.[3,4,14] Overall symptom severity can direct general selection of medical therapy, although therapy should be individualized.

XII. Internet Resources

www.aaaai.org
American Academy of Allergy, Asthma and Immunology. A well-developed web site for both physician and patient information on rhinitis.

www.acaai.org
American College of Allergy, Asthma and Immunology. Another good source for both physician and patient information on rhinitis.

www.jcaai.org
Joint Council on Allergy, Asthma and Immunology. Site has complete text of Joint Task Force Practice Parameters on Rhinitis, including management algorithm, detailed discussion, and extensive references.

www.theallergyreport.org
The Allergy Report. This document was developed by the American Academy of Allergy, Asthma and Immunology in partnership with the National Institute of Allergy and Infectious Diseases and 20 other medical associations, advocacy groups, and government agencies.

XIII. ICD-9 Codes

477.9	Allergic rhinitis
472.0, 477.9, 460	Nonallergic rhinitis syndromes
460	Infectious rhinitis
472.0	Nonallergic rhinitis with eosinophilia syndrome
472.0, 477.9	Occupational rhinitis

XIV. Diagnosis and Management Algorithm (*Fig. 1-10*)

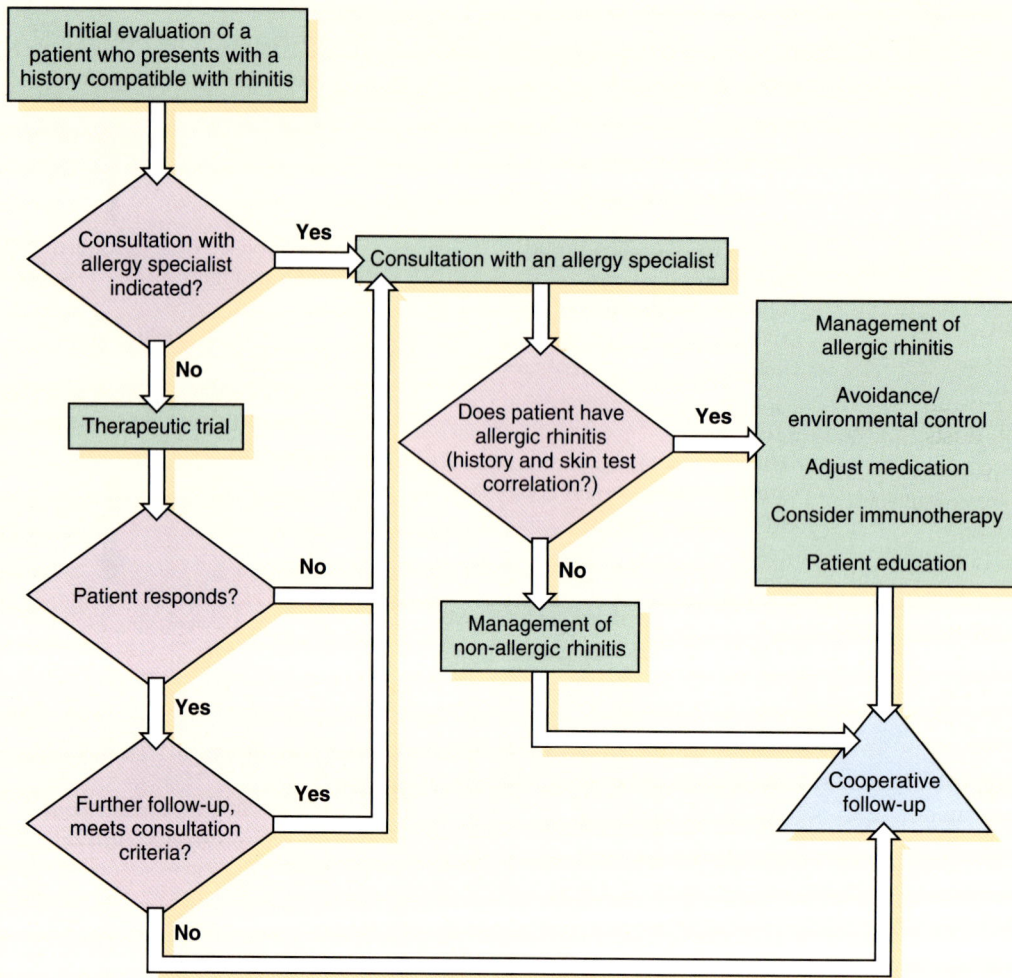

Figure 1-10 Rhinitis management algorithm. (Adapted with permission from Dykewicz MS, Fineman S, Nicklas R, et al: Joint Task Force algorithm and annotations for the diagnosis and management of rhinitis. Ann Allergy Asthma Immunol 1998;81:469–473. © 1998.)

XV. Patient Education Material and Handouts

Rhinitis is an inflammation of the mucous membranes of the nose. This can cause a stuffy, runny nose, postnasal drainage, itching, or sneezing. The nose inflammation may be caused by allergic or nonallergic factors.

A. Allergic Rhinitis

Allergic rhinitis is caused by the body's reactions to allergens such as house dust mites, pollens, molds, furry pets, and cockroaches. Allergens cause the body to produce allergic antibodies, which set off an allergic nose reaction when a person breathes in more of the allergen.

1. *Seasonal Allergic Rhinitis*
Sometimes called hay fever, seasonal allergic rhinitis is caused by allergic reactions to molds or tree, grass, or weed pollens that are present in outside air for only a certain season of the year. The length and time of allergy seasons vary in different regions of the country, depending on climate.

2. *Perennial Allergic Rhinitis*
This is caused by reactions to allergens that are present year-round. These usually are indoor allergens such as house dust mites or furry pets. In some warmer regions of the country, outdoor allergens such as molds can be present year-round and cause perennial allergic rhinitis.

3. ***True Food Allergy***
   A true food allergy involving allergic antibodies can cause rhinitis symptoms, but this is rare in adults unless other problems such as hives or abdominal symptoms are present, and relatively uncommon in children.

B. Nonallergic Rhinitis

In some people, rhinitis occurs without developing allergic antibodies. This usually causes year-round nose symptoms, so it can be difficult to tell whether year-round symptoms are caused by true allergies or not unless allergy testing is done. Nonallergic factors that can irritate or bother the nose without allergic antibodies include strong smells such as cleaning solutions or perfumes, cigarette smoke, or some dusts. Sudden temperature and atmospheric changes can also cause rhinitis symptoms. *Vasomotor rhinitis* is a medical term that is often used to refer to nonallergic rhinitis. Many people may also develop a runny nose or other nasal symptoms when they eat. This is usually caused by changes in the nervous system rather than by a true food allergy and is called *gustatory rhinitis*. Symptoms of nonallergic rhinitis may also occur because of medicines or the hormone changes of pregnancy or an underactive thyroid.

C. Mixed Rhinitis

Some people have a combination of allergic and nonallergic factors that cause rhinitis. Life is not always simple!

D. Treatment of Rhinitis

1. ***Avoid Bothersome Exposures***
   If you have symptoms of allergic rhinitis, the first rule is to try to avoid allergens that give you problems. Although sometimes you will know this from your experience, other times allergy testing is needed to reliably find out what allergies you have.

   - If you are allergic to outdoor allergens, try to reduce time outside, keep doors and windows closed, and use air conditioning whenever possible.
   - If you are allergic to house dust mites, pillows and mattresses should be covered with special covers that do not allow house dust mites to penetrate them; these need not be plastic covers, as there are now special cloth covers available. "Hypoallergenic" polyester pillows are actually no better than feather or down pillows if you are allergic to house dust mites.
   - If you are are allergic to pets and have them in your home, consider finding them a new home. Although keeping pets out of your bedroom at all times might help, this is often unsuccessful.

   - Air cleaners seem to help some people's allergies, but the benefit of air cleaners in scientific studies is usually disappointing, so the money for them may not be worth it.

2. If you are bothered by nonallergic factors, try to avoid exposures that give you problems:
   - If you are using strong-smelling cleaning solutions or paints, use good ventilation.
   - If you have to work with dusts, a filter face mask can reduce exposure.

E. Medications

The following is a brief summary of medications used to treat rhinitis.

1. ***Oral Antihistamines***
   These help reduce allergic nose and eye symptoms, but usually are not very effective for nonallergic rhinitis. Over-the-counter antihistamines, except for Claritin (Alavert), can often cause drowsiness and problems with thinking and driving (even if you don't feel sleepy). Therefore, newer antihistamines that cause fewer of these problems (Allegra, Claritin, Clarinex, Zyrtec) usually are better choices, even though they may not be more effective.
2. ***Oral Decongestants***
   These help reduce nasal stuffiness from allergic and nonallergic rhinitis, and are often combined with antihistamines. They may cause caffeine-like side effects such as nervousness and problems sleeping, and can raise blood pressure.
3. ***Nasally Inhaled Corticosteroids***
   These prescription drugs are generally the most effective drugs for allergic rhinitis, and can often help nonallergic rhinitis. The sprays should be not directed toward the center of the nose, as that can damage the nasal septum. The most common side effects are nose irritation and occasional nosebleeds. In general, these medications are very safe. However, when used in children, the lowest effective dose should be used, and height should be checked periodically because of concern that growth might be affected.
4. ***Nasally Inhaled Antihistamines***
   Azelastine nasal (Astelin) can help symptoms of allergic or nonallergic rhinitis. To avoid getting a bitter taste, the medicine should be sprayed in the nose with the head tilted down toward the feet. Occasional sleepiness can occur.
5. ***Decongestant Nasal Sprays***
   Although these can be used for 3–5 days for relief of nose congestion, longer use should be avoided, as this can result in worsening of nose congestion.

6. ***Intranasal Ipratropium***

   Atrovent is a prescription nose spray that can reduce a runny nose from allergic or nonallergic rhinitis, but it does not help other symptoms such as congestion.

F. Allergen Immunotherapy (Allergy Shots or Vaccines)

If your allergic rhinitis is difficult to control, you have symptoms that are present for many months of the year, or you need several medications in order to feel well, allergen immunotherapy may be a consideration for you. This treatment involves receiving injections over a period of 3–5 years. It helps your immune system react less when exposed to allergens. However, the benefit begins only after many months of treatment; it should be viewed as a long-term approach. Allergen immunotherapy does not help nonallergic rhinitis.

G. Refer to patient education CD, which is provided with this text, for additional patient education information. It has been formatted to provide readily accessible, easy-to-understand handouts for adult patients and the parents of pediatric patients. These handouts can be easily modified to fit specific practice requirements.

REFERENCES

1. Dykewicz MS, Fineman S, Nicklas R, et al: Joint Task Force algorithm and annotations for the diagnosis and management of rhinitis. Ann Allergy Asthma Immunol 1998;81: 469–473.
2. Wright AL, Holberg CJ, Martinez FD, et al: Epidemiology of physician-diagnosed allergic rhinitis in childhood. Pediatrics 1994;94:895–901.
3. Nelson HS, Rachelevsky GS, Bernick J, et al: Rhinitis. In The Allergy Report. Vol. 2. Diseases of the Atopic Diathesis, pp 1–172. Milwaukee: American Academy of Allergy, Asthma and Immunology, 2000. (Text also available on the web, www.aaaai.org.)
4. Bousquet J, van Cauwenberge P, Khaltaev N: Allergic rhinitis and its impact on asthma: ARIA workshop report. J Allergy Clin Immunol 2001;108:S147–S334.
5. Frederick JM, Warner JO, Jessop WJ, Enander I, Warner JA: Effect of a bed covering system in children with asthma and house dust mite hypersensitivity. Eur Respir J 1997;10:361–366.
6. Jen A, Baroody F, de Tineo M, et al: As-needed use of fluticasone propionate nasal spray reduced symptoms of seasonal allergic rhinitis. J Allergy Clin Immunol 2000;105: 732–738.
7. Newson-Smith G, Powell M, Baehre M, Garnham SP, MacMahon MT: A placebo controlled study comparing the efficacy of intranasal azelastine and beclomethasone in the treatment of seasonal allergic rhinitis. Eur Arch Otorhinolaryngol 1997;254:236–241.
8. Stern MA, Wade AG, Ridout SM, Cambell LM: Nasal budesonide offers superior symptom relief in perennial allergic rhinitis in comparison to nasal azelastine. Ann Allergy Asthma Immunol 1998;81:354–358.
9. Mygind N, Borum P: Intranasal ipratropium: Literature abstracts and comments. Rhinol Suppl 1989;9:37–44.
10. Bousquet J, Chanal I, Alquie MC, et al: Prevention of pollen rhinitis symptoms: Comparison of fluticasone propionate aqueous nasal spray and disodium cromoglycate aqueous nasal spray. A multicenter, double-blind, double-dummy, parallel-group study. Allergy 1993;48:327–333.
11. Brooks CD, Karl KJ, Francom SF: Oral methylprednisolone acetate (Medrol tablets) for seasonal rhinitis: Examination of dose and symptom response. J Clin Pharmacol 1993; 33:816–822.
12. Meltzer E, Malmstrom K, Lu S, et al: Concomitant montelukast and loratadine as treatment for seasonal allergic rhinitis: Placebo-controlled clinical trial. J Allergy Clin Immunol 2000;105:917–22.
13. Schatz M: Special considerations for the pregnant woman and senior citizen with airway disease. J Allergy Clin Immunol 1998;101:S373–S378.
14. Dykewicz MS, Fineman S, Skoner DP, et al: Diagnosis and management of rhinitis: Complete guidelines of the Joint Task Force on Practice Parameters in Allergy, Asthma and Immunology. Ann Allergy Asthma Immunol 1998;81: 478–518.

OTHER SUGGESTED READING

Dykewicz M: Rhinitis and sinusitis. J Allergy Clin Immunol 2003;111:S520–529.
Fireman P: Allergic rhinitis. In Fireman P, Slavin RG (eds): Atlas of Allergies, 2nd ed, pp 141–159. London: Mosby-Wolfe, 1996.

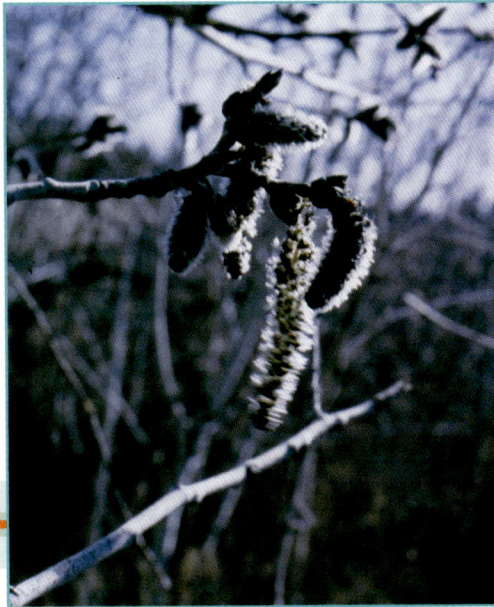

CHAPTER 2
Asthma

Sheldon L. Spector and Ricardo A. Tan

I. Introduction

Asthma is a chronic inflammatory condition of the airways characterized by bronchial hyperresponsiveness and airway obstruction, which are reversible in most patients. The primary goal of managing asthma is to control and diminish the chronic inflammatory process. Symptomatic therapy for acute bronchospasm with bronchodilator medications alone is no longer considered adequate treatment except for patients with mild, intermittent symptoms.

Up to 15 million people suffer from asthma in the United States. Despite better understanding of the pathophysiology of asthma and the introduction of potent anti-inflammatory therapy, the morbidity and mortality from asthma continue to rise, especially in the inner cities. The increasing number of cases of asthma seen in developed countries has led to the hygiene hypothesis, which suggests that decreased exposure to infections during infancy and childhood induces T-helper cells to commit to the Th_2 (T-helper 2) pathway and production of cytokines that promote asthma and allergy. On the other hand, early exposure to infections appears to induce the Th_1 (T-helper 1) pathway.[1]

Based on the frequency and severity of symptoms, asthma can be classified into the following categories:[2] (1) mild intermittent asthma, with daytime symptoms that occur not more than twice a week and nighttime symptoms that occur not more than twice a month; (2) mild persistent asthma, with daytime symptoms that occur more than twice a week but not every day, and nighttime symptoms that occur more than twice a month; (3) moderate persistent asthma, with daytime symptoms that occur daily and nighttime symptoms that occur more than once a week; and (4) severe persistent asthma, in which symptoms are continuous.

Asthmatics are heterogeneous in regard to (1) the triggers that produce symptoms; (2) the primary location of obstruction (i.e., the large airways, small airways, or both); (3) the extent and predominant mechanism of obstruction (i.e., mucous plugging, bronchospasm, or bronchial edema); (4) the percentage of reversible obstruction with treatment; (5) response to medication; and (6) the amount of medication necessary to achieve a satisfactory response. Patient education is therefore as important as comprehensive symptomatic and anti-inflammatory therapy for this serious yet treatable condition. With proper management, most asthmatics can live active lifestyles with few restrictions.

II. Epidemiology

A. Prevalence

The prevalence of asthma in the United States has been reported to range between 3 and 10 per 100,000 population. Despite improved therapy, asthma deaths continue to occur at a rate of 5,000–6,000 each year in the United States.[3] The mortality and morbidity from asthma have been increasing all over the world, especially in developed countries. In the United States, the prevalence of asthma has been increasing especially quickly in inner-city and minority populations. Most cases of asthma have their onset before age 10. There is a 2:1 male-female ratio.

B. Risk Factors

Risk factors for the development of asthma in children and infants include a family history of asthma or allergy, the presence of other atopic conditions (e.g., allergic rhinitis, atopic dermatitis), maternal smoking, viral infections, early exposure to indoor allergens such as house dust mites and molds, diet, and prematurity.[4–8]

III. Etiology and Pathophysiology

A. Acute Asthma

Exposure to a specific trigger (e.g., pollen, cat dander) in a sensitized patient will lead to cross-linking of specific IgE on mast cells and basophils, which causes degranulation of these cells and release of inflammatory mediators such as histamine, leukotrienes, and prostaglandins. Bronchoconstriction, increased vascular permeability, edema, mucous production, and inflammatory cell influx are among the effects of these mediators. Acute asthma symptoms are largely due to bronchial muscle constriction and airway obstruction from mucous production and mucosal swelling. Persistent inflammatory episodes lead to chronic injury and disruption of airway epithelium.

B. Chronic Asthma

Chronic airway inflammation in asthma results from complex interactions of inflammatory cells and their products. Mast cells, eosinophils, macrophages, neutrophils, and the T-helper type 2 subtype of T-lymphocytes are among the most important of these cells. Recent research has focused on identifying the cytokines, cell products that act on other cells, that are involved in asthma. The interaction of these cytokines is very relevant in the search for new asthma therapies. The list of cytokines involved in asthma continues to grow every day and includes pro-inflammatory cytokines (e.g., tumor necrosis factor-alpha [TNF-α], interleukin-1 [IL-1], IL-6, IL-11), anti-inflammatory cytokines (e.g., IL-10, IL-12, IL-18, interferon-gamma [IFN-γ]), chemokines (e.g., MCP-1, MCP-2, MCP-3, eotaxin, RANTES), growth factors (e.g.,transforming growth factor-beta [TGF-β], epidermal growth factor [EGF]), lymphokines (e.g., IL-2, IL-4, IL-5, IL-13, IL-17), and adhesion molecules (e.g., integrins).[9,10]

Genetic and environmental factors determine the initial time of appearance of asthma, which is often in childhood or adolescence but may occur at any age.

Airway remodeling refers to an irreversible component of airway obstruction resulting from chronic inflammation, especially if it is untreated. The concept of airway remodeling, which challenges the long-held belief that reversibility is a hallmark of asthma, is supported by growing evidence. Airway wall thickening results from deposition of fibronectin, collagen I and III, and reticulin in the lamina reticularis and extracellular matrix. Narrowing of the lumen by hypertrophy and hyperplasia of airway smooth muscle cells contributes to the obstruction.[11]

IV. Clinical Manifestations

A. History

1. Episodic shortness of breath, wheezing, chest tightness, and cough are the most common symptoms of asthma. Secondary manifestations or complaints include fatigue, moodiness, changes in breathing pattern, rhinorrhea or other nasal symptoms, itching of the throat or ears, and difficulty sleeping or exercising.

2. Symptoms are usually precipitated by allergens such as pollen or animal dander, irritants such as cigarette smoke or perfume, viral and bacterial respiratory tract infections, or exercise. Strong emotions such as anger, excitement, and laughing can also precipitate symptoms.

3. Seasonal symptoms, especially in the spring and fall, are usually due to pollen sensitivity. Perennial or year-round symptoms are often due to exposure to indoor allergens such as animals, dust mites, or molds. In humid areas such as Florida, outdoor mold allergy can trigger perennial symptoms.

4. *Cough-variant asthma* refers to a kind of asthma in which cough is the sole complaint, but affected individuals show evidence of bronchospasm on pulmonary function testing or bronchial hyperreactivity on a methacholine challenge test.[12]

5. *Nocturnal asthma symptoms* may be a sign of worsening severity. Many asthmatics have constant symptoms despite avoidance of precipitating factors. This may be due to longstanding chronic airway inflammation causing persistent airway obstruction.

6. A *family history* of atopy is usually present. *Atopy* is the tendency to have IgE-mediated allergic responses to environmental allergens. Atopic conditions such as allergic rhinitis and atopic dermatitis are frequently associated with asthma.

B. Physical Examination

1. During an acute asthma attack, the affected individual often has labored and shallow breathing, coughing, flaring of the nostrils, intercostal muscle retractions, hunched shoulders, and audible wheezing. These signs may vary, depending on the degree of severity.
2. Expiratory wheezes may be audible with the unaided ear or heard diffusely over the lung fields on auscultation.
3. Asthmatics may have a normal physical examination when asymptomatic. Signs of associated atopic conditions such as allergic rhinitis and atopic dermatitis, if present, may support the diagnosis of asthma.
4. In *severe asthma* with impending respiratory failure, wheezes may be absent due to the diminished air entry into the lungs. *Pulsus paradoxus*, a difference in systolic and diastolic blood pressure of more than 12 mm Hg, indicates decreased intrathoracic pressure and may be observed. Confusion and deteriorating mental status are signs of hypoxia and respiratory failure.

V. Differential Diagnosis

A. Acute Bronchitis

Acute bronchitis is often a viral infection of the large bronchi with a relatively sudden onset. Symptoms include coughing productive of yellow to green sputum, fever, and shortness of breath. Wheezing is not common. Treatment for purely viral triggers is symptomatic. When secondary bacterial infection occurs, antibiotics may be appropriate.

B. Chronic Bronchitis

Chronic bronchitis is a longstanding infection of the bronchi that lasts for months or years. It is defined as a condition associated with excessive mucous production causing a productive cough for at least 3 months of the year for more than 2 years. It is usually associated with a history of cigarette smoking and is considered a form of chronic obstructive pulmonary disease (COPD). Wheezing is often present due to a bronchospastic component. During acute exacerbations, antibiotics are often indicated. Chronic antibiotic therapy may be useful in some cases. Lack of reversibility in the FEV_1 of at least 12% on inhalation of a β-agonist differentiates COPD from asthma.

C. Emphysema

Emphysema is another form of COPD characterized by permanent distention of air spaces distal to the terminal bronchiole due to loss of elasticity. There is also destruction of alveolar septa. The damaged conduits lose their ability to collapse and force the air out. The condition is invariably caused by many years of cigarette smoking. Symptoms include cough, wheezing, and shortness of breath. Treatment focuses on smoking cessation and supportive medications. Supplemental oxygen may be necessary, especially in the later stages with air trapping and poor air exchange. The hereditary form of emphysema, α_1-antitrypsin deficiency, is not associated with cigarette smoking and occurs in younger individuals. As with chronic bronchitis, lack of reversibility in the FEV_1 of at least 12% on inhalation of a β-agonist differentiates emphysema from asthma.

D. Croup

Croup is a viral infection, especially common in young children, that causes swelling of the vocal cords or surrounding tissue. With progression of the viral infection, there is typically a barking seal-like cough that is often worse at night and is accompanied by fever, runny nose, and nasal stuffiness. Severe cases may require hospitalization and supplemental oxygen. Most patients can be managed at home with mist vaporizers and symptomatic therapy.

E. Bronchiolitis

Bronchiolitis is an acute viral infection usually due to respiratory syncytial virus (RSV) affecting the smaller airways in very young children. Wheezing, cough, and retraction of the chest are common. The clinical picture resembles other viral-induced asthma syndromes.

F. Pneumonia

Pneumonia may affect any age group but is more common in the very young or very old. It is a viral or bacterial infection of the lower airways and alveoli. Common symptoms include high fever, malaise, cough, and shortness of breath. Treatment is aimed at the cause of the infection.

G. Cystic Fibrosis

Cystic fibrosis is an autosomal recessive genetic disorder characterized by recurrent pneumonia, sinusitis, gastrointestinal (GI) problems, and slowed growth resulting from abnormal electrolyte and water transport at the cellular level. Wheezing and cough may accompany respiratory tract infections. The standardized sweat chloride test shows a higher concentration of sodium and chloride in patients with cystic fibrosis. Specific gene therapy may be the treatment of choice in the future.

H. Gastroesophageal Reflux Disease

Gastroesophageal refulx disease (GERD) is a common condition characterized by reflux of gastric contents back into the esophagus, resulting in inflammation, which produces chest tightness and burning. GERD can be either a cause of chest symptoms in nonasthmatics or an aggravating factor worsening asthma resulting from spilling of acid from the esophagus into the airways. A clue is concomitant coughing and choking during recumbency. Treatment of GER may significantly improve asthma symptoms in patients with both conditions.[13]

I. Allergic Bronchopulmonary Aspergillosis

Allergic bronchopulmonary aspergillosis is a chronic inflammatory airway condition resulting from an immunologically mediated response to *Aspergillus fumigatus*. There is no single diagnostic test, but characteristic features include asthma, a positive skin test to *Aspergillus*, elevated total serum IgE >1,000 IU/mL, peripheral eosinophilia >0.5 × 10^9/L, precipitating IgG to *Aspergillus*, elevated serum IgE and IgG to *Aspergillus*, fleeting chest x-ray infiltrates, and central bronchiectasis. Oral steroids are often the treatment of choice.

J. Pulmonary Embolism

Pulmonary embolism (PE) is a life-threatening condition resulting from lodging of thromboemboli in the pulmonary circulation, usually originating from deep vein thrombosis (DVT) in the lower extremities. PE may be silent or associated with sudden shortness of breath, chest pain, cough, wheezing, and hemoptysis. It should be suspected in patients with sudden symptoms who have been immobilized due to disease or have been in a sitting position for long periods of time (e.g., on a long car ride or plane trip). Right ventricular cardiac failure is usually the immediate cause of death.

K. Cardiac Asthma

Cardiac asthma is a general term commonly used to refer to symptoms of wheezing and paroxysmal nocturnal dyspnea due to congestive heart failure (CHF) or PE. It can occur concomitantly with asthma and can complicate diagnosis and treatment. The signs of CHF include basilar rales, leg edema, and congested neck veins. Chest x-ray and cardiac ultrasound often confirm the diagnosis. Treatment of the underlying heart disease ameliorates the symptoms.

L. Hypersensitivity Pneumonitis

Hypersensitivity pneumonitis is an immunologic pulmonary disorder due to inhalation of biologic dusts, chemicals, or even certain medications. The list of organic substances that can be responsible for this order continues to expand and includes mushrooms, grains, wood dust, cheese, bird and mammal proteins, and microbial growth from humidifiers. Coughing, fever, and malaise are often the initial symptoms, followed by shortness of breath, coughing, and weight loss with continued exposure. Avoidance is the best therapy once the agent is suspected and identified, but oral corticosteroids may be necessary for the chronic form.

M. Medication-Induced Cough

Medication-induced cough can occur with such agents as angiotensin-converting enzyme (ACE) inhibitors used for the treatment of hypertension and coronary artery disease. It is rarely associated with wheezing or dyspnea.

N. Foreign Body Aspiration

Foreign body aspiration should be suspected with the sudden onset of shortness of breath, coughing, and wheezing, especially in individuals with no history of previous breathing problems. In children, this may occur while eating or playing with a toy small enough to enter the airways.

O. Vocal Cord Dysfunction

Vocal cord dysfunction is caused by abnormal adduction of the vocal cords leading to episodic choking or shortness of breath. A flow-volume loop obtained during spirometry will show a characteristic flattened inspiratory portion. Patients with vocal cord dysfunction may be mistakenly diagnosed as having severe asthma.[14]

VI. Diagnostic Procedures

A. Peak Flow Meter (see Chapter 18)

Peak flow measurement is a simple, convenient, and inexpensive way to assess airway obstruction in the office and at home. Patients expire forcefully into the peak flow meter, usually a hollow tube, which registers the peak expiratory flow rate (PEFR) in liters per second. The PEFR correlates well with the presence of bronchospasm and is a good estimate of asthma severity. Table 2-1 shows the approximate normal peak flow rate values based on age, height, and sex.

The peak flow meter is recommended for home monitoring for individuals with moderate to severe asthma. Regular once-daily home monitoring, preferably at bedtime when peak flow readings are at their lowest, is useful in following the status of patients, especially those with decreased symptom awareness. An action plan based on peak flow readings that includes specific instructions for using medications and calling the physician should be provided.

Computerized handheld devices that fit easily into a patient's pocket are now available to record peak flow and FEV$_1$ (forced expiratory volume in 1 second) and transmit the results to the doctor's office via a modem (Airwatch). This provides the physician with precise and accurate readings.

B. Spirometry

Spirometry measures lung volumes and flow rates during maximum expiratory effort. Spirometry can be used to determine the reversibility of airways disease and to monitor pulmonary function throughout the course

TABLE 2-1

Approximate Normal Peak Flow Rate Values

Children and Adolescents

Height (Inches)	Males (L/min)	Females (L/min)	Height (Inches)	Males (L/min)	Females (L/min)
40	115	114	55	316	315
41	128	127	56	329	328
42	141	141	57	343	342
43	155	154	58	356	355
44	166	168	59	370	369
45	182	181	60	383	382
46	195	194	61	397	395
47	209	208	62	410	409
48	222	221	63	423	422
49	235	235	64	437	436
50	249	248	65	450	449
51	262	261	66	464	462
52	276	275	67	477	476
53	289	288	68	491	489
54	303	302	69	504	503

Males

Age in Years	Height (Inches) 60	65	70	75	80
15	511	531	548	564	578
20	554	604	624	681	740
25	580	608	636	682	730
30	584	617	627	660	703
35	599	622	643	661	677
40	597	620	641	659	675
45	591	613	633	651	668
50	580	602	622	640	656
55	566	588	608	625	640
60	551	572	591	607	622
65	533	554	572	588	603
70	515	535	552	568	582
75	496	515	532	547	560

Females

Age in Years	Height (Inches) 60	65	70	75	80
15	423	438	451	463	473
20	444	460	474	486	497
25	455	471	485	497	509
30	458	475	489	502	513
35	458	474	488	501	512
40	453	469	483	496	507
45	446	462	476	488	499
50	437	453	466	478	489
55	427	442	455	467	477
60	415	430	443	454	464
65	403	417	430	441	451
70	390	404	416	427	436
75	377	391	402	413	422

These figures are a guideline only. The range of "normal" functions is dependent on many factors that cannot all be included in a table. Data from National Heart, Lung and Blood Institute. Expert Panel Report: Update on Selected Topics 2002. National Asthma Education and Prevention Panel 2002. NIH Publication 02–5075.

of the disease. It is also recommended as part of the initial assessment for all patients with underlying pulmonary disease and as a tool to follow the therapeutic progress.

If performed properly, spirometry can give the clinician much more detailed information about each patient's pulmonary status, including large and small airway diseases, different lung volume measurements, restrictive versus obstructive respiratory disease, and much more. It is important to master the proper use of spirometry because improper use can alter the expected results.

C. Bronchial Challenge Testing or Bronchoprovocation (see Chapter 17)

In some patients with normal spirometry values, asthma may still be suspected. These patients can undergo bronchial challenges, such as the methacholine challenge, which can help determine the degree of airway reactivity.[15] The methacholine challenge is the gold standard for accurate diagnosis of asthma, but because of the risks involved, it is only used for difficult diagnostic dilemmas. Pre- and postspirometric bronchodilatory challenges with albuterol will suffice for most patients in the diagnostic evaluation of reactive airways disease.

D. Allergen-Specific IgE Testing (see Chapters 12 and 13)

Skin testing for allergens should be done to identify allergenic triggers for asthma. Scratch or prick testing is available for approximately 60–70 allergens. Intradermal testing is more sensitive and can be done to detect milder allergen sensitivity. Pollen skin testing should always be directed to the trees, weeds, and grasses in the region where the patient lives. Most antihistamines should be withheld for 3 days prior to testing. A positive control (histamine) and negative (saline) control should always be used.[16]

Serum antigen-specific IgE assays can also be performed for allergen identification. The radioallergosorbent test (RAST) is the most widely known, but there are a variety of assays available. Skin testing correlates better with clinical symptoms than serum assays and is currently the preferred method of testing. Serum assays should be done in patients who refuse skin testing, have extensive skin disease, or have other conditions that prevent skin testing.[16]

VII. Approach to Final Diagnosis

A. Presumptive Diagnosis Based on History

A presumptive diagnosis of asthma can be made with a history of episodic shortness of breath, cough, or wheezing responsive to bronchodilator medications. This diagnosis should be confirmed as soon as it is practical to examine the patient in the office while symptomatic.

B. Spirometry (see Chapter 16)

Spirometry should be done to further support the diagnosis with a finding of a lowered FEV_1 that is at least 12% reversible with inhaled β_2-agonists.

C. Bronchial Challenge (see Chapter 17)

A bronchial challenge or bronchoprovocation testing is usually not necessary for the diagnosis of asthma but may be performed in patients with atypical symptoms or specific triggers such as exercise or occupational allergens.

D. Specific IgE Testing (see Chapters 12 and 13)

Testing for specific IgE through the skin or serum should be done to identify allergenic triggers.

VIII. Therapy and Management

A. Control of Aggravating Factors (see Appendix 7 and patient education CD)

1. *Allergens*
   a. *Pollen.* Pollen from trees, grasses, and weeds results mainly in seasonal exacerbations. Although there are exceptions, and pollination periods overlap, trees generally pollinate in the spring, grasses in the summer, and weeds in the fall. There is usually minimal pollination in the winter. It is helpful to keep windows closed while in the car to minimize pollen exposure. Windows should also be kept closed at home, especially during days with a high pollen count. Hot and windy days generally promote widespread airborne pollen distribution. Air conditioning may be needed in the summer to allow windows to be kept closed. Pollen counts tend to be highest between the hours of 11 a.m. and 3 p.m., and patients should plan their outdoor activities before or after this period. Local pollen counting centers often have toll-free phone numbers or Internet web sites that provide current pollen count and distribution information.
   b. *Dust mites.* Dust mites are very common indoor allergens. *Dermatophagoides farinae* and *Dermatophagoides pteronyssinus* are the two known allergenic species. Dust mites, which are microscopic, thrive in high humidity and are found in pillows, mattresses, and upholstered furniture, especially items containing feathers. One of the most important control measures is to use impermeable covers for pillows and mattresses and to wash sheets and covers in hot water of at least 130°F at least once weekly. Acaricides can kill dust mites, while tannic acid solutions may be used to neutralize allergenic proteins in carpets and upholstered furniture. Occasionally, it may be necessary to remove carpets and install hardwood floors to lessen the dust mite population.
   c. *Animals.* Pets, especially cats and dogs, are often the causes of household allergies and asthma. Removing the animal from the patient's environment is the most effective form of treatment. Patients who consider their pets as part of the family and are unable to give them up should keep pets out of the bedroom to keep symptoms under control. If a pet is removed from the house, the carpets, walls, and sheets should then be thoroughly cleaned, as animal dander has been detected for up to 6 months after removal when this is not done. Cockroach allergy is an important trigger, especially in inner cities. High-efficiency particulate air (HEPA) filters can help remove airborne pollen and animal dander, although they are less effective in removing dust mites, which usually are not airborne.
   d. *Molds.* Mold allergy is a major problem in humid climates, where both outdoor and indoor molds trigger asthma. *Cladosporium* and *Alternaria* are the predominant outdoor molds in many areas and peak in the late summer and autumn. *Aspergillus* and *Penicillium* are often found indoors on bathroom walls, in damp basements, and in trash areas. Old carpets with patches of mold underneath should be removed. Bleach solutions may be used to wash off visible mold on bathroom and basement walls.
2. *Allergic Rhinitis*
   Allergic rhinitis and asthma are often present concomitantly in atopic patients. In recent years, there has been growing evidence that treatment of upper airway inflammation in allergic rhinitis leads to better control of asthma.[17] The mechanism for this relationship is still not completely clear, but the likely possibilities include activation of a nasobronchial reflex, mouth breathing due to nasal congestion causing bronchial inhalation of nonhumidified cold air, postnasal drainage into the bronchi, and the systemic effects of inflammatory mediators released from the nose and sinuses.[18] There is growing evidence that treatment of allergic rhinitis with antihistamines or intranasal steroids can improve concomitant asthma.[19,20]
3. *Sinusitis*
   Chronic sinusitis has often been associated with uncontrolled chronic asthma. It is still not clear whether the two conditions coexist because of similar pathologic mechanisms or whether asthma is triggered by sinus infections. Studies have shown, however, that asthma improves when sinusitis is treated.[21,22] While acute sinus infections have obvious

signs and symptoms such as facial pressure and puru- lent nasal discharge, chronic sinusitis may present only with nonspecific symptoms such as cough or postnasal drip. Acute sinusitis usually responds to 10–14 days of antibiotic therapy, but chronic sinusitis requires a prolonged course of at least 3–4 weeks. A limited four-section CT scan of the sinuses and the osteomeadal complex is a cost-effective imaging procedure for the diagnosis of chronic sinusitis.[23]

4. ***Respiratory Tract Infections***
   Viral respiratory tract infections are common precipitants of acute asthma, especially in children. Bacterial infections such as pharyngitis and bronchitis should be treated promptly with antibiotics. Annual influenza vaccinations are recommended for persons with chronic asthma.[24] These are usually given starting in October and November, with protective immunity present in 2 weeks and lasting for approximately 4 months. A one time pneumococcal vaccine is also recommended for these patients.

5. ***Exercise***
   Most asthmatics experience their first symptoms with exertion. In certain patients, exercise remains the only precipitating or aggravating factor. When tested in the laboratory, exercise-induced asthma (EIA) is defined as a drop in FEV_1 of 10%–15% or more after 10–15 minutes of exertion. Symptoms usually peak after exercise, so the individual may feel fine during exercise. The exact mechanism of EIA is unclear. The two main hypotheses are (1) loss of water due to increased ventilation leads to increased osmolarity, causing mast cell degranulation, or (2) rapid rewarming after exercise causes vasodilation and edema in the airways.[25] After a person exercises for at least 10–15 minutes, whether or not asthma symptoms occur, there is a period of up to 3 hours known as the refractory period when no further symptoms are seen despite continued exercise. Asthmatic athletes use this period to their advantage by warming up before exercise and by increasing the intensity of exertion gradually. Inhaled β_2-agonists (Proventil, Maxair), cromolyn (Intal), or nedocromil (Tilade) may be used 30 minutes to 1 hour before exercise to prevent symptoms.

6. ***Gastroesopheageal Reflux Disease***
   Patients who complain of heartburn should be evaluated for GERD. However, GERD should still be considered even in patients without typical symptoms. Acid reflux can be aspirated and be responsible for refractory asthma.[13] Persons with GERD should keep their heads elevated during sleep and avoid lying down for up to 3 hours after meals. H_2 blockers such as ranitidine (Zantac), 150 mg bid, or proton pump inhibitors such as omeprazole (Prilosec), 20 mg/day,

decrease acid production and improve symptoms. Esophageal pH monitoring is occasionally performed if the diagnosis is not clear.

7. ***Air Pollution and Occupational Exposures***
   Asthmatic patients frequently complain of exacerbations due to air pollution. Ozone, nitrogen dioxide and sulfur dioxide, and total suspended particulates are the likely irritants in the atmosphere.[26] Occupational asthma refers to asthma precipitated primarily in the workplace. Examples of occupational allergens include *Bacillus subtilis* enzymes for detergent workers and soybean dust for farmers. It is important to diagnose occupational asthma conclusively by comparing pulmonary function inside and outside the workplace, as the diagnosis can have far-reaching career and financial consequences for the person. The only effective treatment for occupational asthma is to remove the person or the offending agent from the workplace.

8. ***Aspirin and Other NSAIDs***
   Up to 39% of asthmatics have exacerbations induced by aspirin and nonsteroidal anti-inflammatory drugs (NSAIDs). This association should be considered in patients with nasal polyps as part of the "aspirin triad" (asthma, nasal polyps, sinusitis). The mechanism of aspirin sensitivity is non-IgE-mediated and most commonly attributed to excessive production of leukotrienes from the lipoxygenase pathway due to blockage of the cyclo-oxygenase pathway of arachidonic acid metabolism.[27] The effectiveness of antileukotriene agents in blocking aspirin-induced bronchospasm supports this mechanism. Desensitization with increasing doses of aspirin has been shown in some studies to improve aspirin-sensitive asthma.[28]

9. ***Drugs***
   a. ***β-Blockers.*** Commonly used for hypertension, heart disease, migraine, or glaucoma, β-blockers can worsen asthma by blocking the bronchodilation associated with the adrenergic system. β-blocker eyedrops can trigger asthma attacks. Nonspecific β-blockers can significantly produce both blood vessel constriction and bronchial constriction. Propanolol (Inderal) is the most widely known. Nonspecific β-blockers should be avoided in asthma. Specific β-blockers act primarily on blood vessels, with less effect on the bronchial airways. However, they should be used by asthmatics only if there are no alternatives, as they can still aggravate asthma. Examples include atenolol (Tenormin) and metoprolol (Lopressor).
   b. ***ACE inhibitors.*** ACE inhibitors (e.g., lisinopril [Zestril], enalapril [Vasotec]), commonly indicated in hypertension and heart disease, cause a cough

in 10% of patients.[29] These drugs do not cause bronchospasm directly, but the induced cough can aggravate asthma.

B. Approach to Acute Asthma (Based on NHLBI Guidelines)

1. ***At Home*** (Fig. 2-1)
   a. β_2-agonists provide bronchodilation within minutes and are the first-line medications for acute asthma attacks. During an acute attack, two to four puffs of a metered-dose inhaler (MDI) or a nebulizer treatment may be given every 20 minutes for up to a total of three doses. If there is significant improvement, the patient may continue two puffs from an MDI every 4–6 hours for the next 24 hours.
   b. Oral steroids should be started if there is only partial or temporary relief of symptoms. For adults, prednisone, 40–60 mg/day for 3–10 days or its equivalent, is recommended. For children, the recommended dose is 1–2 mg/kg/day for 3–10 days.
   c. If no improvement is evident, the patient should go to an emergency room for further treatment and evaluation.

2. ***Emergency Room*** (Fig. 2-2)
   a. ***Oxygen therapy.*** Oxygen via nasal cannula or face mask should be given to keep oxygen saturation at ≥90%.
   b. ***Bronchodilator treatment.*** Inhaled β_2-agonists should be given at frequent intervals or continuously until improvement occurs. Alternatively, a subcutaneous β_2-agonist (e.g., epinephrine) may be given for a total of three doses over 60–90 minutes. Anticholinergic agents such as ipatropium may be helpful in severe symptoms or concomitant COPD.
   c. ***Corticosteroids.*** Oral steroids should be started for most patients seen in the emergency room if this has not yet been done. Steroids may be given intravenously (IV) if the patient is nauseous or vomiting. IV methylprednisolone (Solumedrol), 40–60 mg every 4–6 hours, is often used.
   d. ***Aminophylline.*** The usefulness of IV aminophylline continues to be debated. At this time, most experts do not recommend theophylline or aminophylline for emergency treatment because they do not appear to be effective in this setting.

e. ***Antibiotics.*** Routine use of antibiotics for asthma exacerbations is not recommended. Antibiotic therapy should be used only when there is evidence of bacterial infection.
f. ***Response to treatment.*** Frequent reevaluation of the patient's progress by physical examination and spirometry will help guide further treatment. In general, an FEV_1 or peak expiratory flow (PEF) of ≥70% is considered a good response, ≥50% but <70% an incomplete response, and <50% a poor response.

Patients deemed to be ready for discharge should be given instructions to continue and finish the oral steroid course at home. Inhaled β_2-agonist use at regular intervals should be continued for at least 24 hours.

An incomplete response or a poor response (see Status Asthmaticus, following) is an indication for hospital admission.
g. ***Respiratory failure.*** Deteriorating mental status, signs of respiratory fatigue, cyanosis, "silent chest" due to poor air entry, a PCO_2 of >42 mm Hg all point to respiratory failure. These patients should be intubated and started on mechanical ventilation immediately to avoid respiratory or cardiac arrest.

3. ***Status Asthmaticus***
   a. Status asthmaticus refers to severe airway obstruction with no improvement with previously effective bronchodilator therapy. Patients who respond poorly to treatment in the emergency room should be started on IV steroids and hospital admission considered. Status asthmaticus is a life-threatening emergency and is best treated in the hospital intensive care unit, under the careful observation and monitoring of a specialist.
   b. Systemic steroids at the dosage equivalent of 60–240 mg of prednisone in divided doses for adults may be necessary initially. For children, 1–2 mg/kg every 4–6 hours is suggested.
   c. Continuously administered or intermittently used aerosolized β-agonists such as albuterol or levalbuterol are the mainstay of initial therapy.
   d. Epinephrine, 0.25–0.5 mL of 1:1000 solution, may also be used, especially in the younger age group.
   e. IV aminophylline may be useful in a subgroup of patients, aiming for a blood level of 10–18 mg/mL.
   f. Infections should be treated appropriately.
   g. Blood gases, spirometry, or peak flow measurements should be closely monitored.

Assess symptoms/Peak flow

Mild-to-moderate exacerbation
PEF 50-80% predicted or personal best
or
Signs and symptoms:
• Cough, breathlessness, wheeze, or chest
  tightness (correlate imperfectly with severity
  of exacerbation) or
• Waking at night due to asthma, or
• Decreased ability to perform usual activities

Severe exacerbation
PEF <50% predicted or personal best
or
Signs and symptoms:
• Marked wheezing and shortness of breath
• Cyanosis
• Trouble walking or talking due to asthma
• Accessory muscle use
• Suprasternal retractions

Instructions to patient
Inhaled short-acting beta$_2$-agonist
• Up to three treatments of 2–4 puffs by MCI
  at 20-minute intervals, or
• Single nebulizer treatment
Assess symptoms and/or peak flow after 1 hour

Good response
(mild exacerbation)
PEF >80% predicted or personal
best and/or
Signs and symptoms:
• No wheezing, shortness of breath,
  cough, or chest tightness, and
• Response to beta$_2$-agonist
  sustained for 4 hours

Incomplete response
(moderate exacerbation)
PEF 50-80% predicted or personal
best or
Signs and symptoms:
Persistent wheezing, shortness of
breath, cough, or chest tightness

Poor response
(severe exacerbation)
PEF <50% predicted or personal
best or
Signs and symptoms:
• Marked wheezing, shortness of
  breath, cough, or chest tightness
• Distress is severe and
  nonresponsive
• Response to beta$_2$-agonist lasts
  <2 hours

Instructions to patient
• May continue 2–4 puffs
  beta$_2$-agonist every 3–4 hours for
  24–48 hours prn
• For patients on inhaled steroids,
  double dose for 7–10 days
• Contact clinician within 48 hours
  for instructions

Instructions to patient
• Take 2–4 puffs beta$_2$-agonist
  every 2–4 hours for 24–48
  hours prn
• Add oral steroid**
• Contact clinician urgently
  (same day) for instructions

Instructions to patient
IMMEDIATELY:
• Take up to 3 treatments of
  4–6 puffs beta$_2$-agonist every
  20 minutes prn
• Start oral steroid**
• Contact clinician
• Proceed to emergency
  department, or call ambulance
  or 9-1-1

*Patient at high risk for asthma-related death should receive immediate clinical attention after initial treatment. More intensive therapy may be required.
**Oral steroid dosages:
Adult: 40–60 mg, single or 2 divided doses for 3–10 days.
Child: 1–2 mg/kg/day, maximum 60 mg/day, for 3–10 days.

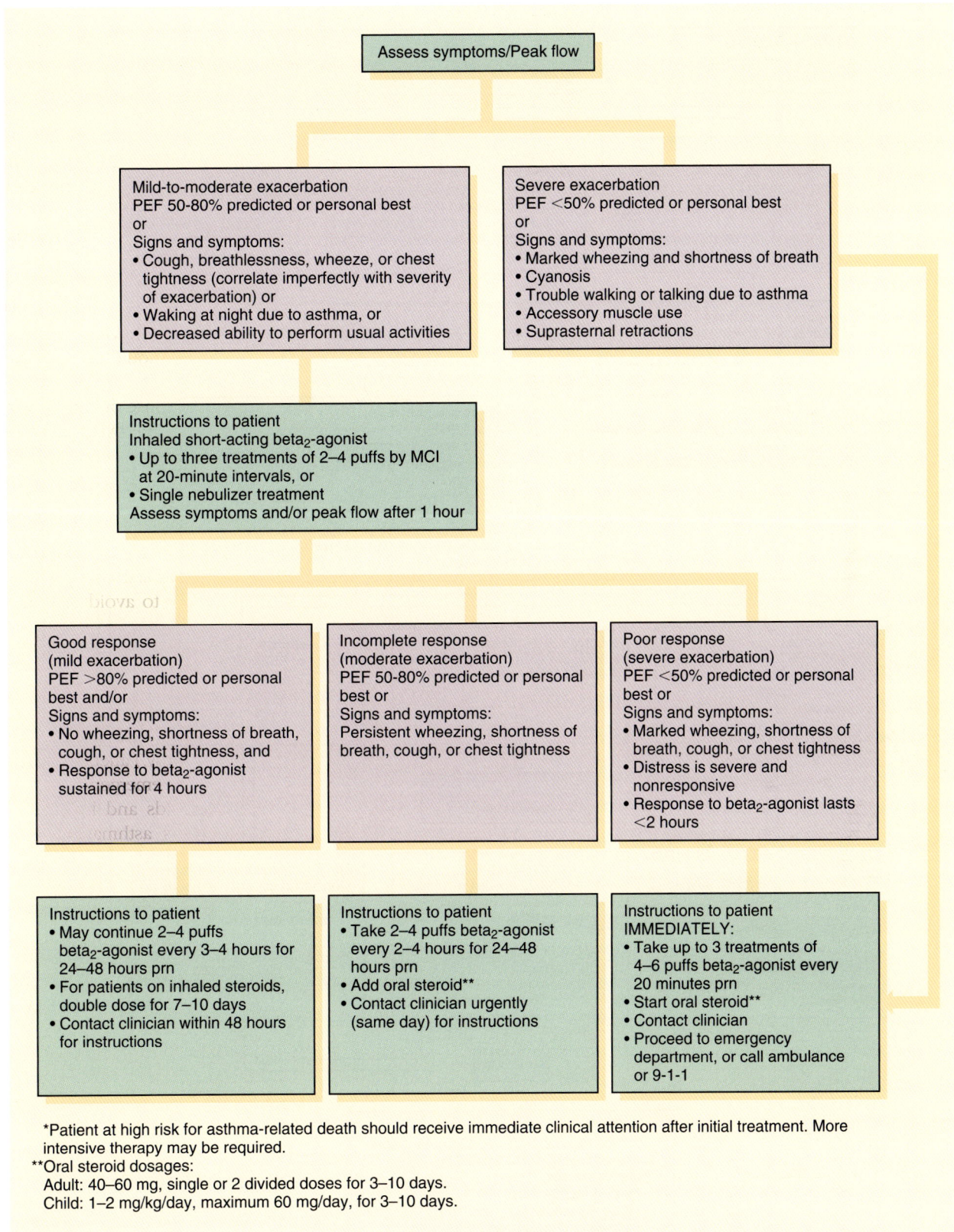

Figure 2-1 Management of asthma exacerbations: home treatment. (From National Heart, Lung and Blood Institute. Expert Panel Report 2. Guidelines for the Diagnosis and Management of Asthma. National Asthma Education and Prevention Program. NIH Publication 97-4051. Bethesda, MD: NIH, 1997.)

Initial assessment
History, physical examination (auscultation, use of accessory muscles, heart rate, respiratory rate), PEF or FEV_1, oxygen saturation, and other tests as indicated

---

FEV_1 or PEF >50%
- Oxygen to achieve O_2 saturation ≥90%
- Inhaled beta₂-agonist by metered dose inhaler or nebulizer, up to three treatments in first hour
- Oral steroids if no immediate response or if patient recently took oral steroid

FEV_1 or PEF <50%
(severe exacerbation)
- Oxygen to achieve O_2 saturation ≥90%
- Inhaled high-dose beta₂-agonist and anticholinergic by nebulization every 20 minutes or continuously for 1 hour
- Oral steroid

Impending or actual respiratory arrest
- Intubation and mechanical ventilation with 100% O_2
- Nebulized beta₂-agonist and anticholinergic
- Intravenous steroid

Repeat assessment
Symptoms, physical examination, PEF, O2 saturation, other tests as needed

---

Moderate exacerbation
FEV_1 or PEF 50–60% predicted/personal best
Physical exam: moderate symptoms
- Inhaled short-acting beta₂-agonist every 60 minutes
- Systemic steroid
- Continue treatment 1–3 hours provided there is improvement

Severe exacerbation
FEV_1 or PEF <60% predicted/personal best
Physical exam: severe symptoms at rest, accessory muscle use, chest retraction
History: high-risk patient
No improvement after initial treatment
- Oxygen
- Inhaled short-acting beta₂-agonist hourly or continuously + inhaled anticholinergic
- Systemic steroid

Good response
- FEV_1 or PEF ≥70%
- Response sustained 60 minutes after last treatment
- No distress
- Physical exam: normal

Incomplete response
- FEV_1 or PEF ≥50% but <70%
- Mild-to-moderate symptoms

Poor response
- FEV_1 or PEF <60%
- PCO_2 ≥42mm Hg
- Physical exam: symptoms severe, drowsiness, confusion

Individualized decision re: hospitalization

Discharge home
- Continue treatment with inhaled beta₂-agonist
- Continue course of oral steroid
- Patient education
  —Review medicine use
  —Review/initiate action plan
  —Recommend close medical follow-up

Admit to hospital ward
- Inhaled beta₂-agonist + inhaled anticholinergic
- Systemic steroid
- Oxygen
- Monitor FEV_1 or PEF, O_2 saturation

Admit to hospital intensive care
- Inhaled beta₂-agonist hourly or continuously + inhaled anticholinergic
- Intravenous steroid
- Oxygen
- Possible intubation and mechanical ventilation

Improve

Discharge home
- Continue treatment with inhaled beta₂-agonist
- Continue course of oral steroid
- Patient education
  —Review medicine use
  —Review/initiate action plan
  —Recommend close medical follow-up

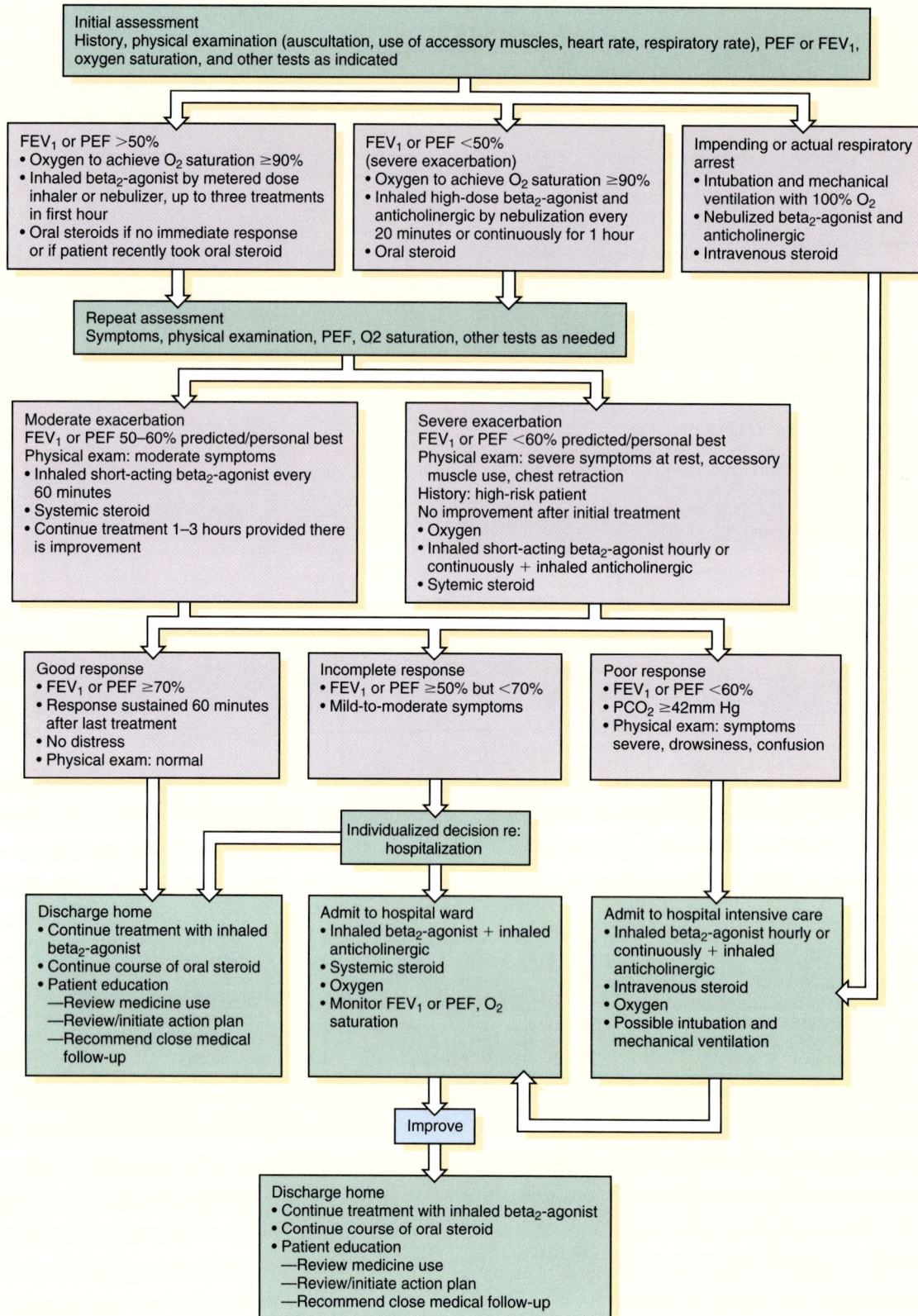

Figure 2-2 Management of asthma exacerbations: emergency department and hospital treatment. (From National Heart, Lung and Blood Institute. Expert Panel Report 2. Guidelines for the Diagnosis and Management of Asthma. National Asthma Education and Prevention Program. NIH Publication 97-4051. Bethesda, MD: NIH, 1997.)

TABLE 2-2

Stepwise Approach for Managing Infants and Young Children (≤5 Years Old) with Acute or Chronic Asthma

Classify Severity: Clinical Features Before Treatment or Adequate Control		*Medications Required to Maintain Long-Term Control*
	Symptoms/Day *Symptoms/Night*	*Daily Medications*

Step 4
Severe persistent
	Continual
	Frequent
		■ Preferred treatment
		   High-dose inhaled corticosteroids
		   and
		   Long-acting inhaled β₂-agonist
		   and (if needed)
		   Corticosteroid tablets or syrup long term (2 mg/kg/d, generally do not exceed 60 mg/d) (Make repeated attempts to reduce systemic corticosteroids and maintain control with high-dose inhaled corticosteroids.)

Step 3
Moderate persistent
	Daily
	>1 night/wk
		■ Preferred treatments
		   Low-dose inhaled corticosteroids and long-acting inhaled β₂-agonists
		   or
		   Medium-dose inhaled corticosteroids.
		■ Alternative treatment
		   Low-dose inhaled corticosteroids and either leukotriene receptor antagonist or theophylline.
		If needed (particularly in patients with recurring severe exacerbations):
		■ Preferred treatment
		   Medium-dose inhaled corticosteroids and long-acting β₂-agonists.
		■ Alternative treatment
		   Medium-dose inhaled corticosteroids and either leukotriene receptor antagonist or theophylline.

Step 2
Mild persistent
	>2×/wk but <1×/d
	>2 nights/mo
		■ Preferred treatment
		   Low-dose inhaled corticosteroid (with nebulizer or MDI with holding chamber with or without face mask or DPI).
		■ Alternative treatment (listed alphabetically)
		   Cromolyn (nebulizer is preferred or MDI with holding chamber)
		   or
		   Leukotriene receptor antagonist

Step 1 *Mild intermittent*	≤2 d/wk ≤2 nights/mo	■ No daily medication needed

Data from National Heart, Lung and Blood Institute: Expert Panel Report: Update on Selected Topics 2002. National Asthma Education and Prevention Panel. NIH Publication 02-5075. Bethesda, MD: NIH, 2002.

C. Approach to Chronic Asthma (Based on NHLBI Guidelines) (Tables 2-2 and 2-3)

1. Avoidance of possible triggers (e.g., allergens) should always be the treatment of choice in order to minimize the use of medications.
2. Chronic asthma treatment should aim at minimizing symptoms, enabling patients to pursue unlimited activities, minimizing use of inhaled short-acting bronchodilators, and avoiding adverse medication effects.

3. The treatment of chronic asthma is a stepwise approach based on asthma severity with early initiation of anti-inflammatory therapy a major goal. The most widely used classification of asthma severity is based on guidelines from the National Heart, Lung and Blood Institute.[2] Asthma can be categorized based on symptom criteria as:
   a. ***Mild intermittent:*** daytime symptoms <2 days/week; nighttime symptoms <2 nights/month.

TABLE 2-3
Stepwise Approach for Managing Asthma in Adults and Children >5 Years Old

Classify Severity: Clinical Features Before Treatment or Adequate Control			*Medications Required to Maintain Long-Term Control*
	Symptoms/Day Symptoms/Night	*PEF or FEV, PEF Variability*	*Daily Medications*

Step 4 *Severe persistent*	Continual Frequent	≤60% >30%	■ Preferred treatment
			  High-dose inhaled corticosteroids
			  and
			  Long-acting inhaled β_2-agonists
			  and (if needed)
			  Corticosteroid tablets or syrup long term (2 mg/kg/d, generally do not exceed 60 mg/d). (Make repeated attempts to reduce systemic corticosteroids and maintain control with high-dose inhaled corticosteroids.)

Step 3 *Moderate persistent*	Daily >1 night/wk	>60%–<80% >30%	■ Preferred treatments
			  Low-to-medium dose inhaled corticosteroids and long-acting inhaled β_2-agonists.
			■ Alternative treatment (listed alphabetically)
			  Increase inhaled corticosteroids within medium-dose range
			  or
			  Low-to-medium dose inhaled corticosteroids and either leukotriene modifier or theophylline.
			If needed (particularly in patients with occurring severe exacerbations):
			■ Preferred treatment
			  Increase inhaled corticosteroids within medium-dose range and add long-acting inhaled β_2-agonists.
			■ Alternative treatment (listed alphabetically)
			  Increase inhaled corticosteroids within medium-dose range and add either leukotriene modifier or theophyline.

Step 2 *Mild persistent*	>2×/wk but <1×/d >2 nights/mo	≥80% 20%–30%	■ Preferred treatment
			  Low-dose inhaled corticosteroids.
			■ Alternative treatment (listed alphabetically)
			  Cromolyn, leukotriene modifier, nedocromil
			    or
			  Sustained release theophylline to serum concentration of 5–15 μg/ml.

Step 1 *Mild intermittent*	≤2 d/wk ≤2 nights/mo	≥80% <20%	■ No daily medication needed. ■ Severe exacerbations may occur, separated by long periods of normal lung function and no symptoms. A course of systemic corticosteroids is recommended.

Data from National Heart, Lung and Blood Institute: Expert Panel Report: Update on Selected Topics 2002. National Asthma Education and Prevention Panel. NIH Publication 02-5075. Bethesda, MD: NIH, 2002.

b. ***Mild persistent:*** daytime symptoms >2×/week but <1×/day; nighttime symptoms >2 nights/month.

c. ***Moderate persistent:*** daily daytime symptoms; nighttime symptoms >1 night/week.

d. ***Severe persistent:*** continual daytime symptoms; frequent nighttime symptoms.

4. For all categories of asthma, the short-acting β_2-agonists can be used as needed for quick relief of symptoms.

5. Persons with mild intermittent asthma do not need regular daily medication.

6. Persons with mild persistent asthma should be started on daily low-dose inhaled steroids (preferred), cromolyn, nedocromil, a leukotriene receptor antagonist, or sustained release theophylline.

7. Persons with moderate persistent asthma should be started preferably on a regimen of low-dose inhaled steroids and long-acting β_2-agonists. Alternatively, medium-dose inhaled steroids alone; or low-dose inhaled steroids with either a leukotriene receptor antagonist or theophylline may be given. For patients with recurrent severe exacerbations, medium-dose inhaled steroids may be used in place of low-dose inhaled steroids in the preceding regimens.

8. Severe persistent asthma should be treated preferably with daily high-dose inhaled steroids and long-acting inhaled β_2-agonists. Oral steroids (2 mg/kg, not to exceed 60 mg/day) may be added if indicated. Leukotriene receptor antagonists may have a place as an additive agent for this category.[30]

9. Recommendations for managing infants and children ≤5 years of age are essentially the same except that theophylline is not recommended as an alternative for children with mild persistent asthma.

10. Table 2-4 shows the recommended low, medium, and high dosages for the available inhaled steroid preparations.

11. The goal of daily maintenance therapy is to improve clinical symptoms and pulmonary function over the long term. If oral steroids are used on a chronic basis, the practitioner should always reduce or taper to the lowest effective dose or discontinue as soon as it is appropriate.

12. Each patient's asthma severity classification may change with time and the treatment should be periodically adjusted (stepped up or stepped down) as needed.

D. Medications (Table 2-5)

1. ***β_2-Agonists***

a. β_2-agonists are the preferred bronchodilator agents, as they act selectively on β_2-adrenergic receptors to counteract bronchoconstriction. The inhaled short-acting β_2-agonists such as Albuterol (Ventolin), levalbuterol (Xopenex), metaproterenol (Alupent) and pirbuterol (Maxair) are the treatment of choice for fast relief of bronchospasm. The long-acting β_2-agonists salmeterol (Serevent) and formoterol (Foradil) are effective for up to 12 hours. Salmeterol has an onset of action of 1 hour and should therefore not be

TABLE 2-4

Estimated Comparative Daily Dosages for Inhaled Corticosteroids

Drug	Low Daily Dose		Medium Daily Dose		High Daily Dose	
	Adult	*Child**	*Adult*	*Child**	*Adult*	*Child**
Beclomethasone CFC 42 or 84 µg/puff	168–504 µg	84–336 µg	504–840 µg	336–672 µg	>840 µg	>672 µg
Beclomethasone HFA 40 or 80 µg/puff	80–240 µg	80–160 µg	240–480 µg	160–320 µg	>480 µg	>320 µg
Budesonide DPI 200 µg/inhalation	200–600 µg	200–400 µg	600–1,200 µg	400–800 µg	>1,200 µg	>800 µg
Inhalation suspension for nebulization (child dose)		0.5 mg		1.0 mg		2.0 mg
Flunisolide 250 µg/puff	500–1,000 µg	500–750 µg	1,000–2,000 µg	1,000–1,250 µg	>2,000 µg	>1,250 µg
Fluticasone MDI: 44, 110, or 220 µg/puff	88–264 µg	88–176 µg	264–660 µg	176–440 µg	>660 µg	>440 µg
DPI: 50, 100, or 250 µg/inhalation	100–300 µg	100–200 µg	300–600 µg	200–400 µg	>600 µg	>400 µg
Triamcinolone ace tonide 100 µg/puff	400–1,000 µg	400–800 µg	1,000–2,000 µg	800–1,200 µg	>2,000 µg	>1,200 µg

*Children ≤12 years old.

Data from National Heart, Lung and Blood Institute: Expert Panel Report: Update on Selected Topics 2002. National Asthma Education and Prevention Panel. NIH Publication 02-5075. Bethesda, MD: NIH, 2002.

TABLE 2-5

Usual Dosages for Asthma Medications

Medication	Dosage Form	Adult Dose	Child Dose
Short-acting β₂-agonists			
Albuterol	MDI 90 µg/puff	1–2 puffs q4h PRN	1–2 puffs q4h PRN
	Syrup 2 mg/tsp	1–2 tsp tid–qid PRN	0.1–0.2 mg/kg up to 2 tsp 3x/d
	2 or 4 mg tablets	1 tab tid–qid PRN	2 mg 3–4x/d (≥6 years)
	4 mg sustained-release tab	1–2 tabs q12h	Not recommended
	Nebulizer 2.5 mg/inh	1 inh tid–qid PRN	1 inh 3–4x/d PRN
Pirbuterol	MDI 200 µg/puff	1–2 puffs q4h PRN	1–2 puffs q4h PRN
Metaproterenol	MDI 0.65 mg/puff	1–2 puffs q4h PRN	Not recommended
	Nebulizer 5% solution	1 inh tid–qid PRN	1 inh tid–qid PRN (≥6 yr)
Anticholinergics			
Ipratropium	MDI 18 µg/puff	2 puffs qid	Not recommended
Cromolyn and nedocromil			
Cromolyn	MDI 1 mg/puff	2–4 puffs tid–qid	1–2 puffs tid–qid
	Nebulizer 20 mg/ampule	1 ampule tid–qid	1 ampule tid–qid
Nedocromil	MDI 1.75 mg/puff	2–4 puffs bid–qid	1–2 puffs bid–qid
Inhaled long-acting β₂-agonists			
Salmeterol	MDI 21 µg/puff	2 puffs q12h	1–2 puffs q12h
	DPI 50 µg/blister	1 blister q12h	1 blister q12h
Formoterol	DPI 12 µg/capsule	1 capsule q12h	1 capsule q12h
Combination preparations			
Fluticasone/salmeterol	DPI (100, 250, or 500 µg/50 µg)/inh	1 inh bid	1 inh bid
Ipratropium/albuterol	MDI (18 µg/90 µg)/puff	2 puffs qid PRN	Not recommended
Leukotriene modifiers			
Zafirlukast	10 or 20 mg tablet	20 mg bid	10 mg bid
Montelukast	4, 5, or 10 mg tablet	10 mg qhs	4 mg qhs (2–5 yr) 5 mg qhs (6–14 yr) 10 mg qhs (>14 yr)
Zileuton	300 or 600 mg tablet	1 tablet qid	Not recommended
Inhaled steroids	(see Table 2-4)		
Methylxanthines			
Theophylline	Capsules, tablets, syrup	10 mg/kg/d, max 800 mg/d	10 mg/kg/d max: <1 yr: 0.2 (age in wks) + 5-mg/kg/d max: >1 yr: 16 mg/kg/d
Systemic steroids			
Prednisone, prednisolone methyprednisolone	Tablets, syrup	Burst: 30–60 mg/d × 3–10 days	Burst: 1–2 mg/kg/d × 3–10 d, max: 60 mg/d
		Long term: 7.5–60 mg/d or qod	0.25–2 mg/kg/d or qod

used for acute attacks. Formoterol has a rapid onset of action, within 15 minutes. β_2-agonists are also available in oral preparations and for nebulizer use. Studies have shown worsening of asthma associated with chronic regular use of β-agonists, but whether it is the cause or effect of worsening asthma is still unclear.[31]

b. Proper technique is of crucial importance in ensuring delivery of drug to the lower airways. Patients who have difficulty with the metered-dose inhaler (MDI) technique should be given spacers or chambers, which improve delivery.[32] New, nonchlorofluorocarbon (CFC) propellants are replacing CFC propellants in older inhalers, which have been shown to damage the ozone layer of the atmosphere. No differences in efficacy have been seen between devices with the two propellants. Diskus and breath-actuated devices (Maxair) require less coordination and are recommended for patients who have difficulty with MDIs. (see Chapter 15)

2. ***Anticholinergic Agents***
Anticholinergic agents can be used in addition to β_2-agonists if symptoms are not completely controlled.[33] These agents are especially effective in patients with concomitant COPD. Ipratropium bromide (Atrovent) is most commonly used and is relatively free of the side effects associated with older agents such as atropine.

3. ***Cromolyn and Nedocromil***
Cromolyn (Intal) and nedocromil (Tilade) are effective anti-inflammatory medications for long-term control of chronic asthma.[34,35] They are associated with the fewest side effects of all the asthma medications and are often used in children. Known as mast cell stabilizers, these agents prevent degranulation and release of inflammatory mediators. Cromolyn and nedocromil can also be used prior to allergen exposure and exercise to prevent symptoms.

4. ***Theophylline***
Theophylline and aminophylline have been part of asthma treatment for decades. These agents improve diaphragmatic contraction and cause bronchodilation by inhibiting phosphodiesterase and adenosine.[36] They also appear to have anti-inflammatory properties, including inhibition of eosinophil infiltration in the airways.[37] The narrow therapeutic index of theophylline and the need for regular serum level evaluations have lessened its use over the years. Adverse effects occuring when the therapeutic dose range is exceeded include seizures and GI distress. There is an increased risk of toxic effects because of reduced clearance, with associated cardiac and respiratory failure, liver disease, high fever, hypothyroidism, viral infections, and use of ciprofloxacin, disulfiram, oral contraceptives, troleandomycin, cimetidine, and erythromycin. Increased clearance with lowering of serum levels occurs with smoking, hyperthyroidism, and the use of phenobarbital, carbamazepine, rifampin, and phenytoin. Theophylline is currently recommended as an alternative for additional maintenance treatment of chronic asthma not controlled with inhaled steroids.[2]

5. ***Inhaled Steroids***
a. Inhaled corticosteroids are the drug of choice for maintenance treatment of chronic asthma and are the most potent anti-inflammatory agents available.[2] Studies show that beclomethasone (Vanceril), triamcinolone (Azmacort), flunisolide (Aerobid), fluticasone (Flovent), and budesonide (Pulmicort) all improve pulmonary function and clinical symptoms when used regularly. Budesonide can be administered by nebulized delivery (Pulmicort respules). This form of delivery may be more efficient and have lower local adverse effects.

b. The anti-inflammatory effects of corticosteroids include decreasing the production of pro-inflammatory cytokines, the chemotaxis of inflammatory cells such as eosinophils, and the release of inflammatory mediators.[38]

c. The various formulations of inhaled steroids are not equivalent on a microgram-per-microgram basis. Instead, each formulation's manufacturer recommends what it considers to be low, medium, and high dose ranges based on individual potency studies (see Table 2-4). Numerous studies have been done to establish the comparative potency of the different inhaled steroid preparations. However, obtaining consistent results in head-to-head comparisons of different preparations is difficult. Studies comparing topical potency by skin blanching do not always imply proportional clinical potency. The comparative efficacy of the different inhaled steroids can only at best be estimated from topical potency tests, comparison of clinical effects, and bioavailability. The NHLBI guidelines provide an estimation, based on topical potency, of the comparative efficacy of the various brands.[39]

d. Unlike systemic steroids, the inhaled steroids have a good safety profile, and the benefits currently outweigh concerns about systemic effects. At the recommended doses, inhaled steroids present a minimal risk for osteoporosis, growth retardation, cataracts or hypothalamic-pituitary axis suppression.[40]

e. While past studies have shown mild dose-dependent decreases in bone density, more recent studies have not shown significant differences in bone mineral density between patients treated with or without steroids for 4 years or more.[41,42] Agertoft and Pedersen[43] studied asthmatic children taking up to 1,300 μg of budesonide per day for 3–6 years and found no significant difference in bone density between steroid and non-steroid groups. Wisnewski[44] studied adults taking inhaled steroids for up to 7–8 years and also found no difference between steroid and nonsteroid groups. However, the cumulative inhaled dose was associated with decreased lumbar density in women. At this time, the risk of osteoporosis from long-term use of inhaled steroids has not been shown to be consistently significant. However, it would be prudent for post-menopausal women, who already have an increased risk of osteoporosis, to take calcium supplements (1–1.5 g/day), vitamin D (400 units/day), or estrogen replacement therapy.[30]

   f. Growth retardation in children remains the main concern for parents. This issue is complicated by the fact that uncontrolled asthma itself can delay growth. Decreases in short-term bone growth measured by knemometry and height velocity have been shown in several studies.[43,44] However, long-term studies appear to show that final adult height, which is the most important outcome, is not affected by prolonged inhaled steroid use.[45,46] In an important prospective study, 142 children who received budesonide showed about a 20% reduction of growth velocity in the first year, but all ultimately attained a normal adult height.[46]

   g. The incidence of cataracts, ocular hypertension, and glaucoma is known to increase with oral steroids, but studies have not established any clear association with inhaled steroids.[47–49]

   h. Local side effects include hoarseness and oral thrush, both of which can be avoided by proper inhaler technique and by mouth rinsing after inhalation.

6. ***Oral Steroids***

   a. Oral steroids should be used if high-dose inhaled steroids do not control a patient's symptoms adequately. Certain severe asthmatics may be on oral steroids for prolonged periods. It is the responsibility of the physician to closely follow the patient's progress and attempt to always taper the steroid dose to the least amount that is effective. Adverse effects of chronic systemic steroid use are well known and include hypertension, hyperglycemia, osteoporosis, glaucoma, cataracts, weight gain, psychiatric disorders, adrenal insufficiency, skin bruising, and many others.

   b. Patients with difficult asthma often receive "bursts" of prednisone or methylprednisolone for exacerbations with initial doses of up to 60 mg of prednisone or its equivalent for 3–10 days. For steroid "bursts" of 10 days or less, slow tapering is not necessary.[50]

   c. Chronic severe asthmatics often are unable to taper off and remain on daily doses for prolonged periods. Once-daily dosing in the morning is preferred because it best approximates the diurnal release of endogenous steroids and therefore causes less hypothalamic-pituitary-adrenal (HPA) axis suppression. The chronic steroid dose should be tapered down as much as possible while maintaining symptom control. Alternate-day dosing has been shown to be associated with less adverse effects and should be attempted. A dose of prednisone (≤10 mg) should be aimed for, as this is associated with the lowest incidence of adverse events.[2]

7. ***Antileukotrienes***

   a. The antileukotrienes or leukotriene modifiers counteract the effects of leukotrienes, which are released by mast cells and eosinophils in response to stimuli and cause bronchoconstriction, increased vascular permeability, edema, mucous production, and influx of inflammatory cells.

   b. The two types of antileukotriene agents are (1) leukotriene synthesis inhibitors, and (2) leukotriene receptor antagonists. Zafirlukast (Accolate) and montelukast (Singulair) are leukotriene receptor antagonists, while zileuton (Zyflo) is a 5-lipoxygenase inhibitor, a type of leukotriene synthesis inhibitor.

   c. Antileukotrienes are effective for long-term control therapy in mild to moderate persistent asthma. Addition of antileukotrienes to the regimen of patients requiring inhaled steroids for control has allowed lowering of inhaled steroid doses. The usefulness of antileukotrienes in severe asthma and their comparative efficacy with inhaled steroids still need to be studied and clarified further.

   d. The antileukotrienes appear to be safe and well-tolerated. Mild, reversible elevation of liver enzyme levels has been seen with zileuton. Reports of Churg-Strauss syndrome seen in patients tapering off systemic steroids while on antileukotrienes are believed to be due to unmasking of the underlying syndrome rather than the effects of antileukotrienes.[51]

8. ***Anti-IgE***

   a. Monoclonal anti-IgE (omalizumab) is a humanized monoclonal antibody against IgE with an IgG1 kappa human framework. By binding to

IgE nonspecifically to form inert anti-IgE:IgE complexes, they have been shown in randomized, controlled studies to improve symptoms and pulmonary function when given subcutaneously once or twice a month.[52]

b. The role of anti-IgE in relation to other asthma medications and immunotherapy remains to be elucidated. It shows great promise in the treatment of both asthma and allergic rhinitis.

9. ***Alternative Medications***

Troleandomycin, methotrexate, gold, cyclosporine, and hydroxychloroquine have been used in asthma with varying success.[53] If effective in certain patients, they can spare the chronic use of systemic steroids.

10. ***Newer Agents***

Promising new treatments include intravenous immune globulin (IVIG)[54] and therapy directed toward cytokines (IL-4, IL-5, IL-13)[55,56] and adhesion molecules (integrins)[57] are all under investigation.

E. Immunotherapy (see Chapter 11 and Appendix 1)

1. Patients with evidence of specific IgE sensitivity by skin or serum specific IgE testing, poor response to pharmacologic therapy, or unavoidable exposure to allergic triggers are candidates for allergen immunotherapy.[58]

2. In studies, immunotherapy has improved chronic asthma due to such allergens as ragweed, dust mites, cat dander, grass, and *Alternaria*.[59]

3. The mechanism of immunotherapy is not completely understood, but IgG "blocking antibodies" are thought to diminish the effects of specific IgE antibodies.

4. Most experts recommend that immunotherapy be administered for at least 3–5 years.[60]

5. Immunotherapy is best administered by an allergy specialist. Injections should always be done in a medically supervised setting with resuscitation equipment available. Self-administration at home or outside a medical setting is strongly discouraged.

IX. Special Considerations in Patient Subsets

A. Risk Factors for Fatal Asthma

1. Risk factors associated with death from asthma include
   a. Poorly controlled asthma
   b. Previous intensive care admissions or intubations
   c. Use of systemic steroids
   d. Poor patient perception of asthma severity
   e. Concomitant systemic diseases
   f. Psychiatric disorders
   g. Low socioeconomic status
   h. Illegal drug abuse
   i. Allergy to *Alternaria*

2. Recognition and close monitoring of patients with these risk factors can prevent unfortunate outcomes.

B. Asthma in Pregnancy

1. Management of asthma during pregnancy requires good communication between the patient, her obstetrician, and the asthma specialist. The aim of treatment throughout pregnancy is to maximize maternal and fetal oxygenation while avoiding potentially harmful pharmacologic therapy (Box 2-1).[61]

2. Relaxation techniques, inhalation of nebulized saline, and avoidance of environmental triggers are important and useful nonpharmacologic measures that should be encouraged in pregnancy.

3. Inhaled or nebulized β_2-agonists remain the drugs of choice for acute, symptomatic treatment throughout pregnancy. Terbutaline is preferred, although other β_2-agonists may be used. For maintenance treatment of chronic asthma, inhaled cromolyn, inhaled beclomethasone, and oral theophylline have all been shown to be safe in pregnancy. Systemic steroids and IV aminophylline may be used for asthma exacerbations. Dosages remain unchanged for the pregnant patient.[62]

4. Immunotherapy may be kept at a maintenance dose throughout pregnancy but should not be initiated or

---

BOX 2-1

Drugs Preferred for Use in Pregnancy

Antihistamines
  Chlorpheniramine
  Tripelennamine
Antibiotic
  Amoxicillin
Anti-inflammatory
  Beclomethasone
  Prednisone
  Cromolyn
Bronchodilator
  Inhaled β_2-Agonist
  Theophylline
Cough
  Guaifenesin
  Dextromethorphan
Decongestant
  Pseudoephedrine
  Oxymetazoline

From National Heart, Lung and Blood Institute: Report of the Working Group on Asthma and Pregnancy: Management of Asthma During Pregnancy. NIH Publication 93-3279. Bethesda, MD: NIH, 1993.

increased during this time, as a systemic reaction with hypoxia would be harmful to the fetus.[63]

5. During pregnancy, a patient's asthma may improve, worsen, or stay the same.[64]

6. There is the greatest chance of improvement, usually in the last 4 weeks of pregnancy. The greatest chance of worsening of asthma usually occurs between weeks 29 and 36 of pregnancy.[65]

7. There is a low incidence of problems during labor and delivery in most asthmatics.[61]

C. Asthma in the Elderly

1. Asthma can frequently go unrecognized in the elderly. Symptoms of shortness of breath or cough are frequently attributed to other diseases or old age. While most asthma starts in childhood, up to 10% of elderly persons in the United States are diagnosed with asthma.[66]

2. COPD is very common in elderly patients with a smoking history. Distinguishing COPD from asthma in the elderly may be complicated by the fact that asthmatic bronchospasm may not be significantly reversible in older patients. Careful history taking and evaluation of factors such as smoking history and symptom triggers are useful for making the correct diagnosis. Episodic symptoms with recognizable triggers are more characteristic of asthma, while persistent symptoms such as a daily productive cough or persistent shortness of breath point more toward COPD. Decreased breath sounds on auscultation and flattened diaphragms on chest radiography are seen in COPD.

3. Allergens do not appear to be as important a factor in the elderly as they are in younger asthmatics.[67]

4. The elderly patient can be on multiple medications for various conditions. A careful review of medications is essential to identify drugs that can worsen asthma.[68] These include β-blockers, aspirin and NSAIDs, opiates, ACE inhibitors, and COX-2 inhibitors.

5. Dosages for medications may need to be adjusted for decreased metabolism or clearance in the elderly.

6. Medications for one condition may cause adverse effects for another. For example, medications taken for heart disease, such as β-blockers and ACE inhibitors, can exacerbate asthma symptoms. On the other hand, β-agonists can cause palpitations and other cardiac effects.

D. Occupational Asthma

1. It is estimated that 2%–15% of patients who present with asthma in the United States have an occupational trigger.[69] Occupational asthma may often be a challenge to diagnose, as the relationship between work and symptoms may not be immediately clear. A history of work-associated asthma symptoms that recede when the patient is not at work is the first clue. The potential consequences for the worker's career make an accurate diagnosis essential.

2. Comparison of serial peak expiratory flow rate (PEFR) or FEV_1 at work and outside of work can determine if the asthma is occupational in nature.

3. Specific bronchial challenge to suspected occupational agents is the gold standard for diagnosis of occupational asthma.

4. Several hundred agents have been identified as causing occupational asthma, and the list grows longer each year as new products and substances in industries ranging from pharmaceutical to automobile manufacturing are reported to be causative agents.

5. Occupational triggers are generally classified into high-molecular-weight or low-molecular-weight agents (Table 2-6).[70] High-molecular-weight agents are primarily proteins from plant or animal sources (e.g., animal proteins, grain and feed dust, flour, latex), while low-molecular-weight agents include organic and inorganic chemicals (e.g., anhydrides in epoxy resins, antibiotics, diisocyanates used for spray painting, precious metals, wood dusts such as western red cedar or plicatic acid, dyes).[71]

X. When to Obtain Consultation

Consultation with an asthma specialist can assist greatly in providing comprehensive care for the maximum improvement of the patient. Subsequent cooperation between the primary care provider and the specialist is essential and will benefit the patient greatly.

The Joint Council of Allergy, Asthma and Immunology recommends referral to a specialist:

• When the diagnosis of asthma is in doubt.
• When identification of allergic or nonallergic triggers is necessary.
• When allergen immunotherapy is being considered.
• When the patient's asthma is incompletely or poorly controlled.
• When patient education and monitoring by a specialist is desired.

XI. ICD-9 Codes

493.0	Asthma, extrinsic
493.1	Asthma, intrinsic
493.1	Asthma with COPD
493.0	Asthma with allergic rhinitis
5th digit: 0	without mention of status asthmaticus with status asthmaticus with acute exacerbation

TABLE 2-6
Selected Occupational Asthma Triggers

Agent	Occupation	Agent	Occupation
High-molecular-weight allergens			
Insects		*Low-molecular-weight allergens*	
Fowl mites	Poultry workers		
Mealworms	Grain workers	Dyes	
Fruit flies	Laboratory workers	Paraphenylenediamine	Fur dyers
		Anthraquinone methyl blue	Cloth dyers
Plant proteins			
Wheat flour	Bakers	Wood dusts	
Hydrolyzed gluten	Bakers	Western and eastern red cedar (plicatic acid)	Carpenters, sawmill workers
Grain dust	Dockworkers, millers		
Latex	Health care workers	Diisocyanates	Paint, plastics, polyurethane foam, foundry workers
Animal proteins			
Chicken	Poultry workers		
Cow	Dairy workers	Metals	
Laboratory animals	Drug and research workers	Chromiun	Cement, tanning workers
		Nickel	Metal plating workers
		Cobalt	Hard metal workers
Plant enzymes			
Papain	Food processors	Anhydrides	
Bromelain	Food processors	Trimellitic anhydride	Epoxy resins, plastics
		Phthalic anhydride	Plastics, drugs
Vegetable gums		Himic anhydride	Fire retardants
Tragacanth	Printers, hairdressers	Antibiotics	
Guar	Carpet workers	Penicillin	Drug manufacturers
Karaya	Food processors, hairdressers	Tetracycline	Drug manufacturers
Microbial enzymes			
Bacillus subtilis	Detergent workers		
Fungal amylase, hemicellulase	Bakers		
Esperase, savinase, alcalase	Detergent workers		

Adapted from Bernstein DI, Bernstein IL: Occupational asthma. In Middleton E Jr, Reed CE, et al (eds.): Allergy: Principles and Practice, 5th ed. St. Louis: Mosby, 1998, with permission.

XII. Internet Resources

www.aaaai.org
American Academy of Allergy, Asthma and Immunology

www.acaai.org
American College of Allergy, Asthma and Immunology

allergy.mcg.edu
Allergy, Asthma and Immunology Online
Source for the public

allergy.mcg.edu/lifeQuality/nasp.html
Nationwide Asthma Screening Program (sponsored by the ACAAI)

www.jcaai.org
Joint Council of Allergy, Asthma and Immunology

www.chestnet.org
American College of Chest Physicians

www.lungusa.org
American Lung Association

www.thoracic.org
American Thoracic Society

www.njc.org
National Jewish Medical and Research Center

www.nhlbi.nih.gov
National Heart, Lung and Blood Institute

www.niaid.nih.gov
National Institute of Allergy and Infectious Diseases

www.nlm.nih.gov
National Library of Medicine

www.aanma.org
Allergy & Asthma Network/Mothers of Asthmatics

www.aafa.org
Asthma and Allergy Foundation of America

www.lungusa.org/asthmacamps/
Consortium on Children's Asthma Camps

XIII. Patient Education

A. Patient education should start at the first visit and continue throughout the patient's treatment. Education and participation of patients and their families in their care is important in achieving maximum control of asthma.

B. The NIH guidelines strongly recommend that patients be given:[30]

1. Basic information about asthma.
2. Information about the role of asthma medications.
3. Instructions on proper inhaler techniques, peak flow monitoring, and other ways to monitor asthma status.
4. Instructions on how to avoid and control environmental triggers.
5. Written action plans for acute exacerbations and long-term maintenance treatment.

C. There is no reason why educated individuals with asthma who participate actively in their own care should not be able to live a full, active, unrestricted life.

D. Refer to patient education CD, which is provided with this text, for additional patient education information. It has been formatted to provide readily accessible, easy-to-understand handouts for adult patients and the parents of pediatric patients. These handouts can be easily modified to fit specific practice requirements.

REFERENCES

1. Busse WW, Lemanske RF: Asthma. N Engl J Med 2001;344:1643–1644.
2. National Heart, Lung, and Blood Institute: Expert Panel Report: Update on Selected Topics 2002. National Asthma Education and Prevention Panel. NIH Publication 02-5075. Bethesda, MD: NIH, 2002.
3. Centers for Disease Control: Asthma mortality and hospitalization among children and young adults—United States, 1980–1993. Morbid Mortal Weekly Rep 1996;45:350–353.
4. Pullan CR, Hey EN: Wheezing, asthma and pulmonary dysfunction 10 years after infection with respiratory syncytial virus in infancy. BMJ 1982;284:1655–1669.
5. Hu FB, Persky V, Flay BR, Zelli A, Cooksey J, Richardson J: Prevalence of asthma and wheezing in public schools children: Association with maternal smoking during pregnancy. Ann Allergy Asthma Immunol 1997;79:80–84.
6. Ingram JM, Sporik R, Rose G, et al: Quantitative assessment of exposure to dog (Can f1) and cat (Fel d1) allergens: Relation to sensitization and asthma among children living in Los Alamos, New Mexico. J Allergy Clin Immunol 1995;96:449–456.
7. Jenkins MA, Hopper JL, Bower G, et al: Factors in childhood as predictors of asthma in adult life. BMJ 1994;309:90–93.
8. Sporik R, Holgate ST, Platts-Mills TAE, Cogswell JJ: Exposure to house-dust mite allergen (Der p1) and the development of asthma in childhood: A prospective study. N Engl J Med 1990;323:502–507.
9. Lemanske RF: Inflammatory event in asthma: An expanding equation. J Allergy Clin Immunol 2000;105:S633–S638.
10. Pearlman DS: Pathophysiology of the inflammatory response. J Allergy Clin Immunol 1999;104:S132–S137.
11. Fahy JV, Corry DB, Boushey HA: Airway inflammation and remodeling in asthma. Curr Opin Pulm Med 2000;6:15–20.
12. Corrao WM, Braman SS, Irwin RS: Chronic cough as the sole presenting manifestation of bronchial asthma. N Engl J Med 1979;300:633–638.
13. Theodoropoulos DS, Lockey RF, Boyce HW Jr, et al: Gastroesophageal reflux and asthma: A review of pathogenesis, diagnosis and therapy. Allergy 1999;54:651–661.
14. McFadden ER, Zawadski DK: Vocal cord dysfunction masquerading as exercise induced asthma: A physiologic cause for choking during athletic activities. Am J Respir Crit Care Med 1996;153:942–947.
15. Tan RA, Spector SL: Lung disease. In Kemp SF, Lockey RF (eds): Diagnostic Testing of Allergic Disease, pp 175–197. New York: Marcel Dekker, 2000.
16. Joint Task Force on Practice Parameters: Practice parameters for allergy diagnostic testing. Ann Allergy Asthma Immunol 1995;75(Pt 2):543–625.
17. Spector SL. Allergic inflammation in upper and lower airways. Ann Allergy Asthma Immunol 1999;83:435–444.
18. Dykewicz MS: Rhinitis and sinusitis: Implications for severe asthma. Immunol Clin North Am 2001;21:427–437.
19. Grant JA, Nicodemus CF, Findlay SR, et al: Cetirizine in patients with seasonal rhinitis and concomitant asthma: Prospective, randomized, placebo-controlled trial. J Allergy Clin Immunol 1995;95:923–932.
20. Foresi A, Pelucchi A, Gherson G, et al: Once daily intranasal fluticasone proprionate (200 mcg) reduces nasal symptoms and inflammation but also attenuates the increase in bronchial responsiveness during the pollen season in allergic rhinitis. J Allergy Clin Immunol 1996;98:274–282.

21. Dunlop G, Scadding GK, Lund VJ: The effect of endoscopic sinus surgery on asthma: Management of patients with chronic rhinosinusitis, nasal polyposis, and asthma. Am J Rhinol 1999;13:261–265.

22. Senior BA, Kennedy DW: Management of sinusitis in the asthmatic patient. Ann Allergy Asthma Immunol 1996; 77:6–15.

23. Joint Task Force on Practice Parameters: Practice parameters for the diagnosis and management of sinusitis. J Allergy Clin Immunol 1998;102(Suppl):S117–S144.

24. Joint Task Force on Practice Parameters: Practice parameters for the diagnosis and treatment of asthma. J Allergy Clin Immunol 1995;96(Suppl):S707–S870

25. Anderson SD, Daviskas E: The mechanism of exercise-induced asthma is. . . . J Allergy Clin Immunol 2000; 106:453–459.

26. Peters J, Avol E, Gauderman W: A study of twelve Southern California communities with differing levels and types of air pollution: Effects on pulmonary function. Am J Respir Crit Care Med 1999;159:768–775.

27. Israel E, Fischer AR, Rosenberg MA, et al: The pivotal role of 5-lipoxygenase products in the reaction of aspirin-sensitive asthmatics to aspirin. Am Rev Respir Dis 1993;148: 1447–1451.

28. Pleskow WW, Stevenson DD, Mathison DA, et al: Aspirin desensitization in aspirin sensitive asthmatic patients: Clinical manifestations and characterization of the refractory period. J Allergy Clin Immunol 1982;69:11–19.

29. Boulet L-P, Milot J, Lampron N, et al: Pulmonary function and airway responsiveness during long-term therapy with captopril. JAMA 1989;261:413–416.

30. Spector SL: Safety of antileukotriene agents in asthma management. Ann Allergy Asthma Immunol 2001;86(6 Suppl 1):8–23.

31. Angell M, Kassirer JP: Inhaled beta2-agonists in the treatment of asthma. N Engl J Med 1996;335:886–890.

32. Barron EN Jr: Proper technique for using inhalers in asthma. N Engl J Med 1987;316:951–952.

33. Rebuck AS, Gent M, Chapman KR: Anticholinergic and sympathomimetic combination therapy in asthma. J Allergy Clin Immunol 1983;71:317–323.

34. Edwards AM, Stevens MT: The clinical efficacy of inhaled nedocromil sodium in the treatment of asthma. Eur Respir J 1993;6:35–41.

35. Eigen H, Reid JJ, Dahl R, et al: Evaluation of the addition of cromolyn sodium to bronchodilator maintenance therapy in the long-term management of asthma. J Allergy Clin Immunol 1987;80:612–621.

36. Weinberger M, Hendeles L: Theophylline in asthma. N Engl J Med 1996;334:1380–1388.

37. Kidney J, Dominguez M, Taylor PM, et al: Immunomodulation by theophylline in asthma. Am J Respir Crit Care Med 1995;151:1907–1914.

38. Barnes N: Relative safety and efficacy of inhaled corticosteroids. J Allergy Clin Immunol 1998;101:S460–S464.

39. National Heart, Lung and Blood Institute: Expert Panel Report 2. Guidelines for the Diagnosis and Management of Asthma. National Asthma Education and Prevention Program. NIH Publication 97-4051. Bethesda, MD: NIH, 1997.

40. Lipworth BJ: Systemic adverse effects of inhaled corticosteroid therapy: A systematic review and meta-analysis. Arch Intern Med 1999;159:941–955.

41. Agertoft L, Pedersen S: Effects of long term treatment with an inhaled corticosteroid on growth and pulmonary function in asthmatic children. Respir Med 1994;88: 373–381.

42. Wisnewski AF, Lewis SA, Green DJ, Maslanka W, Burrel H, Tattersfield AE: Cross section investigation of the effects of inhaled corticosteroids on bone density and bone metabolism in patients with asthma. Thorax 1997;52:853–860.

43. Agertoft L, Pedersen S: Bone mineral density in children with asthma receiving long term treatment with inhaled budesonide. Am J Respir Crit Care Med 1998;157:178–183.

44. Tinkelman DG, Reed CE, Nelson HS, et al: Aerosol beclomethasone diproprionate compared with theophylline as primary treatment of chronic, mild to moderately severe asthma in children. Pediatrics 1993;92:64–77.

45. Doull IJM, Freezer NJ, Holgate ST: Growth of prepubertal children with mild asthma treated with inhaled beclomethasone dipropionate. Am J Respir Crit Care Med 1995;151: 1715–1719.

46. Balfour-Lynn L: Growth and childhood asthma. Arch Dis Child 1986;61:1049–1055.

47. Agertoft L, Pedersen S: Effect of long-term treatment with inhaled budesonide on adult height in children with asthma. N Engl J Med 2000;343:1064–1069.

48. Simons FER, Persaud MP, Gillespie CA, Chang M, Shuckett EP: Absence of posterior subcapsular cataracts in young patients treated with inhaled glucocorticoids. Lancet 1993;342:776–778.

49. Cumming RG, Mitchell P, Leeder SR: Use of inhaled corticosteroids and the risk of cataracts. N Engl J Med 1997;337:8–14.

50. Garb E, Le Lorier J, Boivin JF, Suissa S: Inhaled and nasal glucocorticoids and the risks of ocular hypertension or open-angle glaucoma. JAMA 1997;277:722–727.

51. O'Driscoll BR, Kalra S, Wilson M, et al: Double-blind trial of steroid tapering in acute asthma. Lancet 1993;341: 324–327.

52. Wechsler ME, Finn D, Gunawardena D, et al: Churg Strauss syndrome in patients receiving montelukast as a treatment for asthma. Chest 2000;117:708–713.

53. Milgrom H, Fick RB Jr, Su JQ, et al: Treatment of allergic asthma with monoclonal anti-IgE antibody. N Engl J Med 1999;341:1966–1973.

54. Ziment I, Tashkin DP: Alternative medicine for allergy and asthma. J Allergy Clin Immunol 2000;106:603.

55. Mazer BD, Gelfand EW: An open-label study of high-dose intravenous immunoglobulin in severe childhood asthma. J Allergy Clin Immunol 1991;87:976–983.

56. Borish LC, Nelson HS, Lanz MI, et al: Interleukin-4 receptor in moderate atopic asthma: A phase I/II randomized placebo-controlled trial. Am J Respir Crit Care Med 1999; 160:1816–1823.

57. Lalani T, Simons RK, Ahmed AR: Biology of IL-5 in health and disease. Ann Allergy Asthma Immunol 1999;82:317–332.

58. Lin KC, Ateeg HS, Hsiung SH, et al: Selective, tight-binding inhibitors of integrin a4B1 that inhibit allergic airway responses. J Med Chem 1999;42:920–934.

59. Joint Task Force on Practice Parameters: Practice parameters for allergen immunotherapy. J Allergy Clin Immunol 1996;98:1001–1011.

60. Abramson MJ, Puy RM, Weiner JM: Is allergen immunotherapy effective in asthma? A meta-analysis of randomized controlled trials. Am J Respir Crit Care Med 1995;151: 969–974.

61. Mosbech H, Osterballe O: Does the effect of immunotherapy last after termination of treatment? Follow-up study in patients with grass pollen rhinitis. Allergy 1988;43:523–529.

62. National Heart Lung and Blood Institute: Report of the Working Group on Asthma and Pregnancy: Management of Asthma During Pregnancy. NIH Publication 93-3279. Bethesda, MD: NIH, 1993.

63. Schatz M, Hoffman CP, Zeiger RS: The course and management of asthma and allergic diseases during pregnancy. In Middleton EJ, Reed CE, Ellis EF, et al (eds): Allergy: Principles and Practice, 5th ed, pp 938–952. St. Louis: Mosby, 1998.

64. Metzger WJ, Turner E, Patterson R: The safety of immunotherapy in pregnancy. J Allergy Clin Immunol 1978;61:268–272.

65. Schatz M, Harden K, Forsythe A, et al: The course of asthma during pregnancy, postpartum and with successive pregnancies: A prospective analysis. J Allergy Clin Immunol 1988;81:509.

66. Juniper EF, Newhouse MT: Effect of pregnancy on asthma: A systematic review and meta-analysis. In Schatz M, Zeiger RS, Claman HN (eds): Asthma and Immunologic Diseases in Pregnancy and Early Infancy, p 401. New York: Marcel Dekker, 1998.

67. Barbee RA: Asthma in the elderly. In Middleton EJ, Reed CE, Ellis EF, et al (eds): Allergy: Principles and Practice—Update, pp 1–17. St. Louis: Mosby, 2001.

68. Burrows B, Barbee RA, Cline MG, et al: Characteristics of asthma among elderly adults in a sample of the general population. Chest 1991;100:935

69. Beers MH, Ouslander JG: Risk factors in geriatric drug prescribing: A practical guide to avoiding problems. Drugs 1989;37:105–112.

70. Bardana EJ, Montanaro A: Occupational asthma and allergies. Ann Allergy Asthma Immunol 1999;83:577–630.

71. Blank P: Occupational asthma in a national disability survey. Chest 1987;92:613–617.

American Thoracic Society: Standardization of spirometry: 1994 update. Am J Respir Crit Care Med. 1995;152:1107–1136.

Calls RS, Smith TF, Morris E, Chapman MD, Platts-Mills TAE: Risk factors for asthma in inner city children. J Pediatr 1992;121:862–866.

Corren J: The impact of allergic rhinitis on bronchial asthma. J Allergy Clin Immunol 1998;101:S352–S356.

Crapo RO: Pulmonary function testing. N Engl J Med 1994;331:25–30.

Crapo RO, Morris AH, Clayton PD, Nixon CR: Lung volumes in healthy nonsmoking adults. Bull Eur Physiopathol Respir 1982;18:419–425.

Crapo RO, Morris AH, Gardner RM: Reference spriometric values using techniques and equipment that meet ATS recommendations. Am Rev Respir Dis 1981;123:659–664.

Dockery DW, Ware JH, Ferris BG Jr, et al: Distribution of forced expiratory volume in ione second and forced expiratory vitral capacity in healthy, white, adult never-smokers in six US cities. Am Rev Respir Dis 1985;131:511–520.

Fireman P, Adkinson F, Atwater J, et al: Role of the allergisr/immunologist as a subspecialist. J Allergy Clin Immunol 1997;100:288–289.

Fish JE: Bronchial challenge testing. In Middleton E Jr, et al (eds): Allergy: Principles and Practice, 4th ed, pp 613–627. St. Louis: Mosby, 1993.

Hopp RJ, Bewtra AK, Nair NM, et al: Specificity and sensitivity of methcholine inhalation challenge in normal and asthmatic children. J Allergy Clin Immunol 1984;74: 154.

McFadden ER Jr: Pulmonary structure, physiology, and clinical correlates in asthma. In Middleton ER Jr, et al (eds): Allergy: Principles and Practice, 4th ed, pp 672–693. St. Louis: Mosby, 1993.

Rossiter CE, Weil H: Ethnic differences in lung function: Evidence for proportional differences. Int J Epidemiol 974;3:55–61.

Spector SL: Allergen inhalation challenges. In Spector SL (ed): Provocative Testing in Clinical Practice, pp 325–368. New York: Marcel Dekker, 1995.

Tan RA, Spector SL: Antileukotriene agents. Curr Opin Pulm Med 1997;4:26–33.

Tan RA, Spector SL: Asthma and exercise. In Weisman IM, Zeballos RJ (eds): Clinical Exercise Testing. Progress in Respiratory Research, pp 205–216. Basel: Karger, 2002.

Webster JR Jr, Saadeh GB, Eggun PR, et al: Wheezing due to pulmonary embolism. Exercise N Engl J Med 1966;274: 931–933.

OTHER SUGGESTED READING

American College of Chest Physicians: Committee Report. Criteria for the assessment of reversibility in airways obstruction: Report of the Committee on Emphysema. Chest 1974;65:552–553.

American Thoracic Society: Lung function testing: Selection of reference values and interpretive strategies. Am Rev Respir Dis 1991;144:1202–1218.

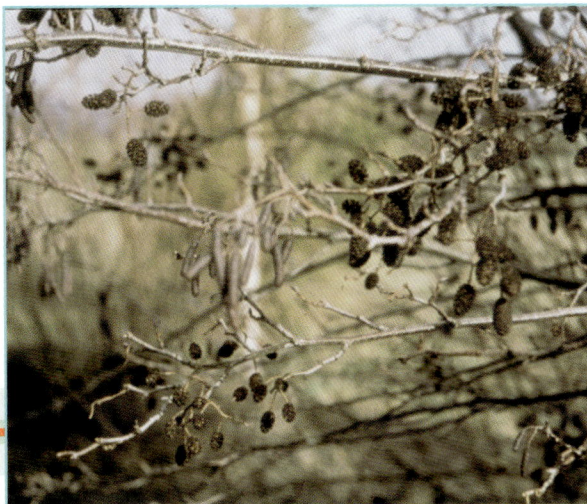

CHAPTER 3
Atopic Dermatitis

Richard P. Usatine

I. Introduction

Atopic dermatitis is a common inflammatory skin disorder that is characterized by itching and inflamed skin. The condition is triggered by the interplay of genetic, immunologic, and environmental factors. It usually begins in early childhood but may persist into adulthood. Many aggravating factors can increase the itching and exacerbate the subsequent rash. If it doesn't itch, it is not atopic dermatitis. Atopic dermatitis is sometimes called the itch that rashes.

Persons with atopic dermatitis often have other allergic conditions, such as asthma and allergic rhinitis. These allergic conditions often run in their families. The exact cause of atopic dermatitis is unknown, although a genetic predisposition and a combination of allergic and non-allergic factors appears to be important in determining disease expression.

Moderate to severe atopic dermatitis can have a profound effect on the quality of life of both the affected individuals and their families. These effects include intractable itching, skin damage, soreness, sleep loss, and the social stigma of a visible skin disease. The burden of disease is increased by the need for frequent visits to doctors and the daily use of messy topical medications.[1]

1. *Atopy* is a genetic predisposition toward the development of immediate (type I) hypersensitivity reactions against common environmental antigens. The most common clinical manifestation is allergic rhinitis. Asthma, atopic dermatitis, and food allergy occur less frequently. The atopic triad is atopic dermatitis, allergic rhinitis, and asthma (Fig. 3-1). Atopic persons have an exaggerated inflammatory response to factors that irritate the skin.

2. *Dermatitis* is a Latin term that means inflammation of the skin. Atopic dermatitis is one of many types of dermatitis.

3. *Eczema* is a Greek term that is used as a synonym for dermatitis. It means "to boil over" and refers to the vesicles seen in acute dermatitis (Fig. 3-2). *Atopic eczema* or *atopic dermatitis* refer to the same condition. There are many other types of eczema.

The use of these terms is confusing because they are not used synonymously in all conditions. For example, seborrheic dermatitis is not usually called seborrheic eczema. Therefore, while dermatitis and

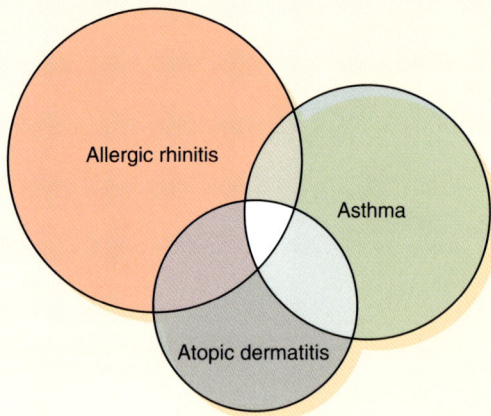

Figure 3-1 Venn diagram of the relative prevalence of atopic diseases after puberty.

eczema both refer to skin inflammation, these terms are not always used interchangeably.

4. *Extrinsic atopic dermatitis* describes the condition characterized by elevated levels of IgE in response to environmental or food allergens, which occurs in 80% of affected individuals. This figure may be above 90% in patients less than 2 years old.

5. *Intrinsic atopic dermatitis* refers to the approximately 20% of cases in which IgE levels are not elevated.

II. Epidemiology

Atopic dermatitis is the most frequent inflammatory skin disorder in the United States and the most common skin condition in children. The prevalence of atopic dermatitis is as high as 7%–15% in the United States and Europe.[2] Fifty-five percent of cases begin during the first year of life. Another 30% develop before the age of 5 years.

Atopic dermatitis is slightly more common in males than females. There is a strong pattern of inheritance. In one series, 60% of adults with atopic dermatitis had children with atopic dermatitis. When both parents had atopic dermatitis, the prevalence in children was 81%.[3] Unfortunately, the exact mode of inheritance is not known.

III. Etiology

Many factors influence the pathogenesis of atopic dermatitis. Atopic dermatitis seems to result from a vicious cycle of dermatitis associated with elevated T-lymphocyte activation, hyperstimulatory Langerhans' cells, defective cell-mediated immunity, and B-cell IgE overproduction.[4] In some cases, the exotoxins of *Staphylococcus aureus* may act as superantigens and stimulate activation of T-cells and macrophages.[2]

Persons with atopic dermatitis may have a primary T-cell defect. This may explain why they are more prone to severe skin infections caused by herpes simplex virus (eczema herpeticum) or bacteria (widespread impetigo). Further, atopic persons have increased susceptibility to skin infections such as molluscum contagiosum and cutaneous fungal infections.

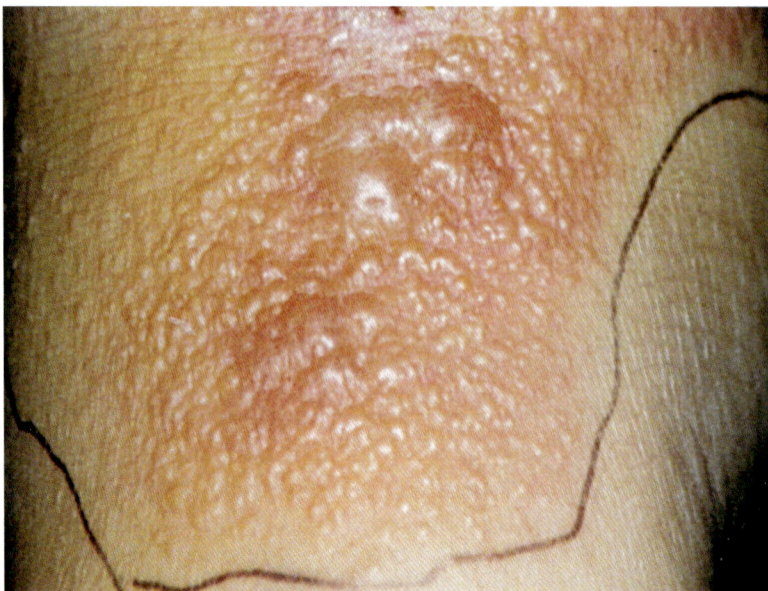

Figure 3-2 *Eczema* means to "boil over," referring to the vesicles seen in any type of acute dermatitis.

Even though research is being done on the immunology of atopic dermatitis, there are no clear mechanisms that provide a unified understanding of this condition. The role of IgE in the pathophysiology is not clear because 20% of individuals with atopic dermatitis do not have elevated IgE levels. Fortunately, the diagnosis and management of atopic dermatitis do not require an in-depth understanding of current allergy and immunology research.

IV. Clinical Manifestations

The essential feature of atopic dermatitis is pruritus. The itch may precede the rash, and scratching the itch may bring on the rash. The itching may be the most disruptive part of this disease because it may keep the individual up at night or distracted during the day.

A. Morphologic Characteristics

The morphologic characteristics of atopic dermatitis are variable.

1. Primary lesions
   a. Vesicles
   b. Scale
   c. Papules
   d. Erythematous patches and plaques
   e. Xerosis (dry and scaly skin)
2. Secondary (or sequential) lesions
   a. Lichenification (thickened skin with accentuation of skin lines)
   b. Pustules and crusts when a secondary infection has occurred
   c. Nodules in prurigo nodularis
   d. Excoriations from scratching
   e. Skin edema

3. Lesions in chronic atopic dermatitis
   a. Follicular hyperaccentuation (more prominent hyperkeratotic follicles) (Fig. 3-3A)
   b. Fissures
   c. Postinflammatory hyperpigmentation (Fig. 3-3B)
4. Summary of major clinical features
   a. Pruritus
   b. Typical morphology and distribution
   c. Flexural lichenification (thickening of the skin) and linearity in adults
   d. Facial and extensor involvement in infants and young children
   e. Chronic or chronically relapsing dermatitis
   f. Personal or family history of atopy (asthma, allergic rhinitis, allergic conjunctivitis, atopic dermatitis)

B. Other Features

Other features, seen around the eyes in atopic dermatitis, include:

1. Infraorbital folds and allergic shiners are seen on the lower eyelids (Fig. 3-4).
2. Loss of the lateral one-third of the eyebrows can occur when patients rub their face with their hands or against their pillow at night.

C. Phases of Atopic Dermatitis

The distribution of the rash varies by age and individual.

1. ***Infant Phase: 0–2 Years***
   Infants tend to start with atopic dermatitis on the cheeks of the face (Fig. 3-5). In the mildest cases, the cheeks look red, flushed, and a bit dry. This is

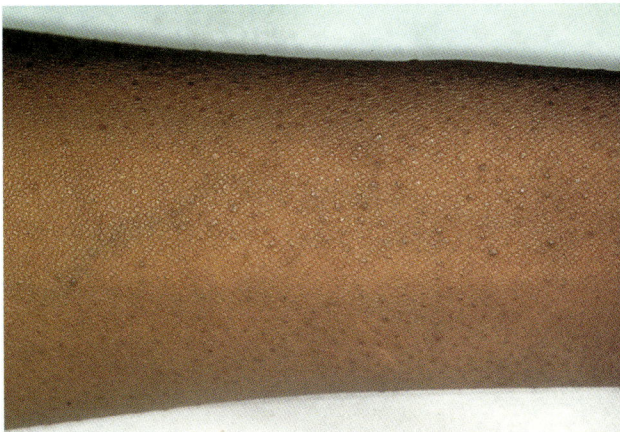

A

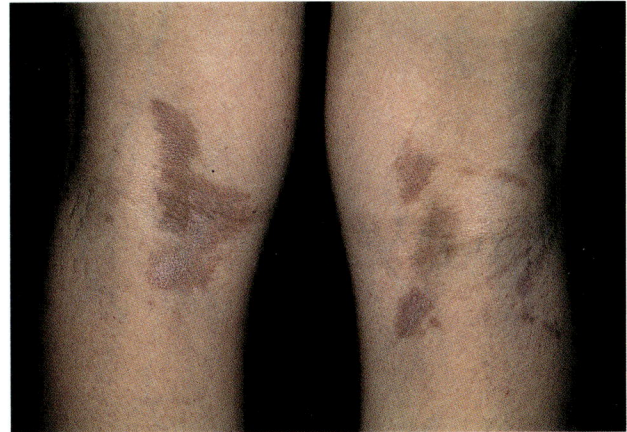

B

Figure 3-3 A, Follicular hyperaccentuation. **B**, Postinflammatory hyperpigmentation in the popliteal fossae.

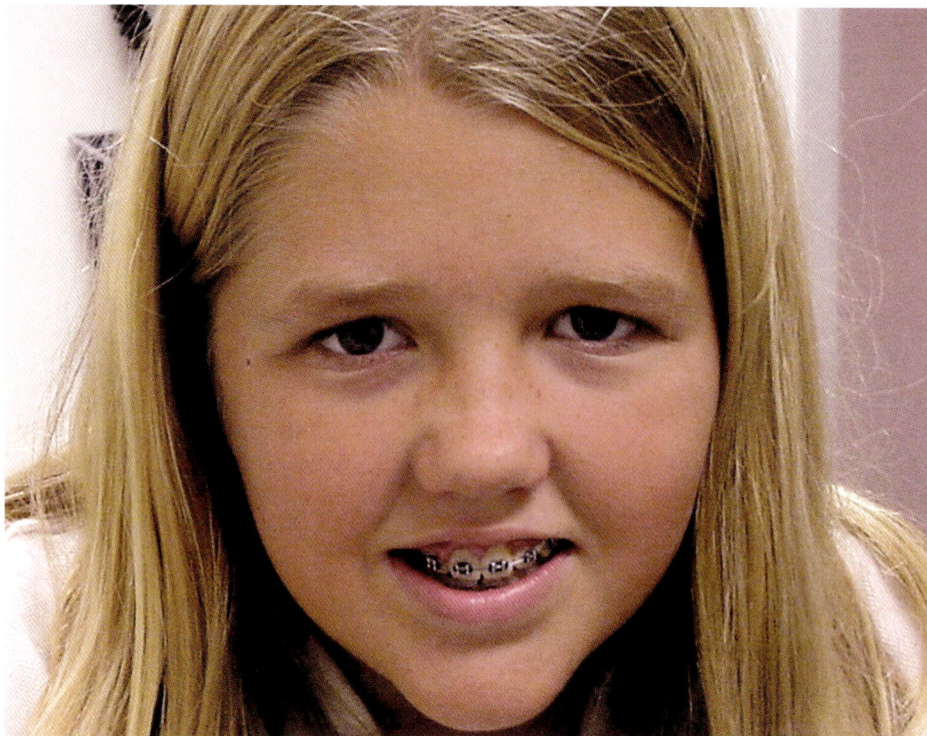

Figure 3-4 Eyelids in atopy. This young girl has allergic shiners and infraorbital folds on her lower eyelids. The infraorbital folds are referred to as the Dennie-Morgan sign.

the same appearance that might occur on exposure to cold. Sometimes the chin is involved, and this may be related to irritation from drooling.

In more severe cases the eruption includes the trunk and extremities. The flexural surfaces may be involved, and patches may even resemble nummular eczema (Fig. 3-6). Secondary infection (Fig. 3-7) will make the case more severe. The infant shown in Figure 3-8 has a severe eruption combined with secondary infection.

Atopic dermatitis resolves in about 50% of infants by age 18 months.

2. ***Childhood Phase: 2–12 Years***
   Children often have atopic dermatitis in the antecubital and popliteal fossa. Involvement of the neck, wrists, and ankles also may occur. Perspiration in these areas may initiate the itch-scratch cycle and aggravate the skin. The eruption may begin with papules that may become widespread or coalesce into plaques (Fig. 3-9).

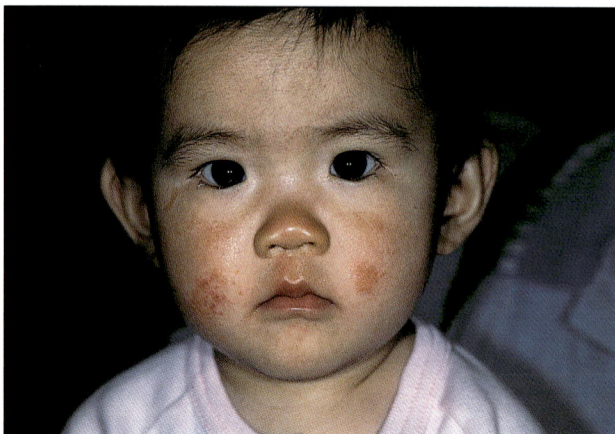

Figure 3-5 Mild atopic dermatitis on the cheeks of an infant.

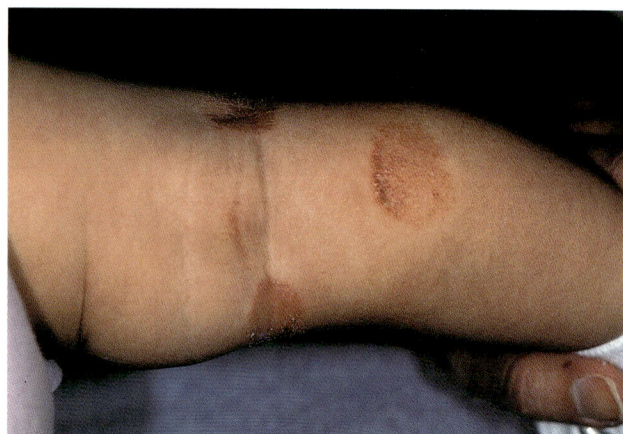

Figure 3-6 The same child in Figure 3-5 with involvement of the flexural surface of the leg in the pattern of nummular eczema.

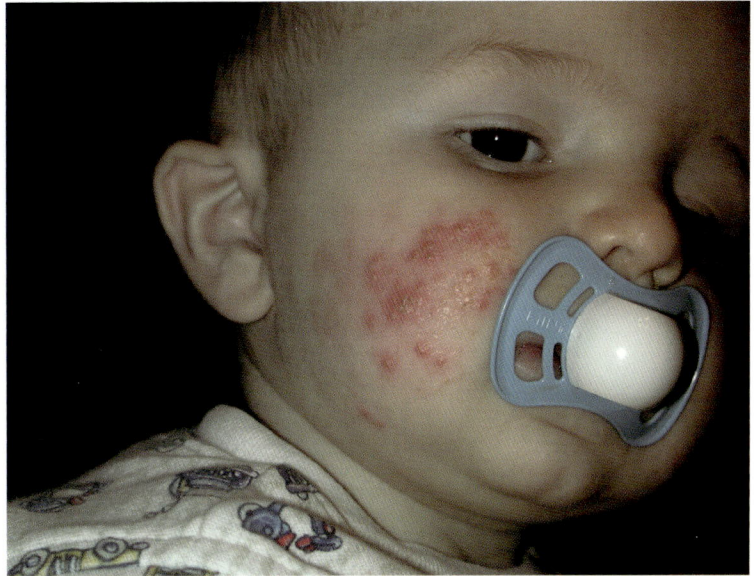

Figure 3-7 More severe atopic dermatitis on the face of a boy showing superinfection with papules and pustules.

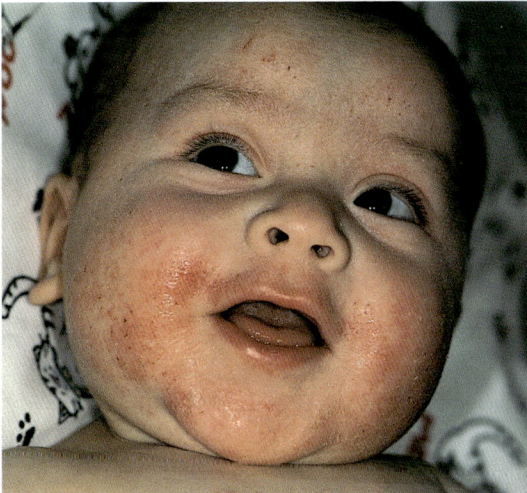

A

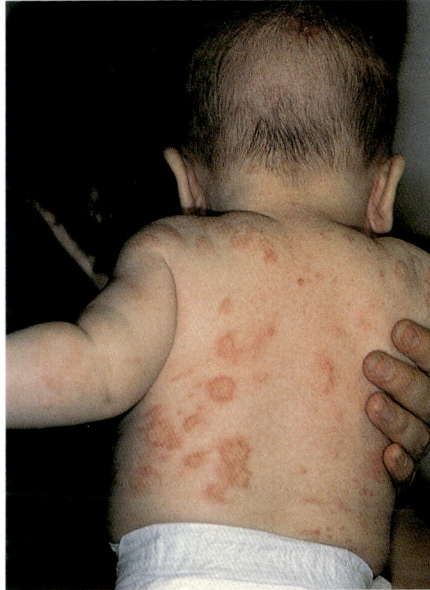

B

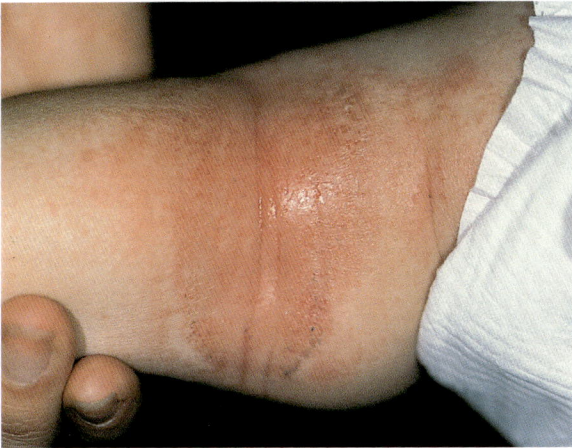

C

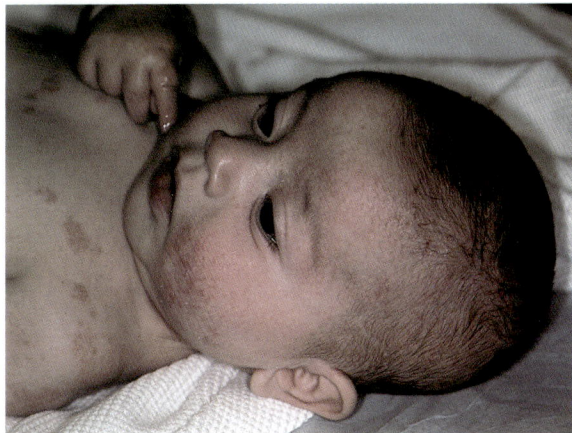

D

Figure 3-8 Severe superinfected atopic dermatitis on the face, trunk and extremities of an infant. **A**, Face. **B**, Back. **C**, Popliteal fossa. **D**, Cheek and shoulder.

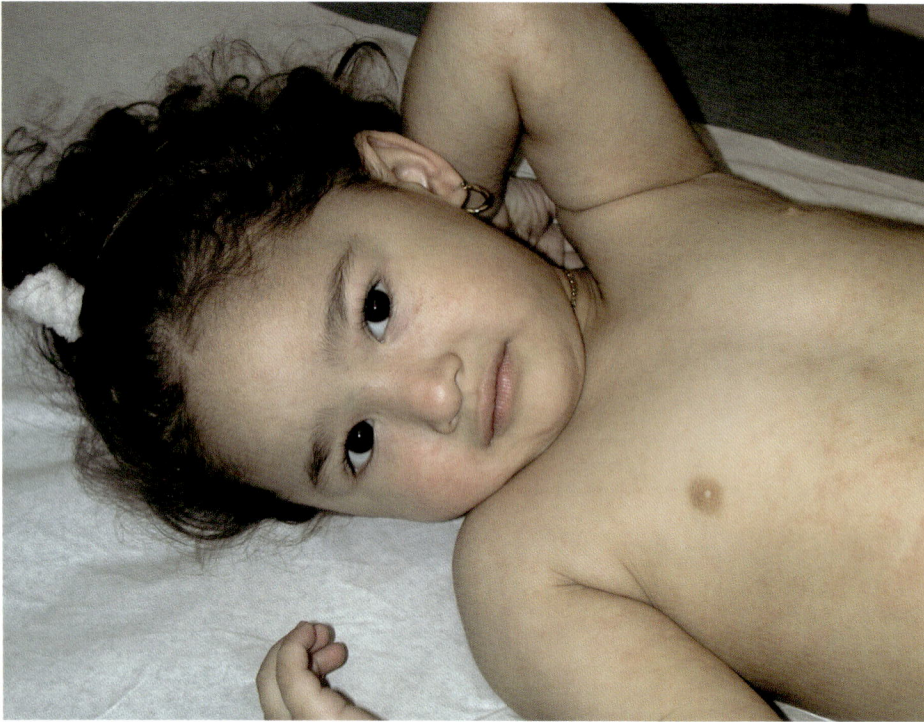

A

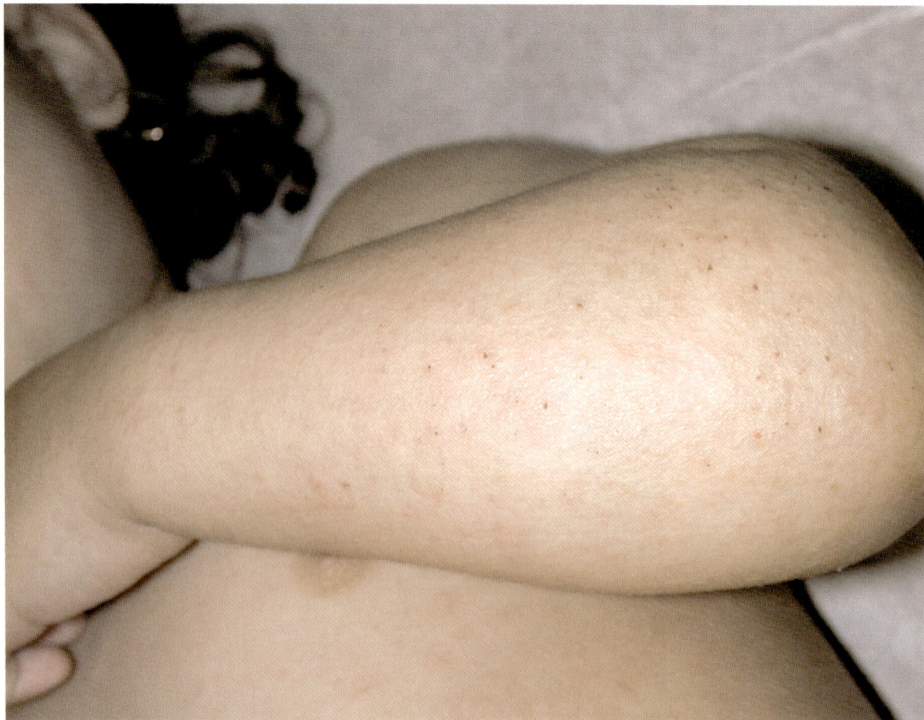

B

Figure 3-9 **A–D**, Widespread atopic dermatitis on the trunk, arm, abdomen, and popliteal fossae of a 2-year-old girl.

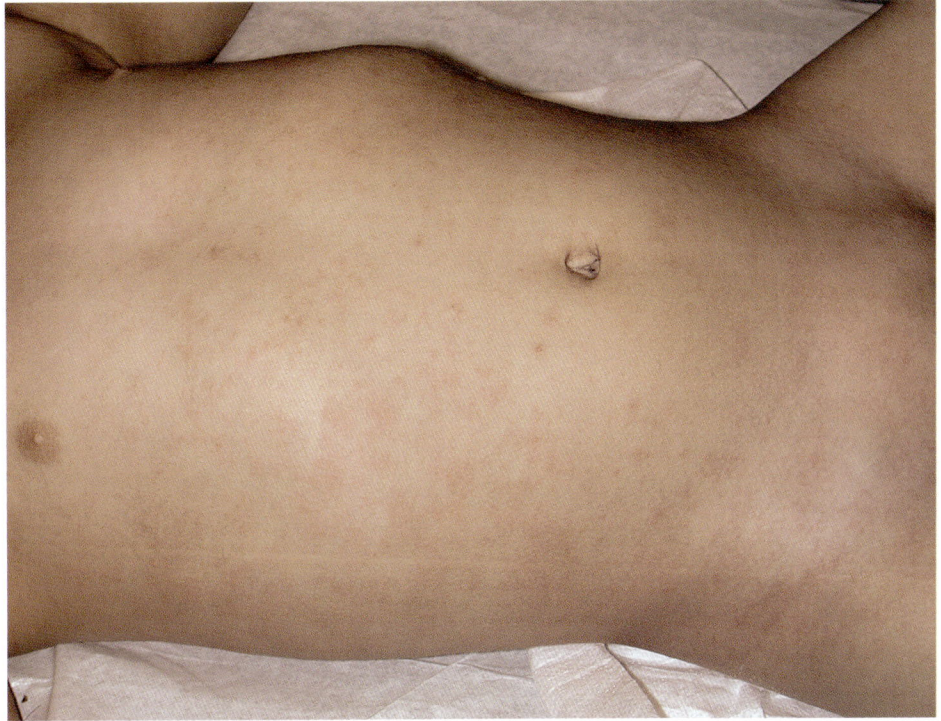

C

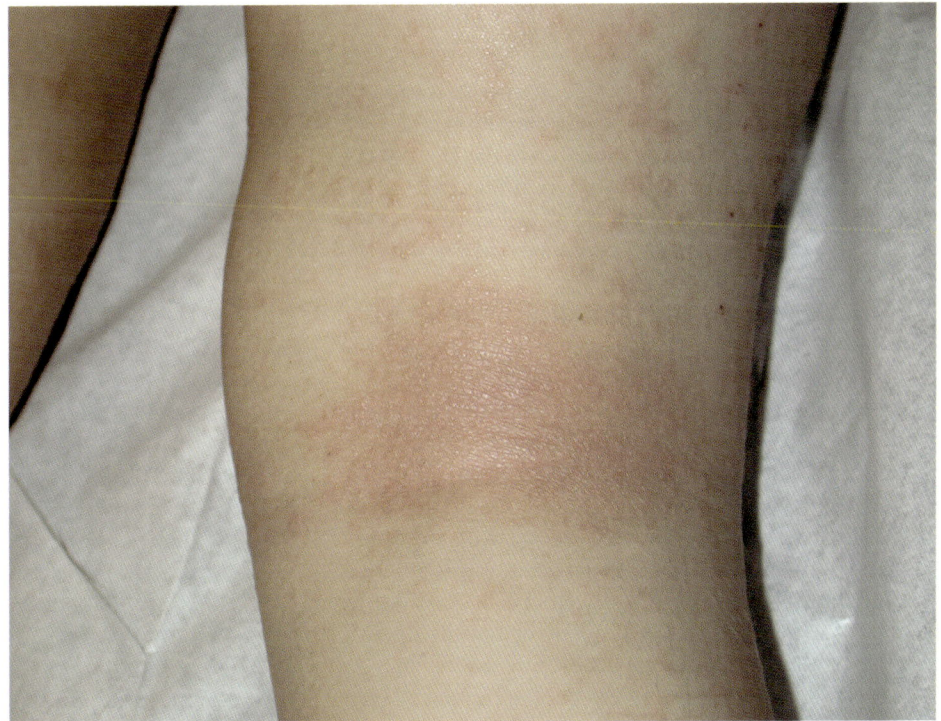

D

Figure 3-9, cont'd.

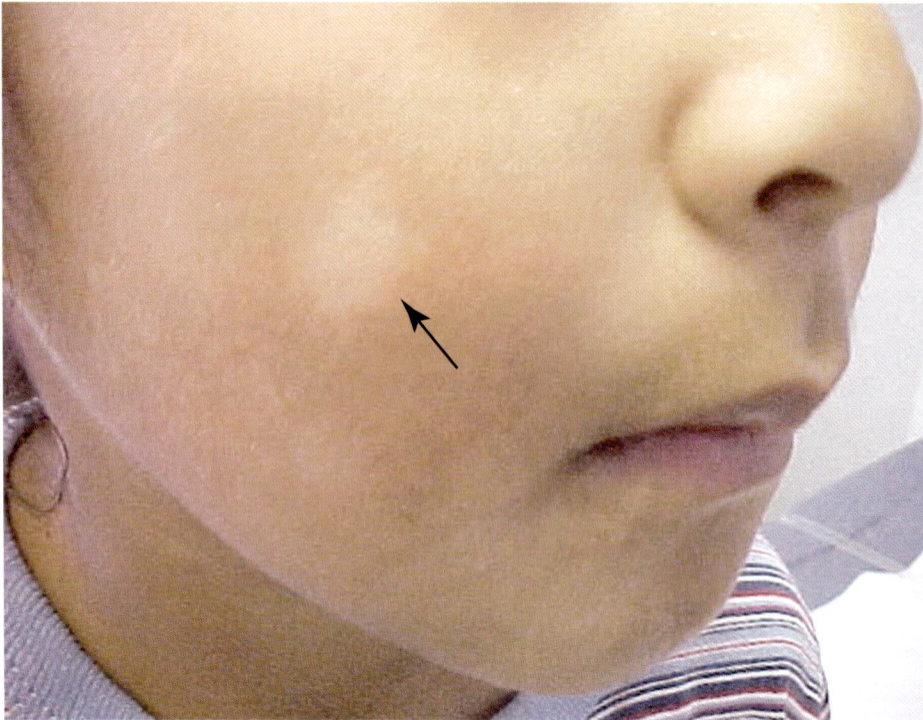

Figure 3-10 Pityriasis alba (white patches) on the face of a Latina girl.

Lichenification occurs after repeated scratching. Associated features may include pityriasis alba (Fig. 3-10) on the face or a follicular eczema (Fig. 3-11). The African-American girl shown in Figure 3-11 has follicular eczema on her face and neck. This pattern shows a hyperkeratotic accentuation of the skin follicles.

3. ***Adult Phase: 12 Years–Adult***
When atopic dermatitis begins in or continues into adulthood, the antecubital and popliteal fossae are usually involved (Fig. 3-12, p. 48). Furthermore, adults are more likely to have atopic dermatitis on the hands and face (Fig. 3-13, p. 49).

Some persons with atopic dermatitis get hand dermatitis or hand eczema. Not everyone who gets hand dermatitis or hand eczema has atopic dermatitis. Any kind of hand dermatitis may be aggravated by repeated washing and exposure to chemicals at work. Doctors and nurses may develop hand eczema by repeated washing between patient contacts (Fig. 3-14*A*, p. 50). Stay-at-home mothers and child-care workers are also at risk for hand dermatitis and dishydrotic eczema because of repeated hand washing (Fig. 3-14*B*). Persons who develop dishydrotic eczema on the hands and feet do not necessarily have atopic dermatitis.

4. ***Exacerbating Factors***
The history is likely to reveal factors believed to exacerbate the patient's atopic dermatitis. The most common factors cited are:
 a. Temperature change and sweating
 b. Decreasing humidity
 c. Excessive washing
 d. Contact with irritating substances
 e. Contact allergy
 f. Aeroallergens
 g. Microbial agents such as *Staphylococcus aureus*
 h. Foods: eggs, peanuts, milk, fish, soy, wheat (especially < age 2)
 i. Emotional stress
 j. Hormonal factors

5. ***Itch Provokers***
The most common provokers of pruritis reported by patients with atopic dermatitis are:
 a. Heat and perspiration (96%)
 b. Wool (91%)
 c. Emotional stress (81%)
 d. Certain foods (49%)

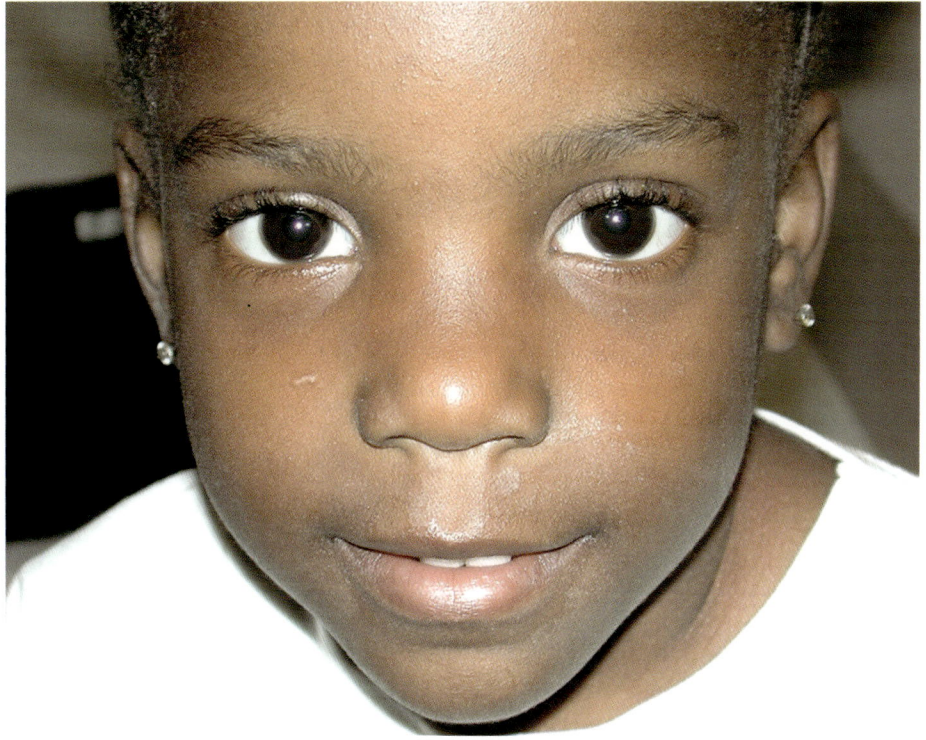

A

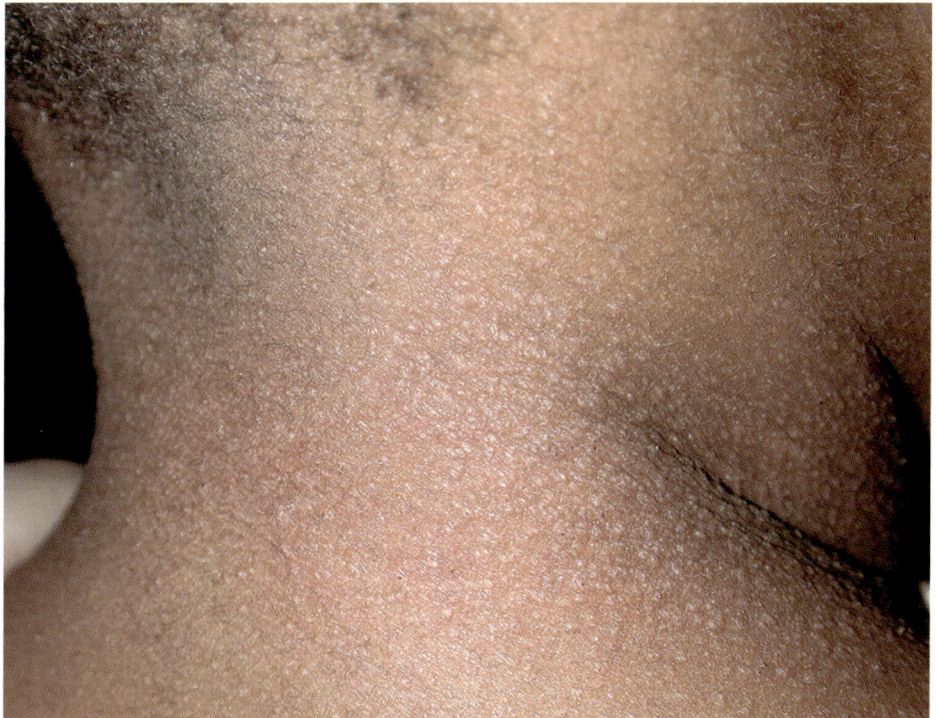

B

Figure 3-11 Follicular eczema or hyperkeratotic atopic dermatitis on a 4-year-old African-American girl: on the face (**A**) and on the neck (**B**).

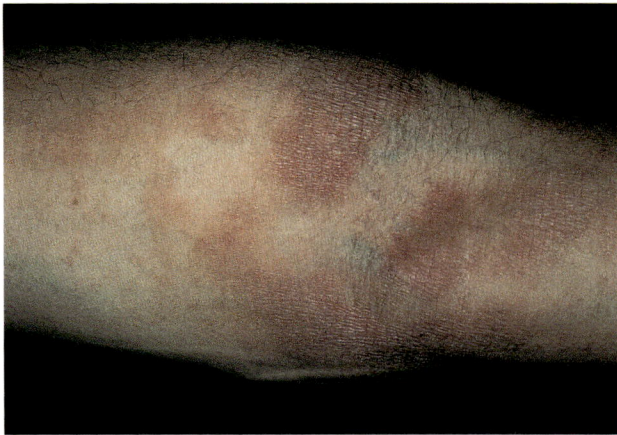

Figure 3-12 Chronic atopic dermatitis in the antecubital fossa in a young adult male partially treated with topical corticosteroids.

e. Alcohol (44%)
f. Common cold (36%)
g. Dust mite (35%)[5]

6. ***Stages of Dermatitis***
   The three stages of dermatitis or eczema are:
   a. ***Acute***—papules and vesicles on a red base.
   b. ***Subacute***—thicker, less red plaques with remnants of the vesicles, more linear excoriations.
   c. ***Chronic***—lichenified, dry, and scaly plaques with excoriations.
   Not all patients with atopic dermatitis manifest all three stages.

V. Differential Diagnosis

A number of other types of dermatitis may be confused with or may coexist with atopic dermatitis. The most common types are seborrheic dermatitis and contact dermatitis. Psoriasis can be confused with atopic dermatitis as well; especially if it is inverse psoriasis located on flexor surfaces. Less common types of dermatitis that may be confused with atopic dermatitis include nummular eczema, dishydrotic eczema, and dermatitis herpetiformis.

A. Differential Diagnosis of Atopic Dermatitis[6]

1. Seborrheic dermatitis (Fig. 3-15, p. 50)—Greasy, scaly lesions on the scalp, face, and chest.
2. Psoriasis (Fig. 3-16, p. 50)—Localized patches on the extensor surfaces, scalp, and buttocks; pitted nails.
3. Lichen simplex chronicus (sometimes called neurodermatitis) (Fig. 3-17, p. 50)—Usually, a single patch in an area accessible to scratching; absence of family history.

4. Contact dermatitis (Fig. 3-18, p. 51)—History of exposure; rash in area of exposure; absence of family history.
5. Scabies (Fig. 3-19, p. 51)—Papules, burrows, finger web involvement, positive skin scraping.
6. Dermatophyte infection (Fig. 3-20, p. 51)—On the hands it can appear like hand dermatitis. A positive KOH preparation for hyphae can help make the diagnosis.
7. Dermatitis herpetiformis (Fig. 3-21, p. 51)—Vesicles over extensor areas; may be associated with nontropical sprue.

Many of the common types of eczematous eruptions can coexist with atopic dermatitis (Fig. 3-22, p. 52). Certain infections and infestations may appear to resemble atopic dermatitis, but their history should be very different. Furthermore, these infections or infestations may be complicating factors on top of a preexisting atopic dermatitis. Rare conditions such as immunodeficiencies, metabolic diseases, or neoplastic diseases may resemble atopic dermatitis. These conditions should have other systemic findings or present with a history of multiple recurrent skin infections.

VI. History and Physical Examination

When the patient presents with a skin rash, the physician should ask questions while inspecting the skin.[7] Ask about itching and any history of skin conditions, asthma, and allergic rhinitis in both the patient and family. Look carefully at the lesions to determine the type of primary (basic or initial) lesions and any secondary (or sequential) lesions that are present (see Appendix 5, Table A5-1, for descriptions of primary and secondary lesions). It is often helpful to touch or palpate the lesions. If there is concern for disease transmission, as in scabies, gloves should be worn.

Next, look at the distribution of the lesions. Look at the local distribution first to determine if the primary lesions are arranged in groups, rings, lines, or merely scattered over the skin. For example, atopic dermatitis is often symmetric and found on the flexor surfaces of older children and adults. Determine which parts of the skin are affected and which are spared.

Observe the remainder of the skin, nails, hair, and mucous membranes. Patients often display one small area and may be reluctant to show the rest of their skin. With many skin conditions it is essential to look beyond the most affected area. Think of yourself as a detective collecting clues. Patients may have lesions on their back or feet that they have not observed. For example, a patient may have an eruption on the hands that is an autosensitization to a fungal infection on the feet. If you don't look

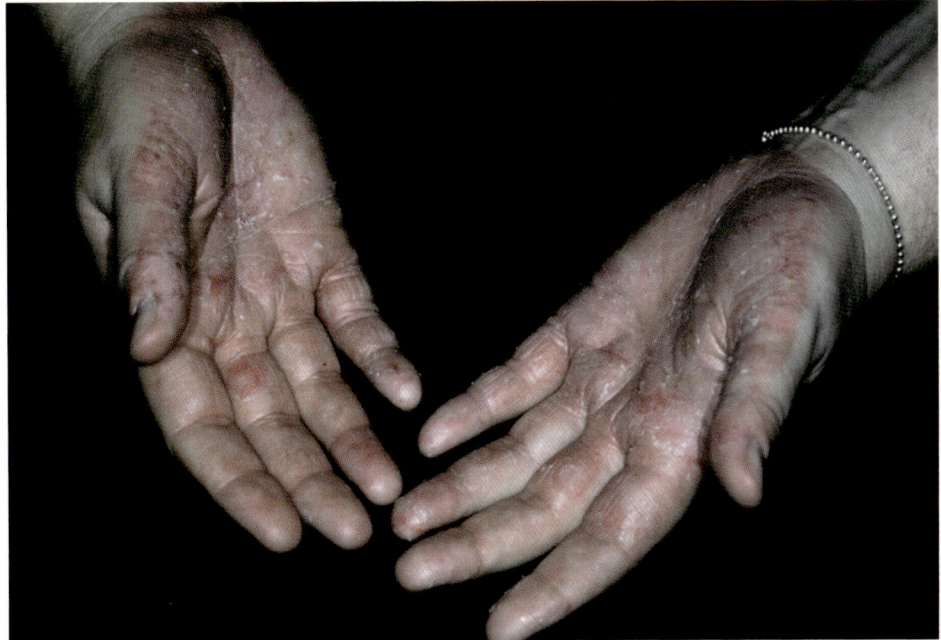

A

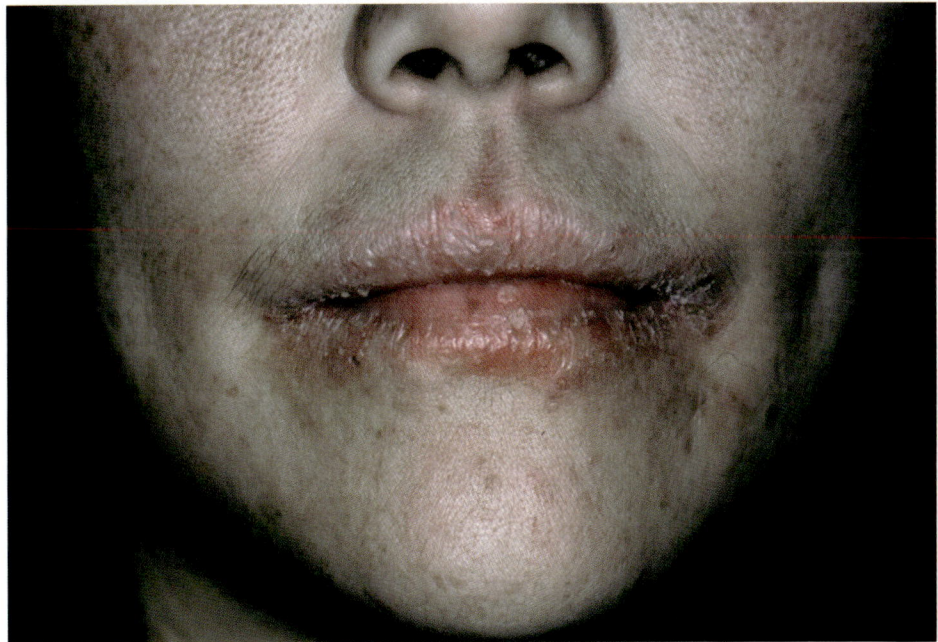

B

Figure 3-13 Atopic dermatitis on the hands (**A**) and face (**B**) of a middle-aged Japanese woman.

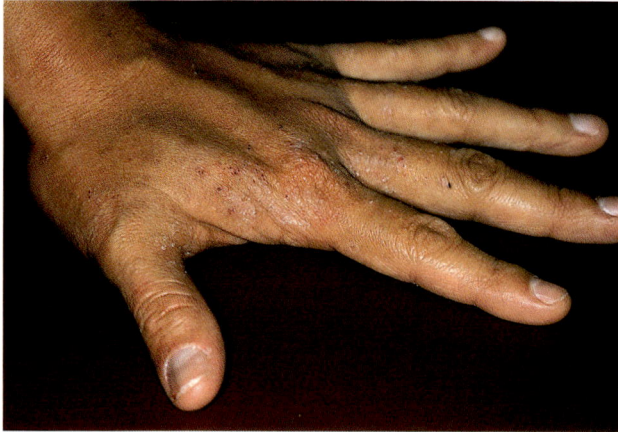
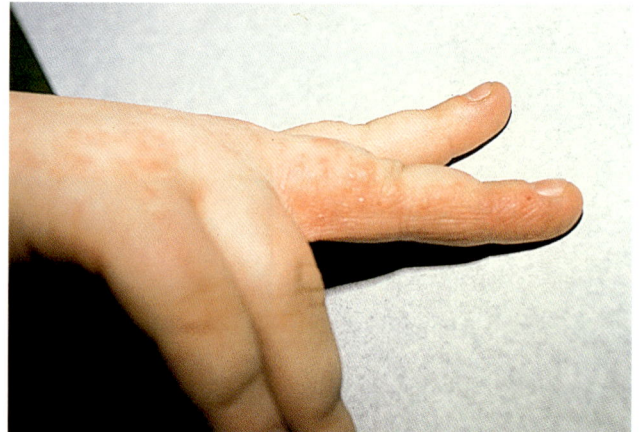

A

B

Figure 3-14 **A**, Atopic dermatitis on the hands of a medical student worsened by hand washing. **B**, Dyshidrotic eczema between the fingers, with small papules and vesicles.

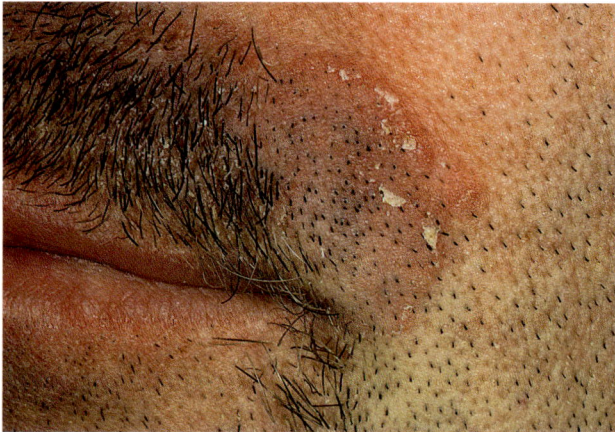

Figure 3-15 Seborrheic dermatitis. Note greasy scaling on the face.

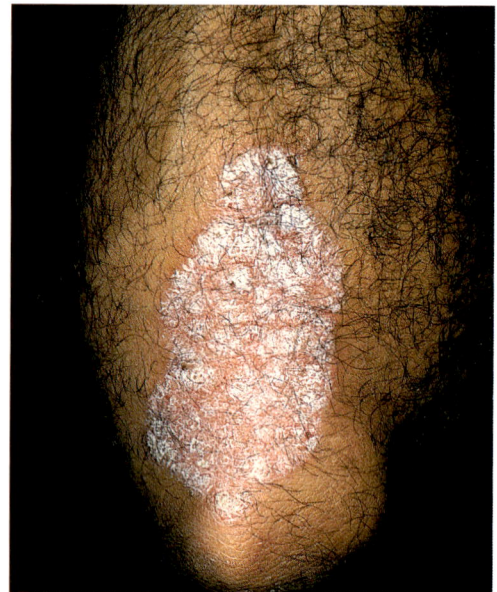

Figure 3-16 Psoriasis, with localized patches on elbow.

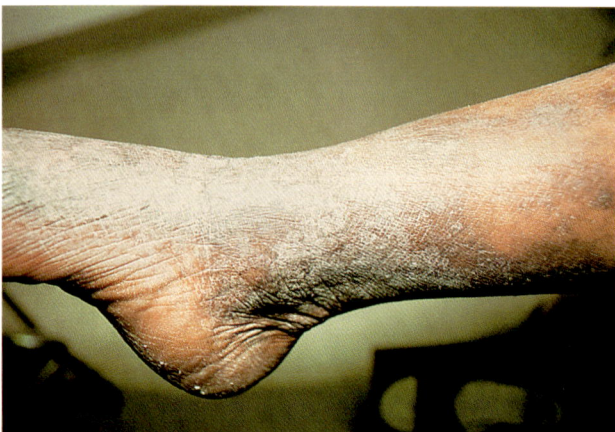

Figure 3-17 Lichen simplex chronicus or neurodermatitis in the ankle area.

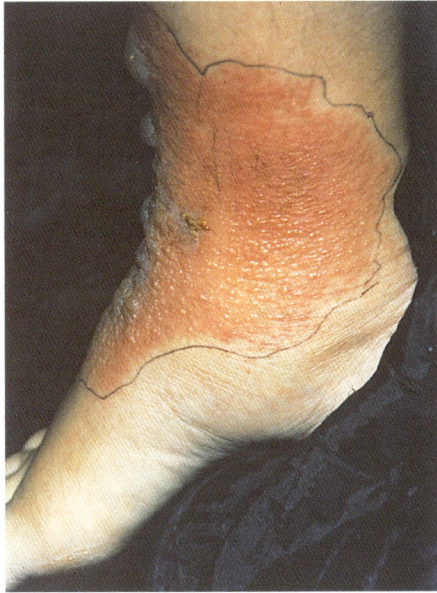

Figure 3-18 Contact dermatitis on the ankle.

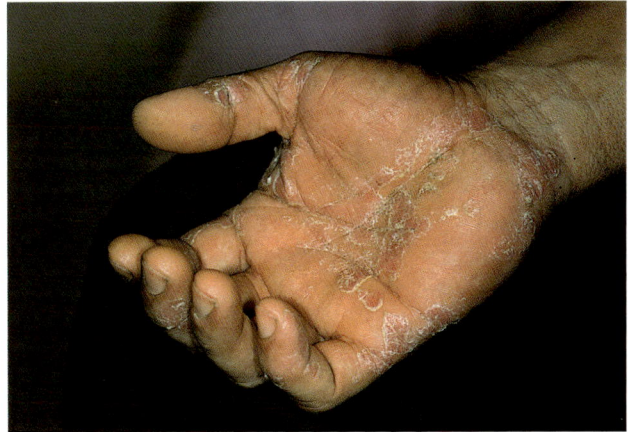

Figure 3-20 Tinea manus with a positive KOH preparation to confirm the diagnosis.

for the fungus on the feet, you will miss the diagnosis. A magnifying glass or loupe is helpful to distinguish the morphology of many skin conditions.

Look at the entire distribution of the dermatitis and characterize the morphology of the lesions. It is helpful to determine which lesions are new and primary and which are secondary to scratching or infection. Although the patient may be able to provide a clear history of the onset and changes over time, much of the same information can be gleaned from knowledge of skin lesion morphology. Initial lesions often involve papules and vesicles, while scaling, crusts, and lichenification develop over time.

Identifying infection is very important because atopic dermatitis often worsens as a result of these infections.

Staphylococcal aureus can act as a superantigen and worsen atopic dermatitis. Furthermore, impetigo and cellulitis can develop as a result of the superinfection of atopic dermatitis. Occasionally, signs of infection are very subtle and lesions can present with a slight exudate of clear to honey-colored fluid from the lesions. Figure 3-23 shows a 13-year-old girl with a superinfection of the left popliteal fossa by *S. aureus*. The right popliteal fossa has papules that are not infected; the left side shows an exudate of honey-colored fluid and increased erythema. Detecting this change allowed successful treatment of this patient with a systemic antistaphylococcal antibiotic. Sometimes the infections are less subtle, and significant crusts and pustules are visible.

The child shown in Figure 3-7 is beginning to develop a superinfection of infantile atopic dermatitis. The following day this child had more prominent pustules and

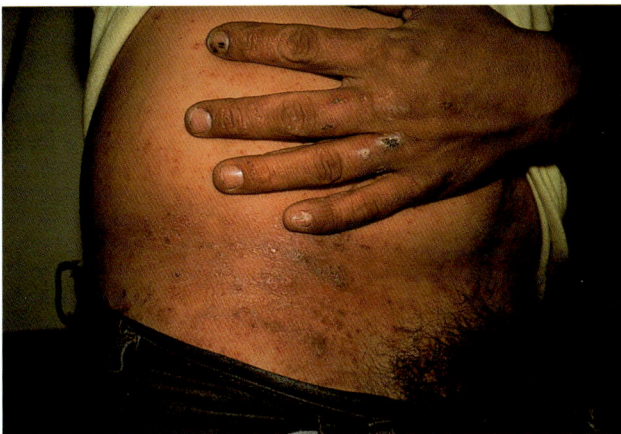

Figure 3-19 Scabies with a burrow on the finger and lesions around the waist.

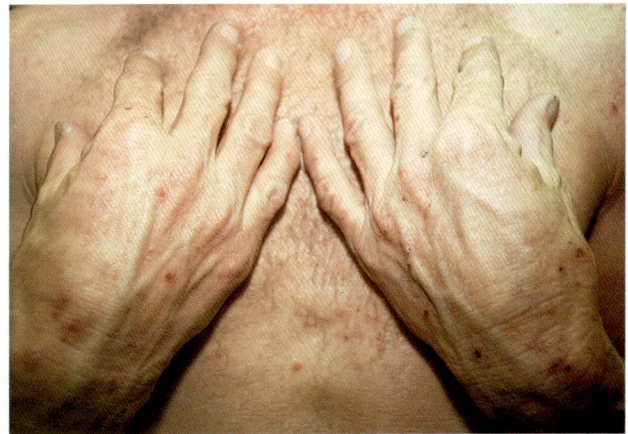

Figure 3-21 Dermatitis herpetiformis with papules, vesicles, and excoriations over extensor areas.

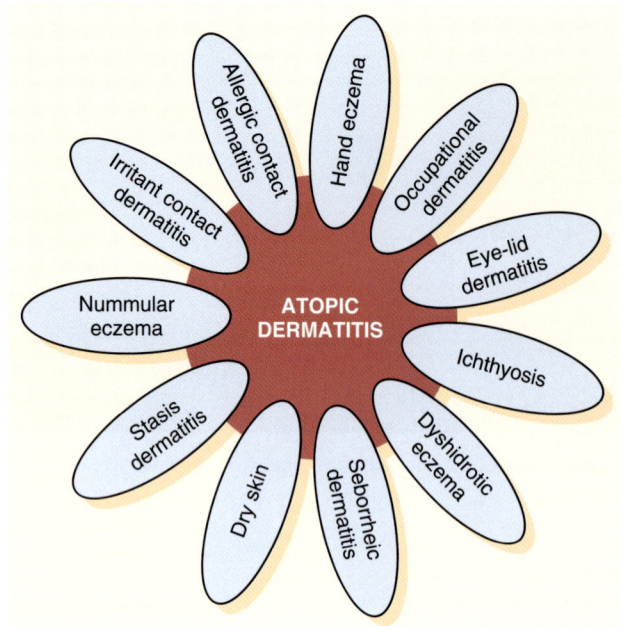

Figure 3-22 Venn diagram of the common eczematous eruptions frequently associated with atopic dermatitis. (Adapted from Altman LC, Becker JW, Williams PV: Allergy in Primary Care. Philadelphia: WB Saunders, 2000, with permission.)

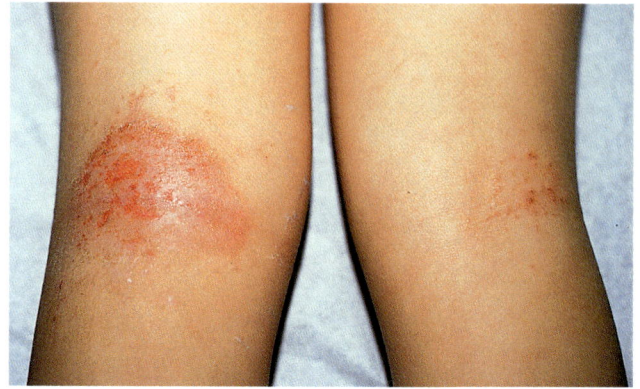

Figure 3-23 Atopic dermatitis with secondary infection in the popliteal fossa of a 13-year-old girl.

weeping exudate. The topical antibiotic administered the day before was not effective but, ultimately, the child responded well.

VII. Laboratory Examination

The diagnosis of atopic dermatitis is based on the history and physical examination findings. There are no laboratory tests that alone can rule in or out atopic dermatitis.

A. Helpful Tests

The following tests may be considered in special circumstances:

1. ***Serum IgE Levels*** (see Appendix 4)
    Serum IgE levels are sometimes measured in atopic dermatitis. Eighty percent of persons with atopic dermatitis have elevated IgE levels (extrinsic atopic dermatitis). Because 20% of individuals with atopic dermatitis (intrinsic atopic dermatitis) have normal or low IgE levels, this is unlikely to be a pathogenic factor. The levels of IgE do not correlate well with the activity of the disease and are rarely useful for diagnosis or management. It is debatable whether distinguishing between extrinsic and intrinsic atopic dermatitis helps management.

2. ***KOH Test*** (see Chapters 19 and 20)
    This test is helpful when a scaling rash is present that could be a fungal infection. The scale is scraped onto a slide using another slide or the edge of a No. 15 scalpel. KOH (preferably with DMSO) is added and the specimen is examined under the microscope for hyphae.

3. ***Skin Testing or Patch Testing***
    The role of aeroallergens in the causation or perpetuation of atopic dermatitis is controversial. "Patients with atopic dermatitis frequently show positive scratch and intradermal reactions to [a] number of antigens. Avoidance of these antigens rarely improves the dermatitis."[4] Therefore, routine skin testing or patch testing is not recommended. The information obtained from these tests is of limited value in managing most cases of atopic dermatitis. In severe atopic dermatitis that does not respond to other therapies, skin testing may serve a purpose.

4. ***Radioallergosorbent Testing*** (see Chapter 13)
    RAST may provide misleading information about the role of food or other allergens. RAST findings correlate with positive findings on food challenge tests in only one-third of cases.[4] If RAST testing is used, it should be correlated with an accurate history.

5. ***Skin Testing and RAST in Infantile Atopic Dermatitis***
    Infants and toddlers (0–3 yrs) with atopic dermatitis are typically allergic to food allergens, in particular, milk, soy, egg, wheat, fish, and peanuts.[11] Skin tests and/or RAST may be used to identify the inciting food allergen that provokes this condition. Infants with infantile atopic dermatitis may respond to strict elimination of the identified skin test or RAST-positive food allergen. In the childhood phase and beyond, this diagnostic and therapeutic approach is usually unhelpful.

B. Tests of Little Value in Atopic Dermatitis

1. *Serum Eosinophilia*
   A mild eosinophilia may be seen in atopic dermatitis but does not help in the diagnosis or management of this condition.
2. *Bacterial Culture*
   Bacterial culture generally is not needed. Approximately 90% of patients with severe atopic dermatitis are secondarily colonized or infected with *S. aureus*. Deciding whether antibiotics are needed should be based on the clinical appearance, and not on the result of a bacterial skin culture.
3. *Skin Biopsies*
   Skin biopsies are not diagnostic for atopic dermatitis and therefore are not recommended.

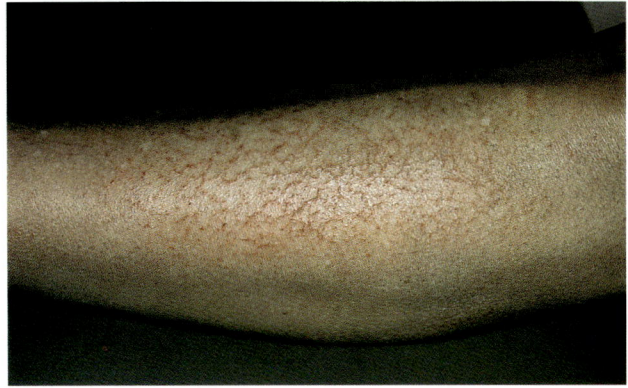

Figure 3-24 Acquired ichthyosis in a person with atopic dermatitis. This is not a case of sex-linked ichthyosis. (Courtesy of Tom Zuber, MD.)

VIII. Approach to Final Diagnosis

The diagnosis of atopic dermatitis is based almost exclusively on the history and physical examination findings.

A. Diagnostic Criteria of Hanifin and Rajka[8]

One accepted method of diagnosing atopic dermatitis is to use the diagnostic criteria of Hanifin and Rajka. This system relies on the presence of three major and three minor criteria to classify a skin disease as atopic dermatitis. While most of the features on the list are based on history and physical examination findings, elevated serum IgE levels and immediate skin test reactivity are two minor features that are included.

1. *Major Characteristics*
   a. Pruritus
   b. Typical morphology and distribution
   c. Flexural lichenification (thickening of the skin) and linearity in adults
   d. Facial and extensor involvement in infants and young children
   e. Chronic or chronically relapsing dermatitis
   f. Personal or family history of atopy (asthma, allergic rhinoconjunctivitis, atopic dermatitis)
2. *Other Characteristics*
   a. Xerosis (dry skin)
   b. Ichthyosis (Fig. 3-24)
   c. Palmar hyperlinearity/keratosis pilaris
   d. Immediate, type I skin test response
   e. Hand or foot dermatitis
   f. Cheilitis
   g. Nipple eczema
   h. Susceptibility to cutaneous infection (especially *S. aureus* and herpes simplex and other viral infections, warts, molluscum, dermatophytes)
   i. Erythroderma
   j. Early age at onset
   k. Impaired cell-mediated immunity
   l. Recurrent conjunctivitis
   m. Infraorbital fold
   n. Keratoconus (protrusion of the cornea)
   o. Anterior subcapsular cataracts
   p. Elevated total serum IgE
   q. Peripheral blood eosinophilia

This list is cumbersome to use in daily practice and encourages the use of unnecessary and expensive laboratory tests. A multicenter study group in the United Kingdom developed a more simplified set of diagnostic criteria that does not require laboratory or skin testing.[9] These criteria are given in the following section.

B. Simplified Diagnostic Criteria for Atopic Dermatitis

1. *Itchy skin condition is obligatory.*
2. *Plus three or more of the following:*
   a. History of flexural involvement
   b. History of asthma/hay fever
   c. History of a generalized dry skin
   d. Onset of rash <2 years
   e. Visible flexural dermatitis.

The simplified criteria make sense in a primary care practice. In severe cases, a referral to an allergist or dermatologist might prompt laboratory tests, skin testing, or patch testing.

C. Associated Diagnoses and Conditions

1. Lichen simplex chronicus (Fig. 3-25)
2. Keratosis pilaris (Fig. 3-26)
3. Molluscum contagiosum (Fig. 3-27)
4. Prurigo nodularis (Fig. 3-28)
5. Chronic eczema (Fig.3-29)
6. Pityriasis alba (see Fig. 3-10)

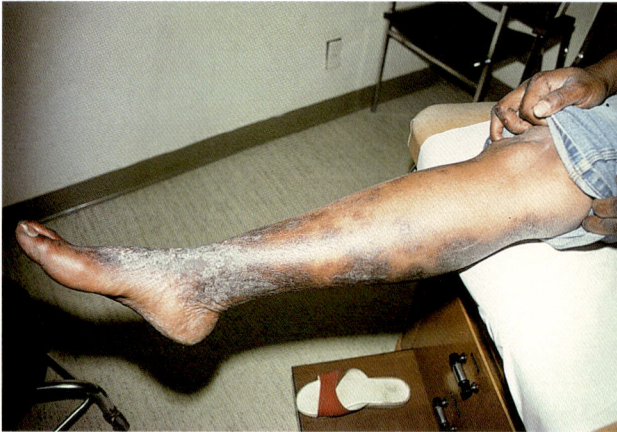

Figure 3-25 Lichen simplex chronicus in an African-American woman.

IX. Therapy and Management

This section reviews the data reported by Charman,[10] who used an evidence-based medicinal approach to look at possible interventions for the treatment of atopic dermatitis. A review of existing evidence indicates that topical steroids are beneficial and the use of emollients is likely to be beneficial.[10]

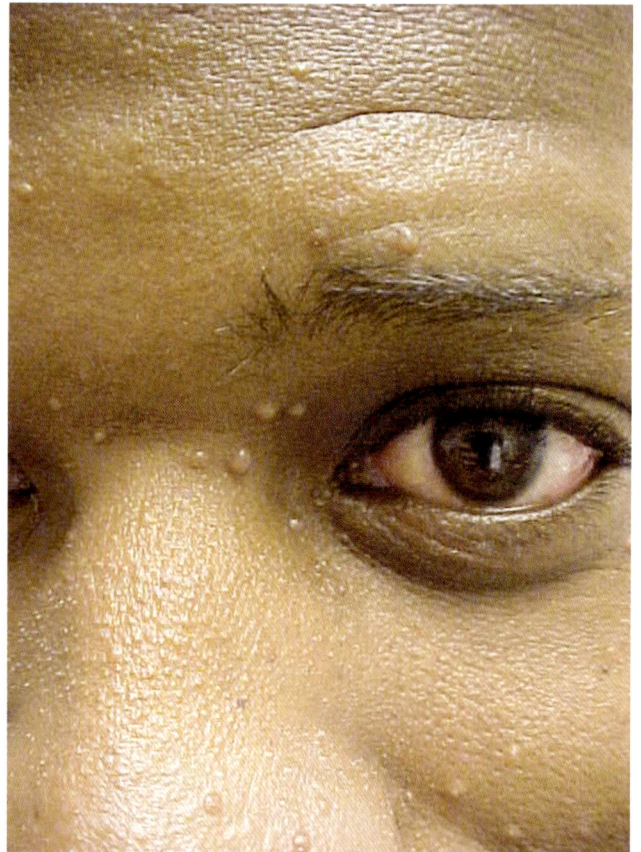

Figure 3-27 Molluscum contagiosum on the face of an African-American man with atopic dermatitis.

Small, randomized, controlled trials have found that topical corticosteroids provide symptomatic relief and are safe in the short term. There is little reliable information on their long-term adverse effects or on effects (if any) on the natural history of atopic dermatitis. Some limited evidence suggests that adding emollients to topical steroid

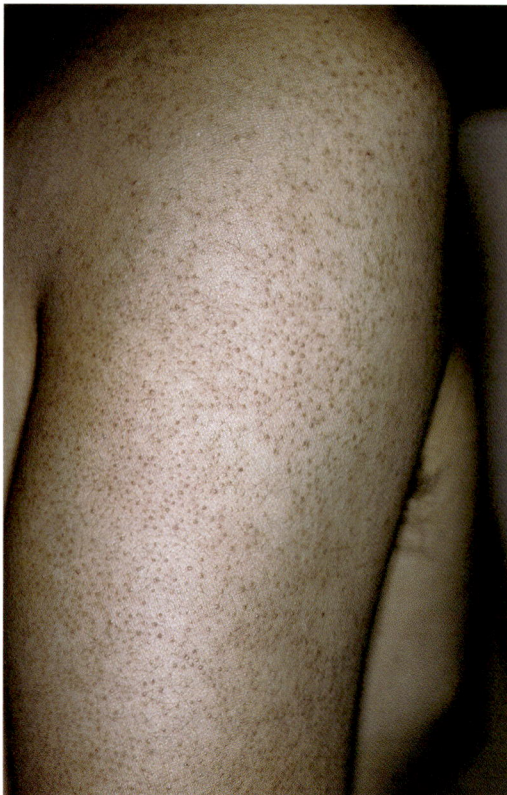

Figure 3-26 Keratosis pilaris.

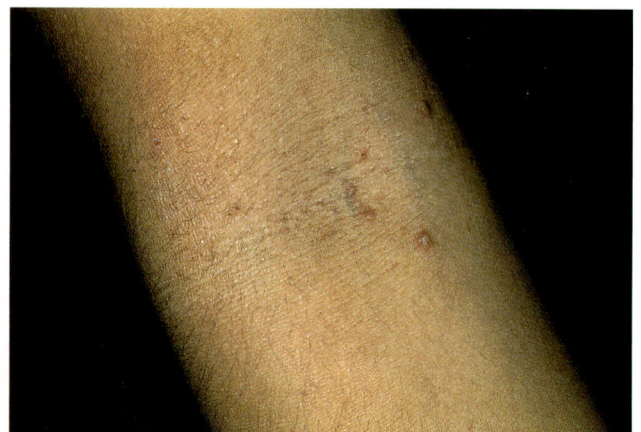

Figure 3-28 Prurigo nodularis in the antecubital fossa.

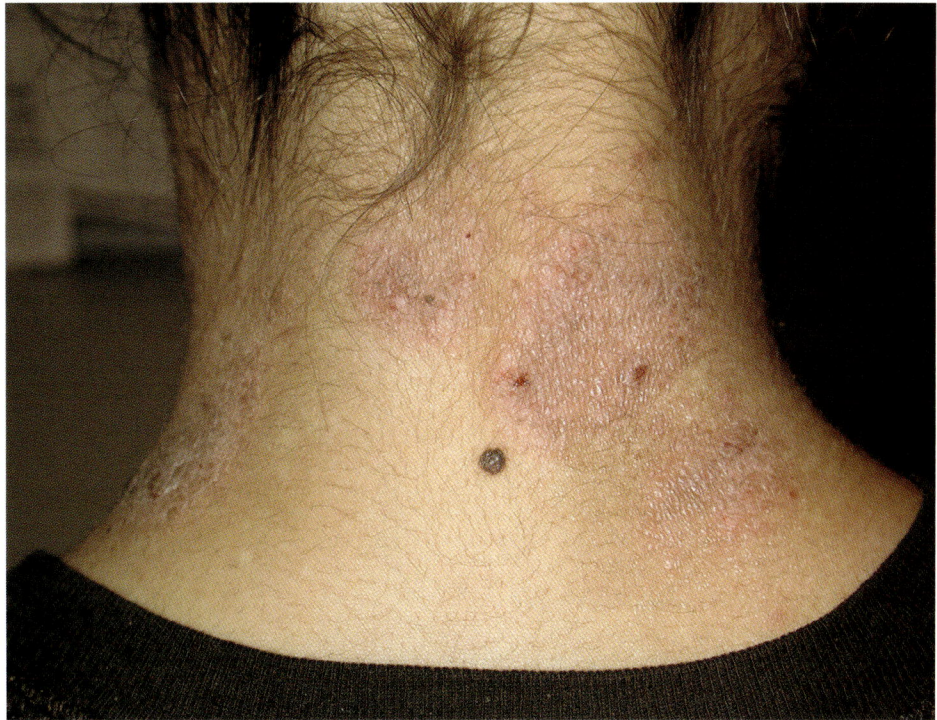

Figure 3-29 Atopic dermatitis on the neck of an adult woman nurse; wearing her stethoscope around her neck exacerbates her eczema.

treatment improves symptoms and signs more than treatment with topical steroids alone.

There is also some limited evidence to suggest that controlling house dust mites reduces the severity of symptoms. Dust mite covers were found to be the most effective method to control dust mites and atopic dermatitis symptoms. There was insufficient evidence that dietary manipulation in adults or children (>3 yrs) reduces symptom severity.

A. Prevention in Predisposed Infants

There is insufficient evidence that either prolonged breast-feeding or maternal dietary manipulation during lactation protects against atopic dermatitis in infants with a family history of atopy.

B. Avoidance of Provoking Factors

1. Charman found no evidence that avoidance of animals, detergents containing enzymes, all washing detergents, or vaccinations is beneficial in atopic dermatitis. Limited evidence was found suggesting that the roughness of clothing textiles is a more important factor for skin irritation than the type of fabric.[10]

2. According to another systematic review of treatments for atopic eczema, there is reasonable evidence from randomized controlled trials to support the use of oral cyclosporin, topical corticosteroids, psychological approaches, and ultraviolet light therapy.[1] There

was insufficient evidence to make recommendations on maternal allergen avoidance for disease prevention, oral antihistamines, Chinese herbs, dietary restriction in established atopic eczema (>3 yrs), homeopathy, house dust mite reduction, massage therapy, hypnotherapy, evening primrose oil, emollients, topical coal tar, and topical doxepin.[10]

3. There was no evidence in randomized controlled trials to support any clear clinical benefit on the use of avoidance of enzyme washing powders, cotton clothing as opposed to soft-weave synthetics, biofeedback, twice-daily as opposed to once-daily topical corticosteroids, topical antibiotic/steroid combinations versus topical steroids alone, and antiseptic bath additives. There was complete absence of evidence from randomized controlled trials regarding the effectiveness of short bursts of potent steroids versus use of longer-term, weaker topical steroids, dilution of topical corticosteroids, oral prednisolone and azathioprine, salt baths, impregnated bandages, wet-wrap bandages, water softening devices, or allergy testing.[10]

4. Two systematic reviews disagree on whether or not dust mite control has sufficient evidence to support its use.[1,10]

It would be helpful if we had large multicenter randomized controlled trials for all the decisions we make in medicine. Unfortunately, many studies in dermatology are conducted on small groups and often lack randomization. Therefore, the sections that follow will try to give reasonable recommendations based on the existing evidence combined with expert opinion.

C. Controlling Atopic Dermatitis

The recommendations are in part based on avoiding the agents that have been observed to exacerbate atopic dermatitis.

1. ***Moisturize***
   a. Avoid frequent hand washing.
   b. Avoid frequent bathing.
   c. Avoid lengthy bathing.
   d. Use tepid water for baths.
   e. Avoid abrasive washcloths.
   f. Apply moisturizer within 3 minutes of leaving the bath.
2. ***Avoid Irritants and Allergens***
   a. Use non-soap cleansers (e.g., Cetaphil), or use soaps only in the axilla, groin, and on the feet. (Good soaps include white unscented Dove and Neutrogena.)
   b. Avoid perfumes or cosmetics that burn or itch.
   c. Avoid fabric softeners.
3. ***Avoid Rough Clothing***
   a. Avoid rough fabrics, including rough wool.
   b. Use 100% cotton.
4. ***Avoid Scratching***
   a. Do not scratch.
   b. Pat firmly, press, or grasp the skin when the itching is severe.
   c. Apply soothing lubricants.
   d. Pat dry with a soft towel after bathing. Do not rub the skin.

D. Control the Environment

1. ***Temperature***
   a. Maintain cool and stable temperatures.
   b. Do not overdress.
   c. Use a limited number of bed blankets.
   d. Avoid sweating.
2. ***Humidity***
   a. Humidify the house in winter, especially when indoor heat dries the air.
3. ***Airborne Allergens and Dust*** (see Appendix 7)
   a. Use special mattress and pillow covers to minimize dust mite exposure (consider in patients who are skin test positive for dust mites).
   b. Avoid tobacco smoke.
   c. Vacuum drapes and clean blankets.
   d. Wet mop floors.
   e. Minimize animal dander, especially if there is a known allergy to a pet or any other animal.

4. ***Emotional Stress***
   a. Learn relaxation techniques such as abdominal breathing and yoga.
   b. Use psychotherapy when indicated. Atopic dermatitis can decrease self-esteem and social interaction.
5. ***Diet***
   a. The role of diet as a precipitating factor in atopic dermatitis is still being debated. The value of elimination diets and testing for food allergy is still questionable. It appears that the younger a child develops atopic dermatitis the more likely food allergy becomes a factor. This is especially true of children younger than 3 years who have generalized atopic dermatitis that responds poorly to routine management.[3] Those children are also more likely to have gastrointestinal symptoms, including colicky abdominal pain, vomiting, and diarrhea.[3] Figure 3-30 shows the relative prevalence of food allergy and other allergic diseases during childhood.
   b. A child younger than 7 years with atopic dermatitis that is unresponsive to routine therapy may have a 50% chance of having food hypersensitivity. The history is of limited value in predicting which patients are likely to have food allergy. Unfortunately, we lack accurate tests for diagnosing food allergy. The existing tests consist of elimination diets, food challenges, skin tests, and RAST specific IgE antibody tests. Skin tests and food challenge tests are more reliable than the RAST tests. A negative food skin test is more accurate at ruling out a food allergy than a positive food skin test is at ruling in a food allergy. Likewise, a positive RAST test is unreliable, but

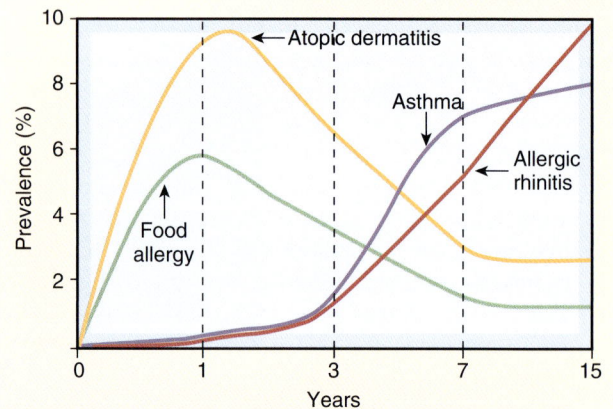

Figure 3-30 Relative prevalence of allergic diseases as they change over time. (Adapted from Altman LC, Becker JW, Williams PV: Allergy in Primary Care. Philadelphia: WB Saunders, 2000, with permission.)

a negative test is quite predictive of a negative food challenge (see Chapters 12 and 13 and Appendix 6).

c. Food hypersensitivity is usually limited to one or two foods, and children often grow out of them. Six foods account for 90% of the positive oral challenges seen in children. In a study of 196 children (45% male; median age 5 years 9 months; atopic dermatitis in 98%, asthma in 62%), there were 513 positive food challenges distributed as follows: egg, 267; milk, 117; soy, 53; wheat, 40; peanut, 24; fish, 12.[11]

d. The most practical and safe food challenge should take place in the office under supervision. The early-phase reaction occurs within 2 hours of ingestion of the food antigen. Symptoms include pruritus, erythema, and edema. The late-phase reaction may involve the recurrence of pruritus 6–8 hours later. Patients may also develop nausea, abdominal pain, emesis, or diarrhea. Respiratory symptoms such as wheezing, sneezing, and nasal congestion may occur. Anaphylactic reactions are uncommon but possible during food challenges (see Chapter 7).

e. Most food allergies disappear after the third birthday. Milk and soy allergies are more likely to disappear, while egg and fish allergies are more likely to remain. According to Sloper et al., an elimination diet of cow's milk, eggs, and tomatoes helped 75% of infantile patients with moderate or severe atopic dermatitis, which relapsed after food challenges.[12] However, according to Werfel, only about 10% of all patients notice a benefit from an elimination diet.[13] Therefore, he cautions that an elimination diet creates a very real danger of malnutrition and should not be used for a prolonged period unless there is also a positive result on an oral provocation test.

f. The lack of consensus on the issue of food allergy and atopic dermatitis necessitates the careful consideration of patient history and clinical judgment to guide the practitioner's use of food testing and elimination diets.

E. Treating Atopic Dermatitis with Medications

1. **Hydration**
Petrolatum is an effective agent for hydration. Other agents include Aquaphor, Eucerin, Lubriderm, and Lac-Hydrin. Lac-Hydrin contains lactic acid, which is keratolytic and can help with xerosis and keratosis pilaris. Most patients will experiment with the different moisturizers and find the agent that works best for them. The timing of the moisturizer application is most important. Patient education includes emphasizing the importance of applying moisturizers within 3 minutes of showering or bathing to maximize skin hydration.

2. **Steroids**
Topical steroids are very effective treatment for atopic dermatitis. There is very strong evidence to support their effectiveness.

a. Choosing the vehicle and strength is an important part of prescribing corticosteroids for atopic dermatitis (see Appendix 5, Tables A5-1 through A5-4, for more descriptions regarding the vehicle and strength of steroids).
   1) The ointments are best for dry and cracked skin.
   2) Creams are easier to apply and are better tolerated.
   3) Use weaker steroids for the face and the groin.
   4) Use weaker steroids for babies and small children to avoid systemic absorption.
   5) Use stronger steroids for thicker skin, such as on the hands and feet.
   6) Use stronger steroids for more severe outbreaks or lesions that have not responded to weaker steroids.

b. Local adverse effects of topical steroids are common with regular use over weeks to months. The most common adverse effect of topical steroid use is skin atrophy, in which the epidermis becomes thin and superficial capillaries dilate. Atrophy can be accompanied by hypopigmentation, telangiectasias, and striae. Although the atrophy is usually reversible over months, striae are irreversible. When fluorinated steroids (the strongest steroids) are continuously applied to the face, perioral dermatitis, rosacea-like eruptions, and acneiform eruptions can occur (Fig. 3-31).

c. Systemic adverse effects, such as hypothalamic-pituitary axis suppression, are rare and occur when large amounts of topical steroids are absorbed systemically. The risk of such absorption increases with stronger steroids, thinner skin, younger patients, longer duration of therapy, and the use of occlusion in therapy. Adverse effects can be prevented by prescribing the minimum strength needed for the shortest duration of time.

d. Choosing and dispensing *topical corticosteroids*.
   The goal in choosing a topical steroid is to maximize benefit and minimize adverse effects. The factors that need to be considered involve the following:
   1) *Skin disorder.* As the severity or chronicity of the disorder increases, the need for higher-potency steroids increases directly. Thicker lesions (e.g., lichen simplex chronicus) need higher-potency steroids.

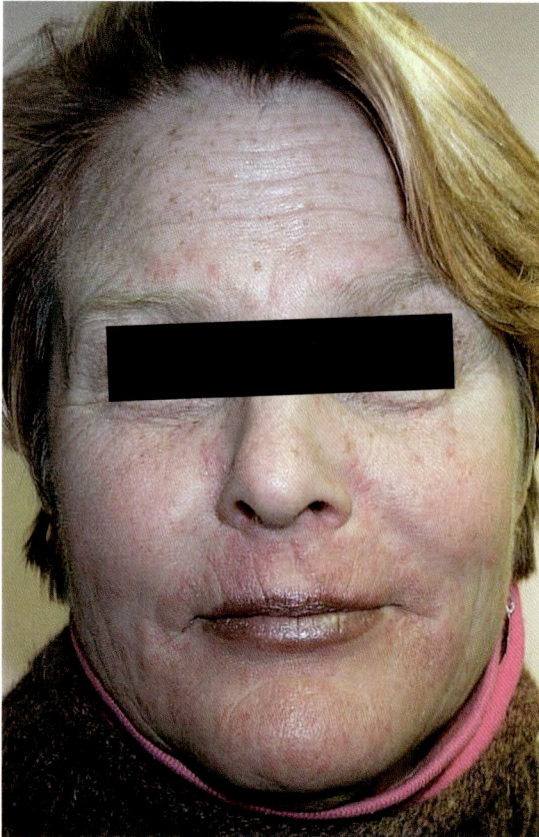

Figure 3-31 Steroid acne on the face of a woman using daily high-potency steroids. (Courtesy of David Elpern, MD.)

2) *Site.* Use only the weakest potency steroids (hydrocortisone) on the face, genitals, and other intertriginous areas (skin folds) where skin is thin and/or moist and skin atrophy and striae occur most rapidly. The skin on palms and soles is so thick that the most potent steroids may be needed.

3) *Age.* Avoid the use of high-potency topical steroids in infants and children because they have greater surface area per body mass than adults, and thus are at greater risk for the adverse effects of systemic absorption.

4) *Steroid potency (strength and concentration).* There are more than 50 types and brands of steroids. It is not necessary to memorize these lists, but the prescriber should know the names of at least one steroid from each of the major levels of potency. To save on costs, the clinician can use generic agents from all the potency groups.
   a) Weakest potency (Group VII): 1% hydrocortisone (OTC) is a good option.
   b) Medium potency (Group III): Consider prescribing 0.1% triamcinolone (generic by prescription).
   c) High potency (Group I): Consider prescribing generic clobetasol or other generic steroids from Group I. (To minimize high-potency steroid use, clinicians can prescribe a lower potency steroid [0.1% triamcinolone] and instruct patients to apply the cream or ointment under an occlusive dressing.)

5) *Vehicle.* The vehicle is the substance in which the steroid is dispersed. The most commonly used vehicles are creams, ointments, gels, solutions, and lotions (see Appendix 5). The choice of vehicle is determined by the characteristics of the lesion (dry or moist), the site involved, and patient preference. Furthermore, the vehicle affects the potency of the steroid because it determines the rate at which the steroid is absorbed through the skin. Ointments are more potent than creams and creams are more potent than solutions.

Most skin preparations can be applied two times a day. This is convenient for working persons to apply at home in the morning and evening. The clinician should try to estimate and prescribe an appropriate amount. Many topical products are supplied in 15-, 30-, 45-, and 60-g sizes. To avoid adverse effects of steroid overuse, do not prescribe large quantities for small lesions, and specify the duration of use. On the other hand, prescribing only 15 g of steroid for a large area of involvement will be frustrating to the patient when the steroid runs out before the prescribed treatment duration is completed.

The duration of therapy should often be limited to the time it takes for resolution of symptoms or lesions.

To avoid adverse effects, the highest potency steroids should not be used for longer than 2 weeks duration. However, they can be used intermittently for recurring atopic dermatitis in a pulse-therapy mode (e.g., apply every weekend, with no application on weekdays).[14]

A study published in the British Medical Journal showed that a short burst of a potent topical steroid for 3 days per week was as effective and safe as prolonged use of a weak preparation (1% hydrocortisone) for mild or moderate atopic eczema.[15] Interestingly, the 1% hydrocortisone worked just as well and is a lot less expensive.

For dry lesions, liberal use of emollients between steroid applications can minimize steroid exposure while maximizing the benefits of therapy.

e. ***Parenteral steroids.*** For extensive disease, consider oral prednisone or an IM shot of triamcinolone (40 mg in 1 mL is an appropriate adult dosage that can be given in the deltoid muscle). Oral prednisone may be prescribed for severe intractable disease at a dose of 60 mg/day for 2 days, then reducing the dose by 10 mg everyday for the next 6 days.[3] Because systemic steroids work so well in atopic dermatitis and can cause major adverse effects if used chronically, it is important to impress upon patients that use of this treatment should be limited to the worst exacerbations of their disease. Otherwise patients with atopic dermatitis are prone to suffer all the long-term side effects of systemic steroids.

3. ***Antibiotics***
Topical and systemic antibiotics are used for atopic dermatitis that has become secondarily infected with bacteria. The most common infecting organism is *S. aureus*. Weeping lesions and crusting during an exacerbation should prompt consideration of antibiotic use.

a. ***Topical antibiotics.*** Mupirocin may be used to treat *S. aureus* infections in small affected areas or applied to the nares to treat nasal carriage of this organism. There are no data to support the use of other topical antibiotics such as bacitracin, Polysporin, or neomycin.

b. ***Oral antibiotics.*** Oral antibiotics more effectively treat superinfection of atopic dermatitis. Antibiotics that are effective against *S. aureus* are prescribed for courses of 5–10 days.

Typical adult dosing includes:

- Dicloxacillin, 250 mg qid or 500 mg bid
- Cephalexin, 250 mg qid or 500 mg bid
- Erythromycin, 250 mg qid or 500 mg bid

Cephalexin suspension is recommended for infants and small children (Fig. 3-32) because of its effectiveness and the suspension is palatable. Dicloxacillin suspension tastes awful, and children will resist the administration of this medicine. Erythromycin is a second-line antibiotic because approximately 20% of cases of *S. aureus* in the community are resistant to it. It is, therefore, reserved for patients who develop allergic reactions to penicillin or cephalosporin. Other alternatives in this situation include clindamycin, the newer macrolides, and the fluoroquinolones.

4. ***Antihistamines***
The role of antihistamines in atopic dermatitis is controversial. The most effective antihistamines in atopic dermatitis are those that are sedating. These include diphenhydramine (Benadryl) and hydroxyzine (Atarax). Diphenhydramine is available over-the-counter, and doses of 25–50 mg may be given three or four times daily or limited to bedtime. Liquid forms of diphenhydramine can be purchased over-the-counter and be given to infants and children. Hydrox-

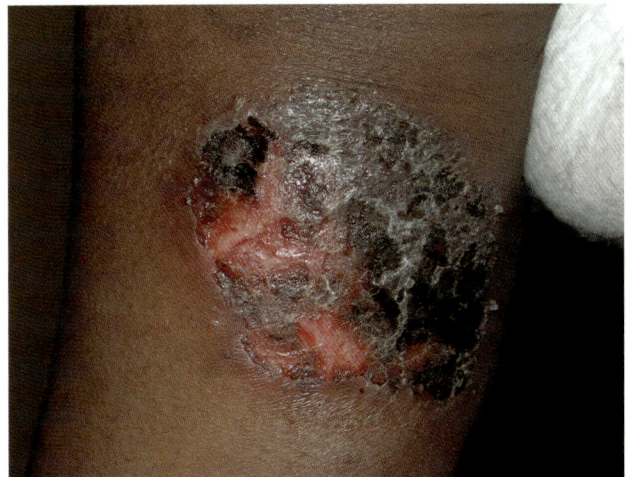

Figure 3-32 Superinfection of atopic dermatitis. The brown crusts represent the exudate of superinfected (impetiginized) atopic dermatitis. See Figure 3-8 for another example.

yzine requires a prescription and should be dosed based on age and weight. These antihistamines are best given at night to provide sedation and improve sleep with the hope that this will decrease itching and scratching. (See Appendix 10.)

There is very little evidence that the newer nonsedating antihistamines help treat atopic dermatitis. Although they may be taken during the day with minimal sedation, it is not clear how effective they are.

a. ***Topical antihistamines.*** Topical diphenhydramine should be avoided because it can be a potent sensitizer. Topical doxepin (Zonalon) cream may be beneficial for short-term management of moderate pruritus in adults with atopic dermatitis and lichen simplex chronicus. Doxepin blocks H_1 and H_2 receptors. It may be used up to 8 days and may be applied four times a day. The most common adverse reactions are drowsiness and burning and/or stinging upon application.

5. ***Tars***

Before the availability of topical corticosteroids, coal tars were used to reduce inflammation in atopic dermatitis. Tar preparations may still be used to minimize topical corticosteroid use during maintenance therapy of atopic dermatitis. While their anti-inflammatory properties are not as potent as corticosteroids, their effects are longer lasting. Newer coal tar products are better tolerated because there is less odor and staining of clothing. Tar preparations are best used at bedtime and washed off in the morning. These preparations should not be used on acutely inflamed skin. Possible adverse effects include folliculitis and photosensitivity.

6. ***New Approaches to Therapy***

a. ***Cyclosporine.*** Cyclosporine is a very effective medication for severe atopic dermatitis. Cyclosporine is a potent inhibitor of T-lymphocyte-dependent immune responses. It is used in doses from 2.5 to 5 mg/kg/day, and clearing of acute eczematous skin lesions may be observed after 4–6 weeks of therapy.[13] Patients being considered for cyclosporin therapy should be referred to a specialist familiar with the use of this medicine.

b. ***Tacrolimus.*** Tacrolimus (Protopic) ointment is the first in a class of topical immunomodulators shown to improve atopic dermatitis through topical treatment. It suppresses antigen-specific T-cell activation and inhibits inflammatory cytokine release.[16] It is the first major advance in the management of atopic dermatitis in 40 years.

1) Topical tacrolimus received FDA approval in 2000 and became available for clinical use in February 2001. It comes as an ointment in two strengths, 0.03% and 0.1%. It is indicated for the short-term or intermittent long-term treatment of moderate to severe atopic dermatitis when conventional therapies are inadvisable, ineffective, or not tolerated.

2) Tacrolimus is not recommended for children less than 2 years old. The 0.03% strength is recommended for children 2–15 years old. Either strength may be used for individuals 16 years of age and older. Tacrolimus should be applied to the affected areas twice daily. It should not be used on infected skin or wet skin. Tacrolimus should be continued for 1 week after resolution of the affected area.

3) In one study of tacrolimus there was marked or excellent improvement or clearance of disease in 54%, 81%, and 86% of patients at week 1, month 6, and month 12, respectively.[17] Hanifin combined the results of two separate studies in which a total of 632 adults with longstanding atopic dermatitis involving 10%–100% of body surface area were randomized in a double-blind fashion (allocation concealment uncertain) to receive either 0.03% tacrolimus ointment, 0.1% tacrolimus ointment, or placebo vehicle.[18] Treatment was applied twice daily to affected skin for up to 12 weeks. A 90% or greater improvement from baseline scores on various eczema evaluation tools was seen for 7%, 28%, and 37% of patients in the vehicle, 0.03% tacrolimus, and 0.1% tacrolimus groups, respectively ($P < 0.001$; number needed to treat [NNT] = 3 for the 0.1% tacrolimus group vs. placebo), and 50% or better improvement was observed for 20%, 62%, and 73% of patients, respectively (NNT = 2). More patients in the placebo groups discontinued use because of adverse events than either active treatment group.

4) Adverse reactions include skin burning, pruritus, headache, flu symptoms, rash, and folliculitis. Most adverse effects were brief and resolved during the first few days of treatment. "Local irritation, adverse events such as burning sensation (47% of patients), pru-

ritus (24% of patients), and erythema (12% of patients) were common but tended to occur only when initiating treatment. Laboratory values showed no marked changes over time. Systemic absorption was minimal, with the maximum tacrolimus blood concentration being less than 1 ng/mL in 76% of patients."[17] Unlike strong topical corticosteroids, tacrolimus ointment does not cause skin atrophy or depigmentation.[16]

    5) Tacrolimus appears to be effective and safe when used for treatment of chronic, severe atopic dermatitis. Unfortunately, no direct comparison studies to more commonly used and less expensive agents (topical steroids) have been reported. Also, there is no data on cost effectiveness, which would be helpful given that topical tacrolimus is at least 10 times as expensive as generic topical steroids.

  c. ***Pimecrolimus.*** Pimecrolimus is the second in a class of topical immunomodulators shown to improve atopic dermatitis through topical treatment. It also suppresses antigen-specific T-cell activation and inhibits inflammatory cytokine release. While Tacrolimus seems to be equivalent to potent topical steroids, Pimecrolimus, when compared with a commonly used potent topical steroid seems to be less effective.[19] Both topical tacrolimus and pimecrolimus are effective in treating atopic dermatitis compared with placebos or the inactive vehicle. They are probably safe, at least in the short term. These new treatments for atopic dermatitis are already being welcomed by patients, parents of patients, and physicians, as another treatment option for atopic dermatitis that does not thin the skin.

 7. ***Interferon and Phototherapy***
Interferon and phototherapy are not within the typical scope of practice for the primary care physician. The data on these therapies are not impressive given the high cost and risks involved.

X. Special Considerations in Patient Subsets

A. Infants

Infants present with atopic dermatitis that is very visible on the face (see Figs. 3-5, 3-7, and 3-8). They have thin skin and need to be treated with low-potency steroids. When they become superinfected they need to be treated with oral antibiotics. Oral cephalexin suspension is

effective, palatable, and relatively inexpensive. Testing for food allergies may be needed when the atopic dermatitis does not respond to first-line measures such as emollients and low-potency steroids.

B. African Americans

Atopic dermatitis may look different in individuals with darker skin. As seen in Figures 3-3*A*, 3-11*A*, and 3-11*B*, it is common to see a follicular hyperaccentuation rather than the erythema and scale that are so common in lighter-skinned individuals. The treatment and management are not different; the appearance of the condition is the most unusual aspect. The response to treatment may also be different in that there is a higher incidence of post-inflammatory hyperpigmentation in persons with darker skin (see Fig 3-3*B*).

XI. When to Obtain Consultation

The vast majority of cases of atopic dermatitis are within the scope of primary care practice. Referral to an allergist or dermatologist should be considered in the following situations:

A. When skin or patch testing are being considered. (See Chapters 12 and 20 for further discussion about these procedures.)

B. When the atopic dermatitis does not respond despite multiple attempts at treatment.

C. In cases of severe unresponsive atopic dermatitis.

D. Based on the practice guideline given in Section XII, consultation with a specialist is recommended for:

   1. Severe or persistent atopic dermatitis (i.e., 20% general skin involvement or 10% skin involvement affecting eyelids, hands, intertriginous areas, and not responsive to first-line therapy)
   2. Erythroderma or extensive exfoliation
   3. Patients requiring more than one course of systemic corticosteroids
   4. Hospital treatment of atopic dermatitis
   5. Identification of triggers and allergens
   6. Intensive education, including control of allergenic triggers, coexisting asthma, rhinitis-impaired quality of life (lost work days, lost school days, sleep disturbance, and poorly controlled pruritus)
   7. Infectious complications
   8. Ocular complications
   9. Psychosocial complications
  10. When the diagnosis of atopic dermatitis is in doubt.

XII. Practice Guidelines

Diagnosis and Management of Atopic Dermatitis: Parameter Documents of the Joint Task Force on Practice Parameters in Allergy, Asthma, and Immunology. (www.jcaai.org/Param/Eczema.htm.)

XIII. Internet Resources

www.jcaai.org/Param/Eczema.htm
Diagnosis and Management of Atopic Dermatitis: Parameter Documents of the Joint Task Force on Practice Parameters in Allergy, Asthma, and Immunology.

dermis.net
An extensive Dermatology Information System (DermIS) from two universities in Germany.

fm.mednet.ucla.edu/derm
An interactive dermatology atlas with over a thousand images that can be searched by many different parameters. This site includes interactive cases and a quiz mode. It was developed by Drs. Usatine and Madden at UCLA.

XIV. ICD-9 Codes

691   Atopic dermatitis and related conditions
691.8   Other atopic dermatitis and related conditions

XV. Patient Education Materials and Handouts

familydoctor.org/handouts/176.html
Patient information from the American Academy of Family Physicians.

www.skincarephysicians.com/eczemanet/
EczemaNet from the American Academy of Dermatology.

www.eczema.org
The British National Eczema Society.

Refer to patient education CD, which is provided with this text, for additional patient education information. It has been formatted to provide readily accessible, easy-to-understand handouts for adult patients and the parents of pediatric patients. These handouts can be easily modified to fit specific practice requirements.

REFERENCES

1. Hoare C, Li Wan Po A, Williams H: Systematic review of treatments for atopic eczema. Health Technol Assess 2000;4(37):1–191.
2. Fitzpatrick BF, Johnson RA, Wolff K, Suurmond D: Color Atlas and Synopses of Clinical Dermatology, 4th ed. New York: McGraw-Hill, 2001.
3. Beltrani VS: Atopic dermatitis. In Altman LC, Becker JW, Williams PV (eds): Allergy in Primary Care. Philadelphia: WB Saunders, 2000.
4. Habif T: Clinical Dermatology: A Color Guide to Diagnosis and Therapy, 3rd ed. St. Louis: Mosby, 1996.
5. Kay J, Gawkrodger DJ, Mortimer MJ, Jaron AG: The prevalence of childhood atopic eczema in a general population. J Am Acad Dermatol 1994;30:35–39.
6. Correale CE, Walker C, Murphy L, Craig TJ: Atopic dermatitis: A review of diagnosis and treatment. Am Fam Phys 1999;60:1191.
7. Usatine R: Skin problems. In Sloane P, Slatt L, Ebell M (eds): The Essentials of Family Medicine, 3rd ed. New York: Williams and Wilkins, 1998.
8. Disease management of atopic dermatitis: A practice parameter. Joint Task Force on Practice Parameters in Allergy, Asthma, and Immunology website. Available at: www.jcaai.org/Param/Eczema.htm.
9. Williams HC, Burney PG, Pembroke, AC, Hay RJ: Validation of the U.K. diagnostic criteria for atopic dermatitis in a population setting. U.K. diagnostic criteria for Atopic Dermatitis Working Party. Br J Dermatol 1996;135(1):12–17.
10. Charman C: Atopic eczema. Clin Evidence 2000;4: 944–956.
11. Sicherer SH, Morrow EH, Sampson HA: Dose-response in double-blind, placebo-controlled oral food challenges in children with atopic dermatitis. J Allergy Clin Immunol 2000;105:582–586.
12. Sloper KS, Wadsworth J, Brostoff J: Children with atopic eczema: I. Clinical response to food elimination and subsequent double-blind food challenge. Q J Med 1991;80: 677–693.
13. Werfel T, Kapp A: Atopic dermatitis and allergic contact dermatitis. In Holgate ST, Church MK, Lichtenstein LM (eds): Allergy, 2nd ed. London: Mosby, 2001.
14. Van Der Meer JB, Glazenburg EJ, Mulder PG, Eggink HF, Coenraads PJ: The management of moderate to severe atopic dermatitis in adults with topical fluticasone propionate. The Netherlands Adult Atopic Dermatitis Study Group. Br J Dermatol 1999;140:1114–1121.
15. Thomas KS, Armstrong S, Avery A, et al: Randomised controlled trial of short bursts of a potent topical corticosteroid versus prolonged use of a mild preparation for children with mild or moderate atopic eczema. BMJ 2002;324:768.
16. Bekersky I, Fitzsimmons W, Tanase A, Maher RM, Hodosh E, Lawrence I: Nonclinical and early clinical development of tacrolimus ointment for the treatment of atopic dermatitis. J Am Acad Dermatol 2001;44(1 Pt 2):S17–S27.

17. Reitamo S, Wollenberg A, Schopf E, et al: Safety and efficacy of 1 year of tacrolimus ointment monotherapy in adults with atopic dermatitis. The European Tacrolimus Ointment Study Group. Arch Dermatol 2000;136:999–1006.

18. Hanifin JM, Ling MR, Langley R, Breneman D, Rafal E: Tacrolimus ointment for the treatment of atopic dermatitis in adult patients: Part I. Efficacy. J Am Acad Dermatol 2001;44:S28–S38.

19. Luger T, Van Leent EJ, Graeber M, et al: SDZ ASM 981: An emerging safe and effective treatment for atopic dermatitis. Br J Dermatol 2001;144:788–794.

OTHER SUGGESTED READING

Williams H: New treatments for atopic dermatitis. BMJ 2002;324:1533–1534. (Article and responses available at www.bmj.com.)

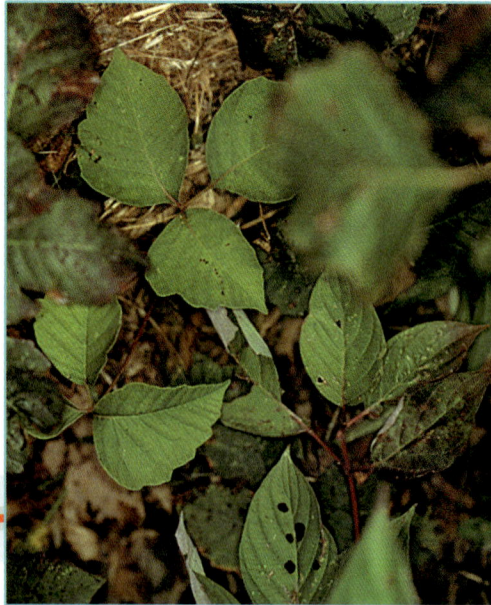

CHAPTER 4
Contact Dermatitis

Brian Halstater and Richard P. Usatine

I. Introduction

Contact dermatitis is a common inflammatory skin condition characterized by erythematous and pruritic skin lesions resulting from the contact of skin with a foreign substance. The term contact dermatitis is actually a descriptive term for two diagnostic categories, allergic contact dermatitis and irritant contact dermatitis. Irritant contact dermatitis is more common than allergic contact dermatitis.

II. Epidemiology

A. Prevalence in Young Children

In children younger than 11 years old, allergic dermatitis is the most commonly diagnosed skin disorder. The incidence has been rising, increasing from 3% in the 1960s to 10% in the 1990s.[1]

B. Overall Prevalence

Contact dermatitis or exzematous disease was diagnosed in more than 7.1 million office-based physician visits and 430,000 hospital-based outpatient physician visits in 1996 in the United States.[2]

III. Etiology

A. Irritant Contact Dermatitis

Irritant contact dermatitis is caused by the non-immune-modulated irritation of the skin by a substance, resulting in a skin rash. Irritant and allergic contact dermatitis most frequently affect the hands (Fig. 4-1). For example, "dishpan hands" are an example of irritant contact dermatitis caused by repeated exposure to soap and water. Whether a substance will evoke a dermatitic reaction of the skin in a specific person depends on several factors:

1. The pH and concentration of the irritant: stronger acids or bases are more irritating than mild soaps and solvents.
2. The duration of contact with the skin: the longer the duration, the more likely the skin is to have a reaction.
3. Physical conditions: several exposures to the same irritant increase the likelihood of a reaction; arid, hot, or cold environments make irritation more likely.
4. The physical integrity of the skin: skin damaged by dehydration or previous injury is more susceptible.

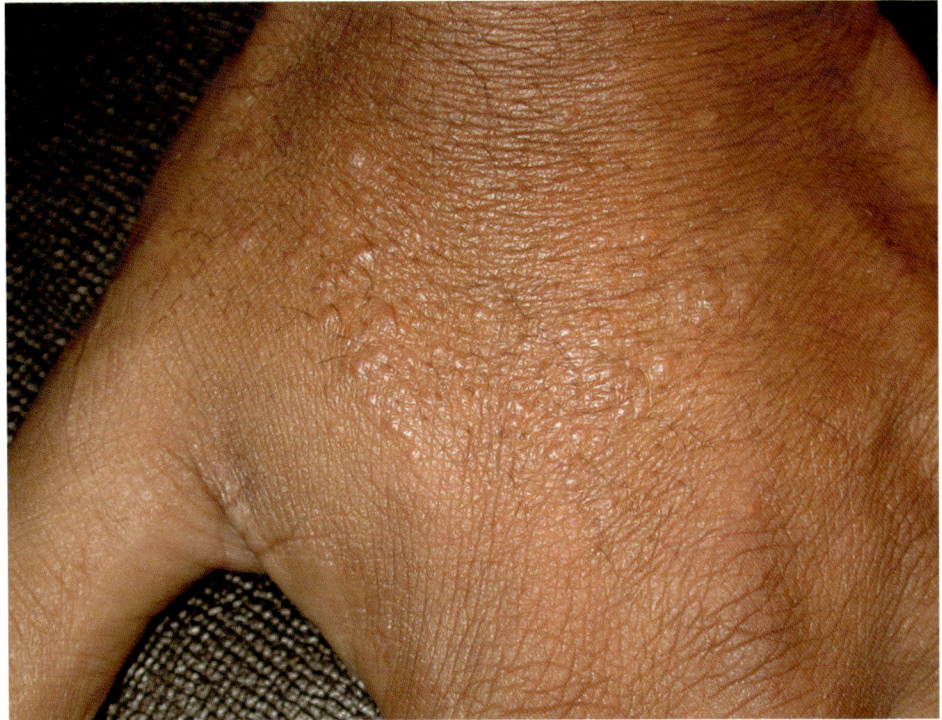

Figure 4-1. This case of hand dermatitis could be irritant contact dermatitis or allergic contact dermatitis.

5. Genetic factors: people with atopic dermatitis are more likely to manifest an irritant contact dermatitis reaction.

Examples of common irritants include strong acids (industrial workers, chemical workers), strong alkalis (industrial workers, chemical workers), solvents (mechanics, industrial workers), soaps (dishwashers, health care professionals, housekeepers), urine (diaper area in infants; Fig. 4-2), stool or urine (ostomy sites), and saliva (lip licking; Fig. 4-3).

B. Allergic Contact Dermatitis

The mechanism of allergic contact dermatitis is a delayed-type hypersensitivity reaction. A foreign substance comes into contact with the skin and is linked to skin protein, forming an antigen complex that is recognized by the immune system. In the skin, the major antigen-presenting cell is the Langerhans cell. The antigen complex is processed by Langerhans cells in the epidermis and is then presented to T-cells, leading to the proliferation of antigen-specific T-cells. This occurs in both the integumentary and the lymphatic systems. This initial process results in sensitization of the individual to the antigen such as the oleoresin in the poison ivy and poison oak plants (Fig. 4-4).

Upon reexposure of the epidermis to the antigen, which may be a single second contact or after multiple repeated exposures, the sensitized T-cells initiate an inflammatory cascade, leading to the skin changes seen in allergic contact dermatitis. The reaction generally occurs within 12–48 hours in a previously sensitized person.

Cross-sensitization may occur in this type of dermatitis as a result of hapten cross-sensitization. A hapten is an antigen that can only trigger an antibody response when combined with a protein. If two haptens are of such similar molecular structure that the immune system is not able to distinguish between them, a person sensitized to one specific antigen may have an allergic contact dermatitis

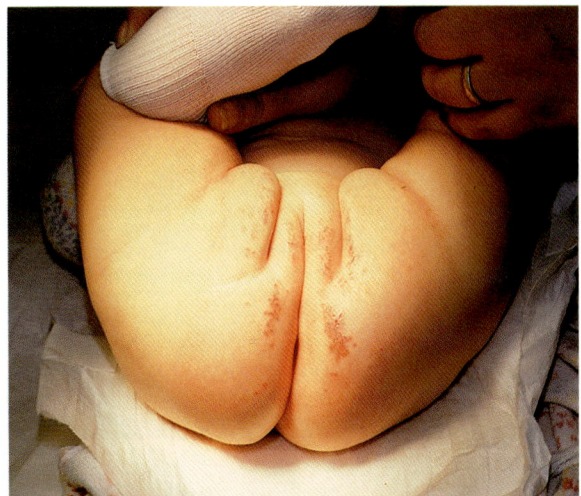

Figure 4-2. Diaper dermatitis caused by urine irritation.

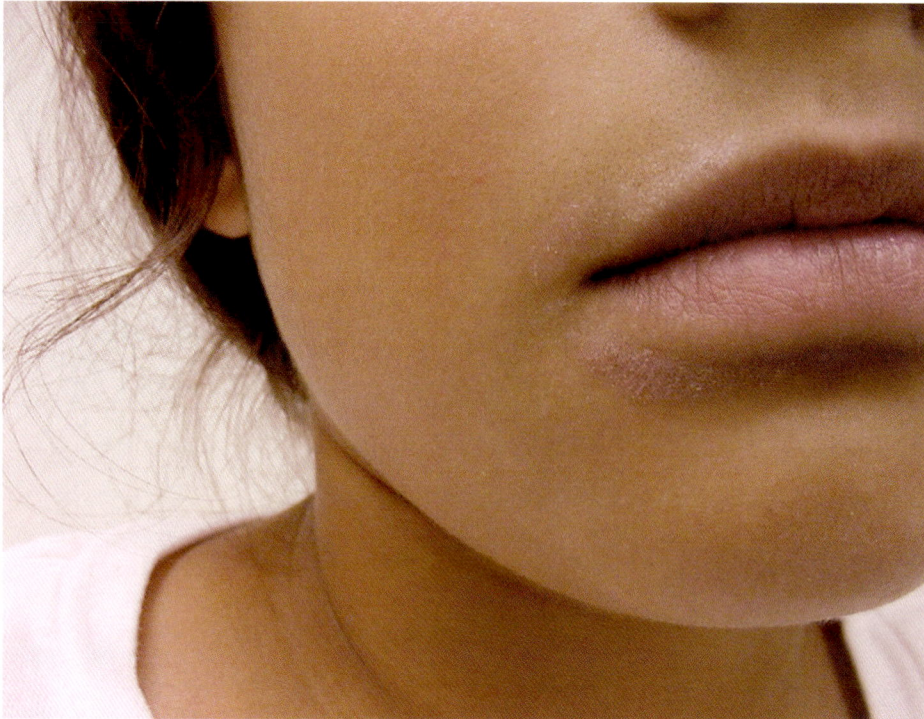

Figure 4-3. Irritation around the mouth caused by lip licking and saliva irritation of the skin.

reaction when first exposed to the similar compound. An example is cashew nuts, which are similar antigenically to the allergic component of poison ivy. A diffuse allergic skin exanthem may result when a person sensitized to poison ivy first ingests cashew nuts.

Often it is difficult to distinguish between irritant contact dermatitis and allergic contact dermatitis. Table 4-1 lists common irritants and allergens that cause contact dermatitis. Table 4-2 is helpful in distinguishing between the two types of contact dermatitis.

IV. Clinical Manifestations

A. Irritant Contact Dermatitis

Irritant contact dermatitis may manifest in a variety of ways. The vast majority of cases of irritant contact dermatitis involve the hands, thus leading to the term "hand dermatitis." Most cases of irritant contact dermatitis exhibit the following characteristics:

1. Location usually on the hands
2. Dryness

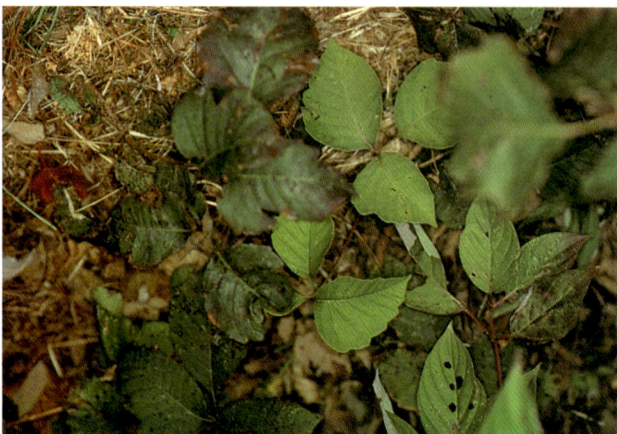

A

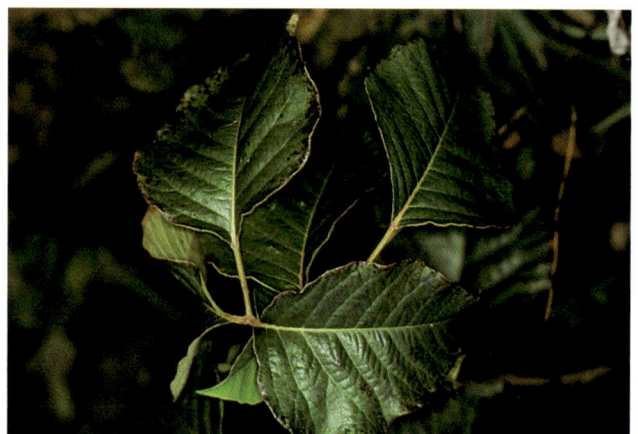

B

Figure 4-4. Poison ivy (**A**) and poison oak (**B**) are members of the same plant family and have leaves in groups of three. (Courtesy of Tom Zuber, MD.)

TABLE 4-1

Causes of Irritant and Allergic Contact Dermatitis

Common Irritants	Common Allergens
Soaps	Poison ivy
Urine	Poison oak (and poison sumac)
Stool	Neomycin
Saliva	Skin tapes
Strong acids	Nickel and other metals in jewelry
Strong bases	Hair dye, cosmetics
Solvents	Fragrances

3. Fissured skin
4. Erythema
5. Indistinct borders
6. Burning
7. Pruritus
8. Pain

B. Allergic Contact Dermatitis

Allergic contact dermatitis usually has a type of distribution on the body that suggests direct contact of the skin with an allergen. Most cases of allergic contact dermatitis exhibit the following characteristics:

1. Location usually on exposed area of skin, often the hands
2. Pruritus as the dominant symptom
3. Vesicles (Fig. 4-5)

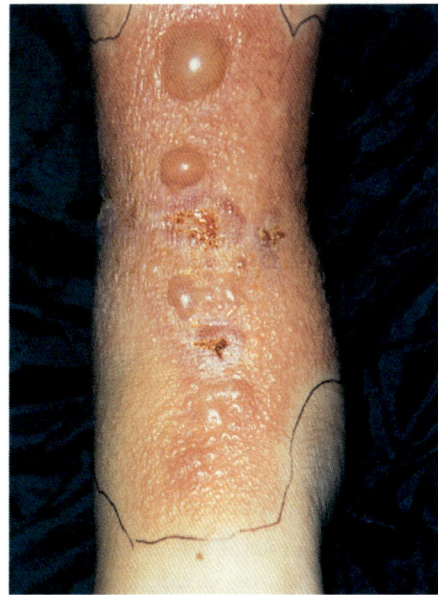

Figure 4-5. Allergic contact dermatitis of the ankle. Note fluid-filled vesicles (<5 mm) and bullae (≥5 mm).

4. Bullae
5. Erythema
6. Edema
7. Distinct angles, lines, and borders

C. Superinfection

Both irritant and contact dermatitis may be complicated by bacterial superinfection.

TABLE 4-2

Contact Dermatitis: Irritant versus Allergic

	Irritant	Allergic
People at risk	Everyone	Genetically predisposed
Mechanism of response	Nonimmunologic; a physical and chemical alteration of epidermis	Delayed hypersensitivity reaction
Nature of substance	Organic solvent, soaps	Low-molecular-weight hapten (e.g., metals, formalin, epoxy)
Concentration of substance required	Usually high	May be very low
Mode of onset	Usually gradual as epidermal barrier becomes compromised	Once sensitized, usually rapid; 12–24 h after exposure
Distribution	Borders usually indistinct	May correspond exactly to an item in contact with the skin (e.g., watchband, elastic waistband)
Investigative procedure	Trial of avoidance	Trial of avoidance, patch testing, or both
Management	Protection and reduced incidence of exposure	Complete avoidance

From Habif T: Clinical Dermatology: A Color Guide to Diagnosis and Therapy, 3rd ed. St. Louis: Mosby, 1996. Reprinted with permission.

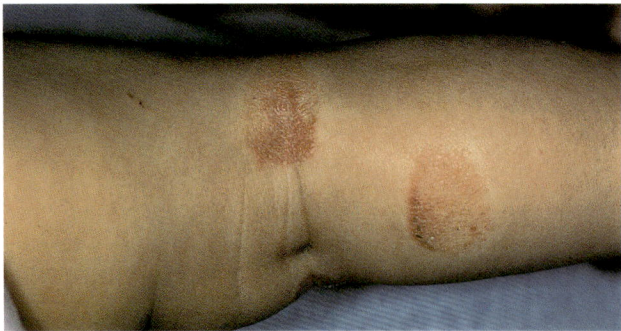

Figure 4-6. Nummular eczema with coin-shaped lesions.

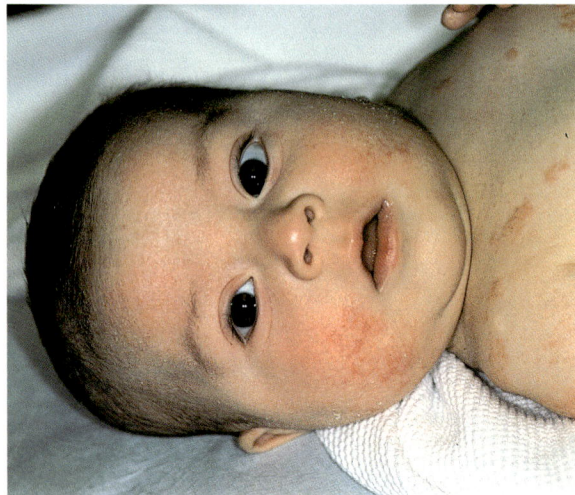

Figure 4-8. This child has atopic dermatitis on the face.

D. Morphologic Characteristics

The morphologic characteristics of allergic and irritant contact dermatitis can be divided into primary and secondary lesions (see Table 4-2; see also Appendix 5, Table A5-1).

V. Differential Diagnosis

A. Other Diagnoses

While it is often difficult to distinguish allergic and irritant contact dermatitis, other diagnoses to consider are as follows.

1. ***Nummular Eczema*** (Fig. 4-6)
   Lesions tend to be coin-shaped and are not necessarily related to contact with any exposure.
2. ***Drug Reaction*** (Fig. 4-7)
   Typically there is an antecedent drug ingestion, with resolution of the rash after the drug is discontinued.

3. ***Atopic Dermatitis*** (Fig. 4-8)
   This disease is more commonly found in children and is characterized more by pruritus, with secondary lichenification.
4. ***Neurodermatitis***
   Lesions tend to be associated with a significant degree of excoriation in areas the patient can reach. Lesions resolve when the itch-scratch cycle is broken.
5. ***Xerosis*** (Fig. 4-9)
   Dry skin that improves with emollients. While it can occur as a sole entity, xerosis can be a prominent feature of atopic dermatitis.
6. ***Dishydrotic Eczema*** (Fig. 4-10)
   Red, itchy, flaky skin that itches and is associated with small vesicles; not related to contact.

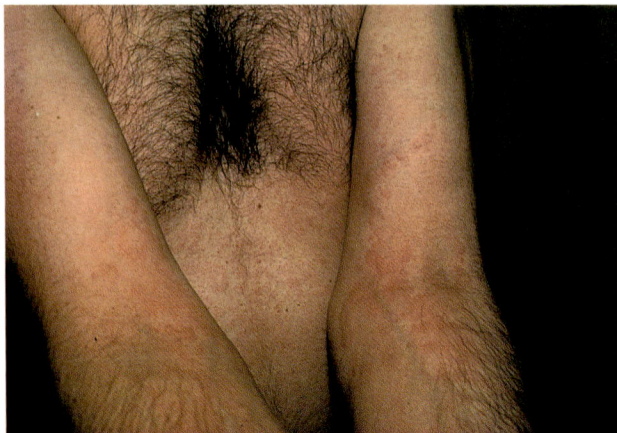

Figure 4-7. Acute urticaria on the extremities and trunk secondary to sulfa allergy.

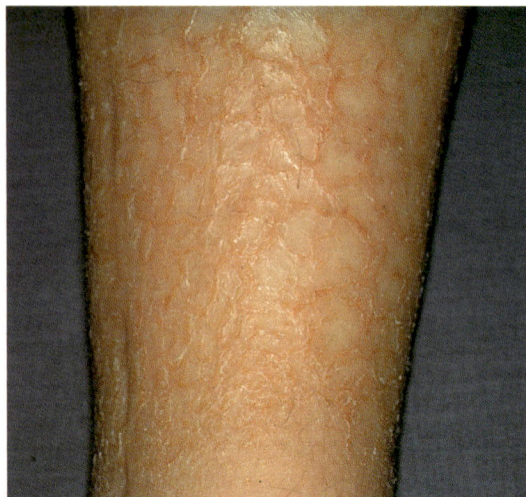

Figure 4-9. This xerosis now looks like fish scales and can be called icthyosis. (Courtesy of Tom Zuber, MD.)

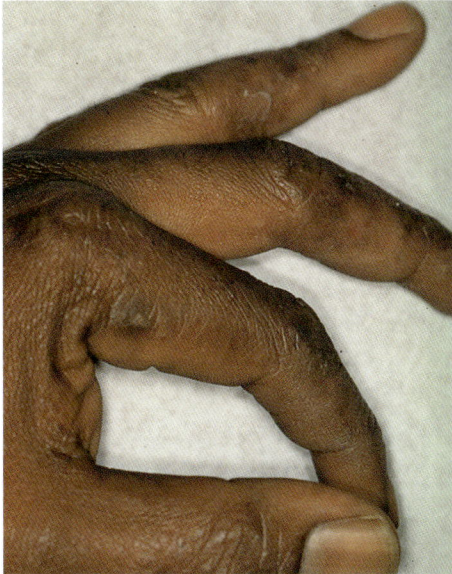

Figure 4-10. Dishydrotic eczema, like contact dermatosis, is found most often on the hands, but tends to be greatest between the fingers. (Courtesy of Tom Zuber, MD.)

7. ***Psoriasis*** (Fig. 4-11)
   Thick-scaled lesions, typically located over the elbows, knees, and sites of trauma.
8. ***Immediate IgE Contact Reaction*** (e.g., latex glove allergy)
   Immediate erythema, itching, and possibly systemic reaction after contact with a known or suspected allergen.

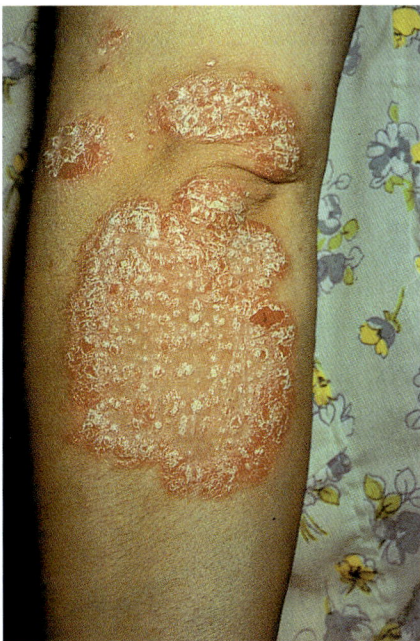

Figure 4-11. This plaque of psoriasis on the elbow demonstrates the thick scaled lesions.

9. ***Fungal Infection*** (Fig. 4-12)
   Positive KOH preparation. Typically will not improve or worsen with the use of corticosteroids.
10. ***Urticaria*** (see Fig. 4-7)
    Red, itchy hives that may be associated with drug or allergen exposure. May be associated with dermatographism.

VI. History and Physical Examination

In addition to the area in which the patient has noted the skin changes or skin symptoms, it may be necessary to examine the hands and feet to get clues to the diagnosis. The physician should note any macules, papules, vesicles, scaling, erythema, and any other skin change. Box 4-1 provides a sample patient history form.

VII. Laboratory Evaluation

Typically the diagnosis of contact dermatitis is made clinically, based on the patient's history and physical examination results. The following tests may also be considered:

A. KOH Preparation

A KOH preparation is used to investigate for fungal infection. This test has a low sensitivity, so a negative test result does not rule out fungal infection.

B. Latex Allergy Testing

Latex allergy testing is performed when the history suggests that the latex allergen is the specific antigen. This type of reaction is neither irritant (nonimmunologic) nor allergic contact dermatitis. The latex allergy type of reaction is a type I or IgE-mediated response to the latex allergen. It can be diagnosed by one of three methods.

1. The first is by the clinical presentation of an allergic-type reaction after latex exposure.

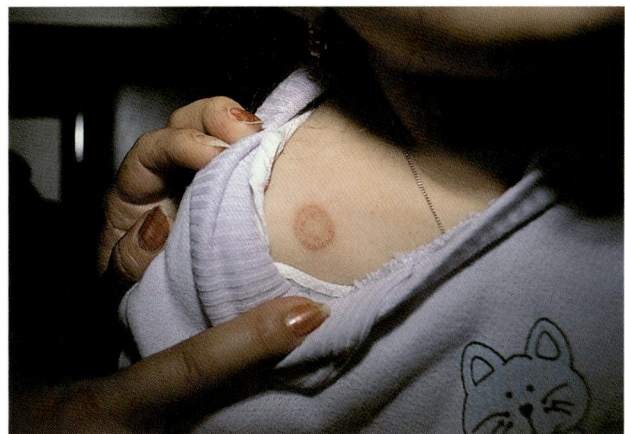

Figure 4-12. Fungal infections often have a ringlike structure with a central clearing.

BOX 4-1

Patient History

Patient's Age: _____   **Sex: M ❏ F ❏**   **Children:** _____   **Ages:** _____   **Patient's Name: ❏**

Current Dermatologic Complaint
Date of onset or approximate duration: _____
Areas(s) affected at onset: _____
Area(s) affected now: _____
Type and pattern of eruption: _____

Severity:	Mild ❏	Moderate ❏	Severe ❏	
Present state:	Stable ❏	Increasing ❏	Decreasing ❏	
Frequency:	No pattern ❏	Seasonal ❏	Weekly ❏	Monthly ❏ Annual ❏
Timing:	Worse during week ❏	After weekend ❏		

Other Known Conditions (Past and Present)
Allergic disease:	Infantile eczema ❏	Asthma ❏	Hay fever ❏	Urticaria ❏
Food allergy:	Suspected ❏	Proven ❏	Type _____	
Known allergies:	Nickel ❏	Flowers ❏	Perfume ❏	Other (name) ❏
Suspected allergies:	Medications ❏	Cosmetics ❏	Other (name) ❏	
Previous drug reactions:	Never ❏	Yes (drug/date) _____		

Family History
Allergic disease: Relationship (name) _____
　　　　　　　　　　　Disease (name) _____
Other relevant disease: Relationship (name) _____
　　　　　　　　　　　Disease (name) _____

Current Medications
Prescription: Name _____   Type _____   Period(s) of use _____
OTC: Name _____   Type _____   Period(s) of use _____
Alternative: Name _____   Type _____   Period(s) of use _____

Occupation(s)
Type _____
Duration _____
Environment _____
Materials involved _____
Other workers with similar complaint _____

Residence
Type _____
Location _____
Duration _____
Environment _____

Sports/Hobbies/Housework
Type _____
Duration _____
Frequency _____
Environment _____
Materials used _____

Pets
Type/number: Dogs _____   Cats _____
　　　　　　　　Horses _____   Birds _____
　　　　　　　　Other (name) _____
Contact: Daily ❏   Regular ❏   Occasional ❏   Rare ❏
Health: Treatment (if any) _____

Cosmetics/Toiletries
Type:	Hair dye ❏	Nail cosmetics ❏	Makeup ❏	Fragrance ❏
Frequency:	Never ❏	Daily ❏	Occasionally ❏	Rarely ❏

Jewelry
Earrings ❏   Rings ❏   Bracelets ❏

Vacations
Exacerbations ❏   No change ❏   Remissions ❏

Unusual Events or Changes in Lifestyle
No ❏   Yes (specify) _____

Courtesy of Allerderm Laboratories, Inc. www.truetest.com/physician-clin.htm. 2001–2003.

2. The second is via epicutaneous skin prick testing, whose sensitivity is close to 100%. The major drawback to epicutaneous skin prick testing is anaphylaxis. Chapter 12 covers this topic in greater detail.

3. The third is via RAST testing, an in vitro technique whose sensitivity and specificity for diagnostic purposes are between 80% and 90%. Chapter 13 covers this topic in greater detail.

C. Patch Testing

Patch testing (Fig. 4-13) entails placing a known concentration of common antigens on the skin of a patient. The antigen is left in place for a period of time, usually 48 hours, at which time the skin where the antigens were placed is examined for a dermatitis reaction. These same sites are examined another time, at least 24 hours after the removal of the patch tests. This allows for two common situations:

1. The first is that the dermatitis is caused by an irritant, and the reaction should subside with the removal of the offending antigen.

2. The second is that some antigens that cause allergic contact dermatitis do not cause a reaction until after 48 hours, so if the second examination is not performed, a positive patch test can be missed.

   Patch testing is a skill that can be learned with experience. However, the physicians skilled in this technique are allergists and dermatologists. Unless you have the skills, the patient should be referred to a physician who is experienced in both the performance and interpretation of the test. See Chapter 20 for greater detail on this topic.

D. Punch Biopsy

A punch biopsy may be performed when another underlying disorder (e.g., psoriasis) is suspected but the diagnosis is unclear. It is rarely performed in the diagnosis of contact dermatitis.

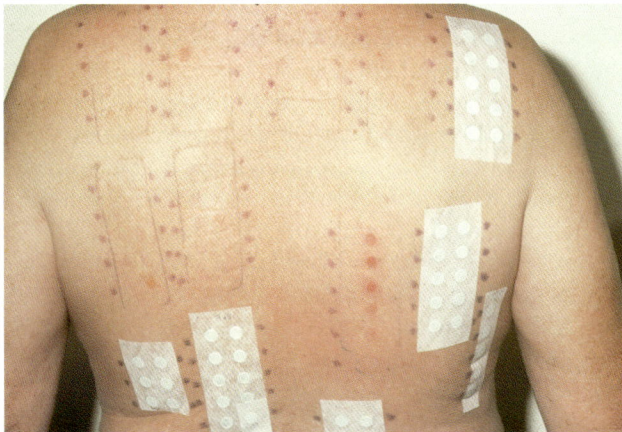

Figure 4-13. Patch testing on the back. (From Holgate ST, Church MK, Lichtenstein LM: Allergy, 2nd ed. St. Louis: Mosby, 2001. Reproduced with permission.)

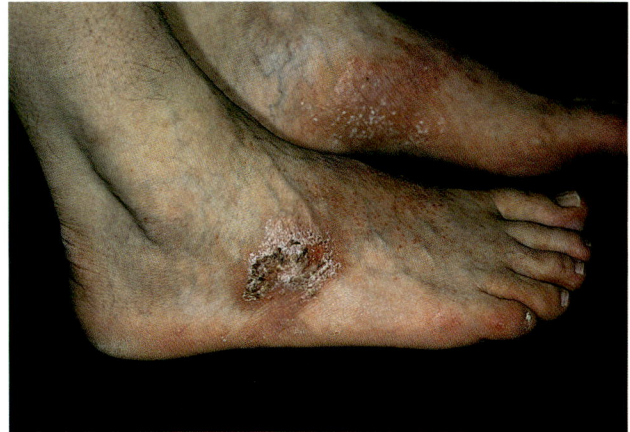

Figure 4-14. Contact dermatitis on the dorsum of the feet.

VIII. Approach to the Final Diagnosis

A. The patient history and clinical presentation help the clinician make the diagnosis of *irritant contact dermatitis*. A history form is provided for your benefit to use with your patients (see Box 4-1). Pertinent points from the history include:

- Use of new soap, shampoo, or cosmetic product.
- History of atopy.
- Worse with frequent hand washings.
- Burning and pain tend to be greater than itching.

1. Chronic use of the same chemicals does not rule out this disease, for two reasons:
   a. Formulations may change.
   b. Small exposures can lead to irritation over time, especially if the skin is chapped or the protective layer of oils is disrupted.

2. The physical examination in *irritant contact dermatitis* tends to show the following:

- Erythematous, ill-defined lesions that may be macular, papular, or vesicular.
- Lesions usually located on the dorsum of the hands or feet, more often than the palm or the sole (Fig. 4-14).
- Dry, cracked skin.
- Patch testing will be negative with this condition at the 48-hour reading. It is important that this 48- and 72-hour examination be performed because there may be an initial irritant reaction (see explanation under Laboratory Evaluation and Chapter 20).

B. Likewise, the diagnosis of *allergic contact dermatitis* is made largely based on the history and physical examination findings. Pertinent information in the history includes the following:

- Contact with known allergens (e.g., nickel, poison ivy, poison oak). Nickel exposure is often related to the wearing of rings or jewelry. Poison ivy and poison

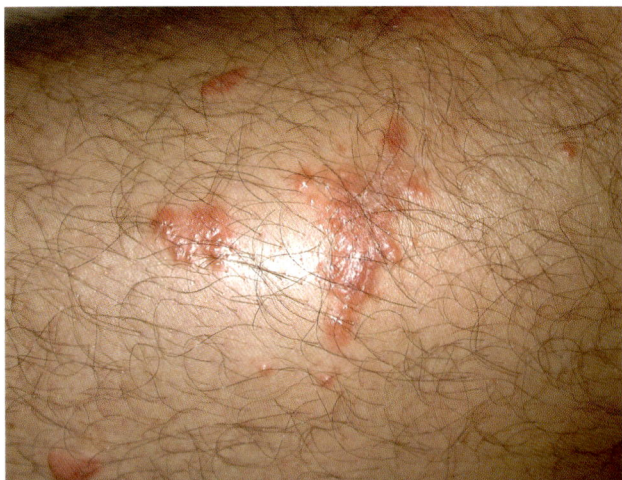

Figure 4-15. A localized case of poison oak in which the lesions are linear.

oak are members of the same plant family and have leaves in groups of three (see Fig. 4-4).
• Lesions spread.
• Itching is usually greater than pain.
• Vesicles are often present.
• If allergen is in the workplace, the condition may improve on weekends.
• The dermatitis usually occurs on the hands, but it may occur on any exposed skin.

The physical examination for *allergic contact dermatitis* may include:

• Vesicles (<5 mm) and bullae (≥5 mm).
• Well-demarcated lesions.
• Lesions that may appear linear (Fig. 4-15).
• Swelling of the skin.
• Positive results on patch testing (see Chapter 20).

IX. Therapy and Management

A. The therapy and management of both types of contact dermatitis are similar. Moderate to severe cases of irritant contact dermatitis should be treated the same as allergic contact dermatitis. Mild cases of irritant contact dermatitis may be treated as follows:

1. *Avoid* the irritant.
2. Use emollients to protect the skin. While in theory this is a very simple and effective intervention, when studied, most people when applying a topical emollient had inadequate coverage to provide a sufficient barrier protection.[2]
3. Wear vinyl gloves when working with potentially irritating substances such as soaps and detergents, and consider using cotton liners under the vinyl gloves both for comfort and to absorb sweat.
4. If possible, wash dishes and clothing in machines, not by hand.
5. Keep hands clean, dry, and well moisturized.
6. Protect the skin from cold or harsh weather.
7. Use mild, unscented soaps.
8. Cool compresses are useful in acute cases of contact dermatitis.

B. For the management of moderate to severe irritant contact dermatitis and allergic contact dermatitis, the treatment is as follows:

1. Follow the preceding principles for the treatment of mild irritant contact dermatitis.
2. Use the appropriate strength topical corticosteroid preparation based on the severity of the dermatitis, the location and thickness of the skin, and the age of the patient. Stronger topical steroids will be needed for acute allergic contact dermatitis on the hands. (A list of topical steroids organized by strength is found in Appendix 5, Table A5-2.)
3. Steroid ointments are more potent than creams and lotions because they penetrate more deeply into the skin. (See Appendix 5, Table A5-3, for descriptions of the differences between ointments, creams, and lotions.)
4. Oral steroids may be appropriate when large areas of skin are involved, mucous membranes are involved, the lesions are progressing, or there is severe local dermatitis.
5. Oral steroids should be prescribed over at least 10 days to prevent rebound dermatitis.
6. For patients who cannot tolerate oral steroids there is some evidence that cyclosporin A may be used as an alternative.[3]
   a. However, cyclosporin A has a significant side effect profile, which includes nephrotoxicity, hypertension, liver toxicity, and systemic immune suppression.
   b. Cyclosporin A has been found efficacious in contact dermatitis when taken by the oral route. The topical application of cyclosporin A has not been found efficacious.[4]
7. Bacterial superinfection should be treated with an appropriate antibiotic that will cover *Streptococcus pyogenes* and *Staphylococcus aureus*. (Cephalexin and dicloxacillin are first-line agents. Erythromycin, azithromycin, or clarithromycin may be used for patients with severe allergic reactions to penicillins or cephalosporins.) Small areas of mild superinfection can be treated with topical mupirocin (Bactroban).
8. Oral H$_1$-blocking antihistamines (diphenhydramine, hydroxyzine) provide both relief from itching and help with sleep. These sedating antihistamines are more effective than the nonsedating antihistamines

but may not be tolerated by patients during the day.

9. Oral H$_2$-blocking antihistamines (ranitidine, cimetidine) may also be added for patients who obtain inadequate relief with the oral H$_1$-blocking antihistamines.

X. Special Cases and Considerations

A. Poison Oak (*Rhus* Allergy)

1. Poison ivy and poison oak are two of the most common contact allergies seen in the United States. In fact, these types of plant dermatitis are more common than all other contact allergies combined. Poison ivy tends to occur on the East Coast, while poison oak tends to be found more on the West Coast. Both plants are members of the genus *Rhus* and both produce an oleoresin that is very allergenic. Once the oleoresin binds to the skin, it is difficult to wash off. Washing the skin within 10 minutes of exposure is most effective. Any soap can be used. The purpose of washing is to remove the oleoresin before it adheres to the skin. Although there are special soaps marketed for this purpose, it is not clear that they work better than any other soap on the market.

2. Plant dermatitis can be relatively mild, as seen in Figure 4-16*A*. It tends to occur with linear features because the plant brushes across the skin or a person rubs the oleoresin in linear fashion. It can become superinfected, as shown in Figure 4-16*B*. Some of the worst cases of poison ivy or oak involve the face or genitals. Most cases of mild plant dermatitis can be treated with topical calamine lotion, Aveeno baths, or oral antihistamines to help control the annoying

pruritus. Unfortunately, topical steroids do not adequately penetrate the lesions to decrease inflammation in plant dermatitis. High-potency topical steroids can control some of the pruritus if other topical measures do not work. Cold wet compresses can be helpful in the acute blistering stage.

3. Systemic steroids provide the most effective relief of symptoms and most rapid resolution of lesions in plant dermatitis. However, oral steroids have known risks and should be reserved for the most severe cases, such as patients with refractory dermatitis or dermatitis associated with extensive involvement or pronounced edema. A common error among physicians is to prescribe too short a course of oral steroids to patients with plant dermatitis. While a short burst of oral steroids may be helpful for asthma or urticaria, there is a significant risk of rebound lesions if the oral steroids are not given for at least 10 days in poison ivy or oak. One typical dosage is prednisone, 20 mg twice a day for 10 days. Some physicians prescribe a tapering dose of steroids over 2 weeks. Commercially available steroid dose packs do not provide an adequate amount of steroids and should be avoided. Another typical regimen consists of prednisone administered daily orally (1 mg/kg initially) and tapered slowly over 2–3 weeks.

B. Tape Dermatitis

Many people react with erythema and itching to skin tape. It is not unusual for patients to have this reaction to tape after surgery. Sometimes the tape is purely an irritant and the reaction is mild. The patient shown in Figure 4-17 had a severe reaction to the tape that was used to hold on her postoperative dressing after an abdominal hysterectomy. By the time she removed the tape, her

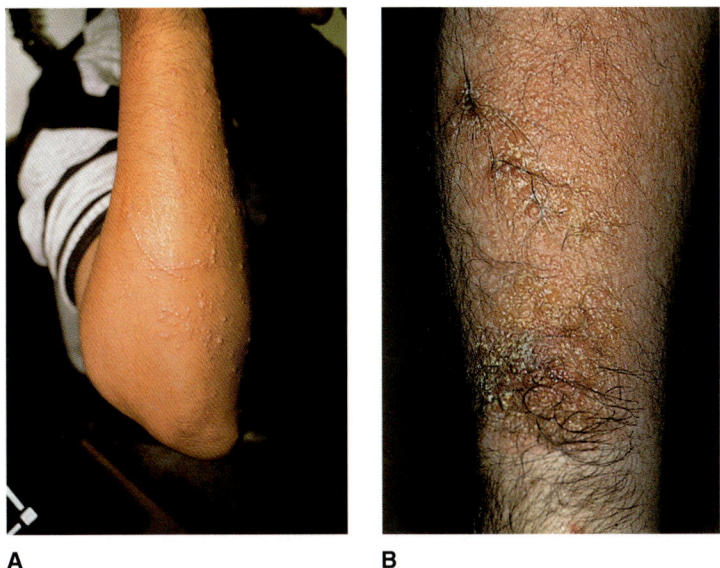

Figure 4-16. Poison oak (*Rhus* allergy) with linear lesions on the arm (**A**) and with superinfection and honey crusts on the legs (**B**).

A   **B**

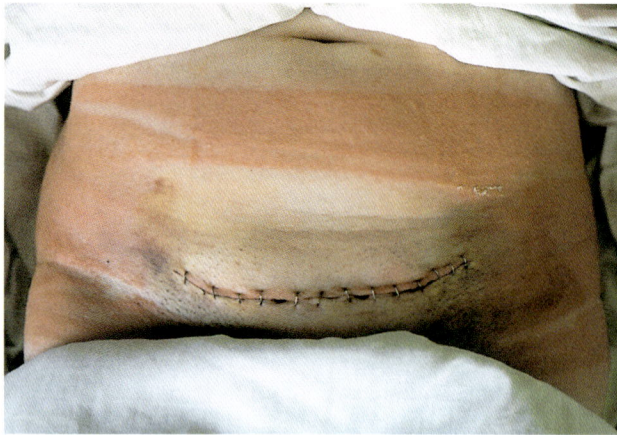

A

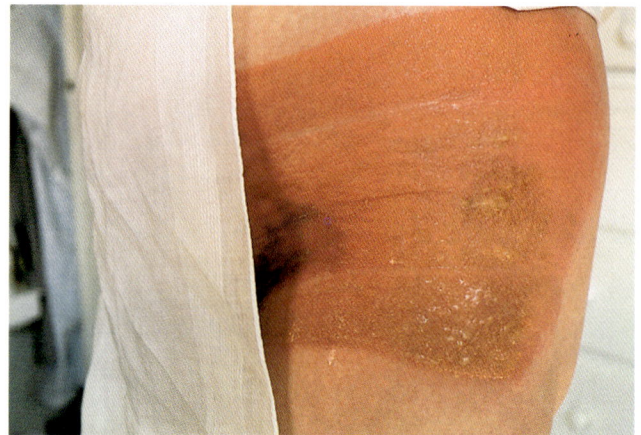

B

Figure 4-17. Tape dermatitis (allergic contact dermatitis) in a woman after an abdominal hysterectomy. **A**, The erythema is initially limited to the areas of the skin covered by tape. Note the absence of erythema under the area previously covered by gauze. **B**, Side view showing the acute vesicles.

skin had become bright red and developed vesicles. The most important part of the treatment involves removing the offending agent. Topical or systemic steroids may be used, depending on the severity of the reaction and the patient's preference.

C. Neomycin Contact Dermatitis

Neomycin is the one topical antibiotic to which people commonly demonstrate a contact allergy. The patient shown in Figure 4-18 had a mild episode of herpes zoster on the back and chose to treat it with a triple antibiotic preparation that included neomycin. She presented for urgent care, wondering why her rash was getting worse rather than better. A careful history disclosed that the patient had developed a contact allergy to the neomycin-containing preparation. The treatment was to remove the

offending agent and to make sure the patient never used neomycin again. A high-potency topical corticosteroid was prescribed for a short course to minimize itching and erythema.

D. Contact Dermatitis to Other Topical Medicines

1. The patient shown in Figure 4-19 had a severe contact dermatitis to a topical Chinese medicine.[5] She had twisted her right ankle by inverting it while walking. Believing that it was a minor sprain, she applied a

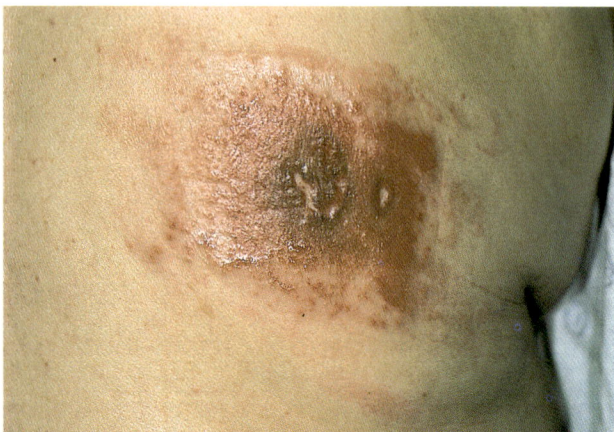

Figure 4-18. Neomycin contact dermatitis after the patient applied topical neomycin on a patch of healing zoster.

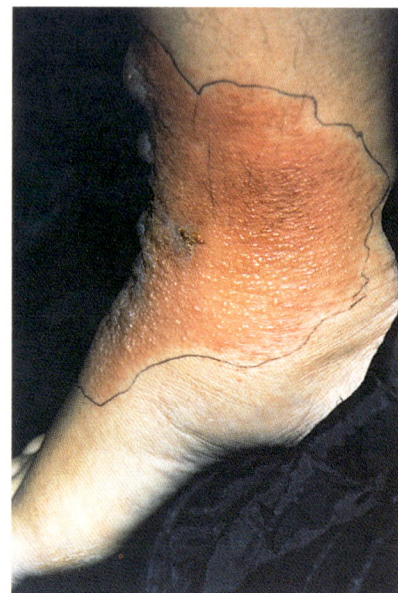

Figure 4-19. Contact dermatitis to other topical medicines. Severe contact dermatitis on the ankle of a woman after application of a Chinese topical medicine.

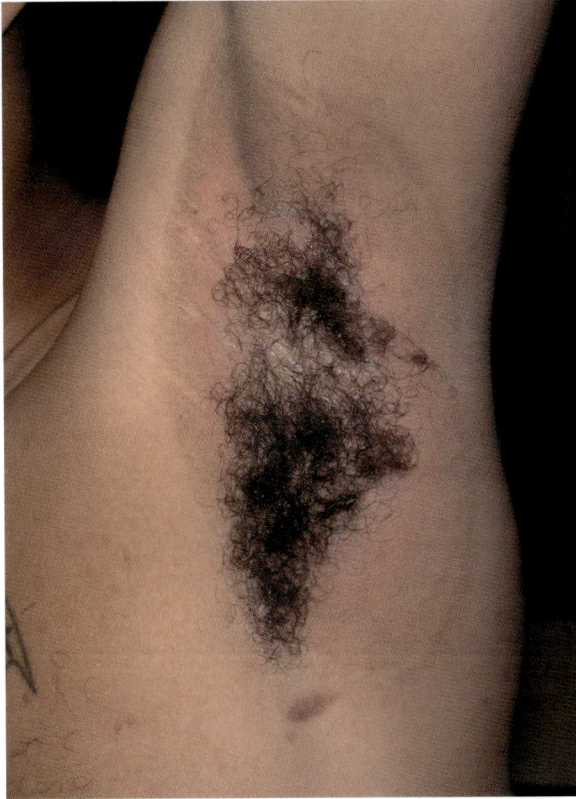

Figure 4-20. Axillary contact dermatitis to a new deodorant.

E. Axillary Contact Dermatitis

Allergic contact dermatitis can occur with deodorants and antiperspirants. The patient in Figure 4-20 noted burning and itching in both axillae. It wasn't until the physician seeing him asked about the use of new deodorants that the patient realized he had just begun using a new stick deodorant prior to the onset of the symptoms. The offending agent was removed and the axillary dermatitis resolved.

F. Contact Dermatitis to Jewelry

Contact dermatitis to nickel and other metals in jewelry is not uncommon. Less expensive jewelry is more likely to cause an allergic contact dermatitis because gold in more expensive jewelry is not a common allergen. The patient shown in Figure 4-21 has lesions on his wrist and ring finger from a watchband and a ring. The hyperpigmentation and thickening of the skin are evidence of a chronic allergic contact dermatitis to the metal involved. The treatment is avoidance of these products. A moderate-potency topical corticosteroid was prescribed to decrease the inflammatory skin changes that had occurred.

G. Shoe Dermatitis and Rubber Allergy

Shoe dermatitis typically appears on the dorsa of the feet and is often mistaken for tinea pedis. However, shoe dermatitis, in contrast to tinea pedis, spares the interdigital spaces. The condition is most often bilateral and spares the soles, which have thick skin more resistant to allergens.

Chinese medicine patch that was given to her by her mother, who had recently immigrated from China. The patient applied the medicine, which was impregnated in a patch, to the anterior medial and lateral portions of her ankle, leaving the posterior portion uncovered. The following day the patient broke out in a red and painful rash with blisters. Because the ingredients of this medicine are unknown, it is difficult to pinpoint the exact allergen causing the contact dermatitis. Although this patient reported no previous occurrences of contact dermatitis, the recent history and physical examination represent a classic pattern for contact dermatitis.

2. The patient stopped using the Chinese medication immediately. Cold compresses and a topical steroid were prescribed. Oral prednisone prescription was considered but not given on the first visit. The patient had no signs of secondary infection that would require antibiotic therapy. She was asked to follow up 2 days later. When the patient showed no improvement despite use of a Class 1, highest-potency topical steroid, she was given a 2-week course of prednisone, starting with 60 mg/day and tapering down to 5 mg/day. The patient responded rapidly and the condition fully resolved.

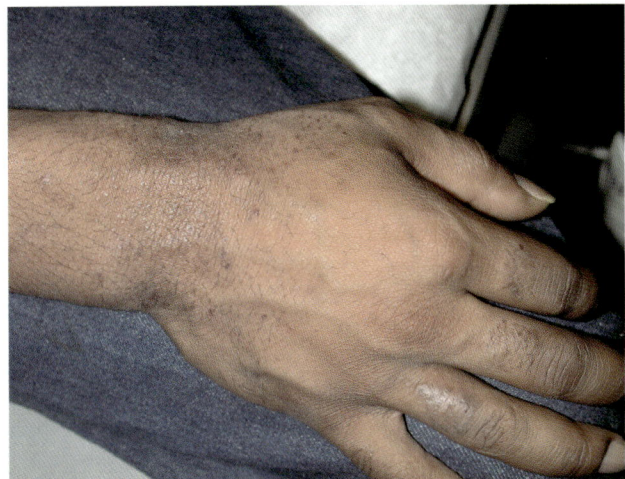

Figure 4-21. Contact dermatitis to jewelry around the wrist and on the ring finger.

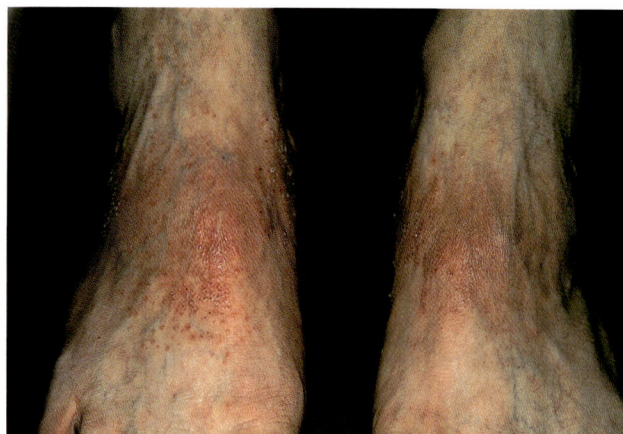

Figure 4-22. Shoe dermatitis and rubber allergy in a man with very sweaty feet.

1. The patient in Figure 4-22 shows bilateral erythema and scaling over the dorsa of both feet. This patient also had a problem with hyperhidrosis, and the sweat causes leaching out of the chemicals from the shoe uppers to create this condition. Two common chemicals that promote contact dermatitis of the feet are mercaptobenzothiazole, a rubber component of adhesives used to cement shoe uppers, and potassium bichromate, a leather tanning agent.

2. Treatment of this patient involved treating the hyperhidrosis with aluminum chloride topically and using different shoes that did not contain the chemicals that could cause this dermatitis. Topical corticosteroids were also prescribed until the inflammation resolved.

XI. When to Obtain Consultation

The vast majority of cases of contact dermatitis are within the scope of primary care practice. Referral to an allergist or dermatologist should be considered in the following situations:

A. When patch testing is being considered and the clinician lacks the expertise to perform this procedure. See Chapter 20, Allergen Patch Testing, for more information on this procedure.

B. When the contact dermatitis does not respond despite multiple attempts at treatment.

C. If a biopsy was performed and revealed a disease that the practioner is unfamiliar with.

D. In cases of severe unresponsive dermatitis.

XII. Practice Parameter

Practice parameters are not yet available for atopic dermatitis. See the following section on internet resources.

XIII. Internet Resources

www.jcaai.org/Param/Aller.htm
Information on allergy testing from the Joint Council of Allergy, Asthma, and Immunology, 2002.

dermis.net
An extensive Dermatology Information System (DermIS) from two universities in Germany.

fm.mednet.ucla.edu/derm
An interactive dermatology atlas with over a thousand images that can be searched by many different parameters. This site includes interactive cases and a quiz mode. It was developed by Drs. Usatine and Madden at UCLA.

XIV. ICD-9 Codes

373.32	Contact and allergic dermatitis of eyelid
692	Contact dermatitis and other eczema
692.2	Dermatitis due to solvents
692.3	Dermatitis due to drugs and medicines in contact with skin
692.4	Dermatitis due to other chemical products
692.5	Dermatitis due to food in contact with skin
692.6	Dermatitis due to plants
692.81	Dermatitis due to cosmetics
692.83	Dermatitis due to metals

XV. Patient Education Materials and Handouts

www.truetest.com/patient/skin.htm
Created by Allerderm Laboratories (producer of patch testing kits), this site contains good patient information about contact dermatitis.

Refer to patient education CD, which is provided with this text, for additional patient education information. It has been formatted to provide readily accessible, easy-to-understand handouts for adult patients and the parents of pediatric patients. These handouts can be easily modified to fit specific practice requirements.

REFERENCES

1. United States Centers for Disease Control and Prevention, National Center for Health Statistics: Vital and Health Statistics Series, vol. 13, No. 134, 1996.
2. Wigger-Alberit W, Maraffio B, Wernli M, Elsner P: Self-application of a protective cream: Pitfalls of occupational skin protection. Arch Dermatol 1997;133:861–864.
3. Higgins EM, MaLelland J, Friedmann PS, Matthew JN, Shuster S: Oral cyclosporin inhibits the expression of contact hypersensitivity in man. J Dermatol Sci 1991;2:79–83.
4. Surber C, Itin P, Buchner S, Maibach HI: Effect of a new topical cyclosporin formulation on human allergic contact dermatitis. Contact Dermatitis 1992;26:116–119.
5. Usatine RP: A red twisted ankle. Western J Med 1999;171: 361–362.

SUGGESTED READINGS

Altman L, Becker J, Williams P: Allergy in Primary Care.
Habif T: Clinical Dermatology: A Color Guide to Diagnosis and Therapy, 3rd ed. St. Louis: Mosby, 1996.
Werfel T, Kapp A: Atopic dermatitis and allergic contact dermatitis. In Holgate ST, Church MK, Lichtenstein LM (eds): Allergy, 2nd ed. London: Mosby, 2001.
Williford P, Sherertz E: Poison ivy dermatitis. Arch Intern Med 1994;3:184–188.

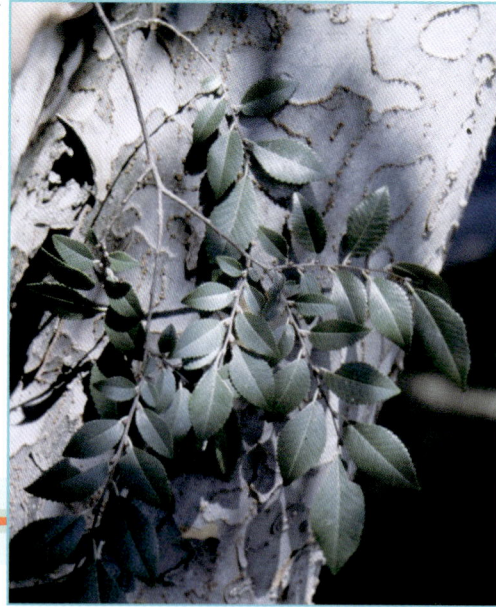

CHAPTER 5
Urticaria and Angioedema

Richard P. Usatine

I. Introduction

Urticaria is the medical term for what is commonly known as hives. A hive or wheal is an erythematous, skin-colored or white, nonpitting, edematous plaque that changes in size and shape by peripheral extension or regression during the few hours or days that the individual lesion exists.

A. *Urticaria* is a dynamic process in which wheals evolve as old ones resolve. These wheals result from localized capillary vasodilation, followed by transudation of protein-rich fluid into the surrounding skin. The wheals resolve when the fluid is slowly reabsorbed.[1] These wheals are usually pruritic but do not have to itch. Urticaria can be found anywhere on the body and is often on the trunk and extremities (Fig. 5-1).

B. *Angioedema* is a large edematous area that involves transudation of fluid into the dermis and deeper subcutaneous tissue (Fig. 5-2). Angioedema is seen more often on the face, especially around the mouth and eyes (Fig. 5-3).

C. Most episodes of urticaria disappear within a few days to weeks. *Acute urticaria* is defined as urticaria lasting less than 6 weeks. *Chronic urticaria* is defined as urticaria lasting 6 or more weeks. Occasionally, a person continues to have urticaria for many years.

II. Epidemiology

It is estimated that 20% of the population may have urticaria sometime during their lifetime. Acute urticaria occurs more commonly in children and young adults, whereas chronic urticaria is more common in middle-aged women.[2] Chronic urticaria may occur in up to 25% of all patients with urticaria. Urticaria is more common in patients who are atopic.

Chronic idiopathic urticaria is a common skin condition that affects 0.1%–3% of people in the United States and Europe.[3] Chronic urticaria is twice as common in women as in men. Chronic urticaria predominantly affects adults. More than 50% of cases of hives resolve spontaneously in about 6 months. More patients will have their urticaria resolve with time, so that by a few years, many patients are cured. However, up to 40% of patients with chronic urticaria of more than 6 months' duration still have urticaria 10 years later.[4]

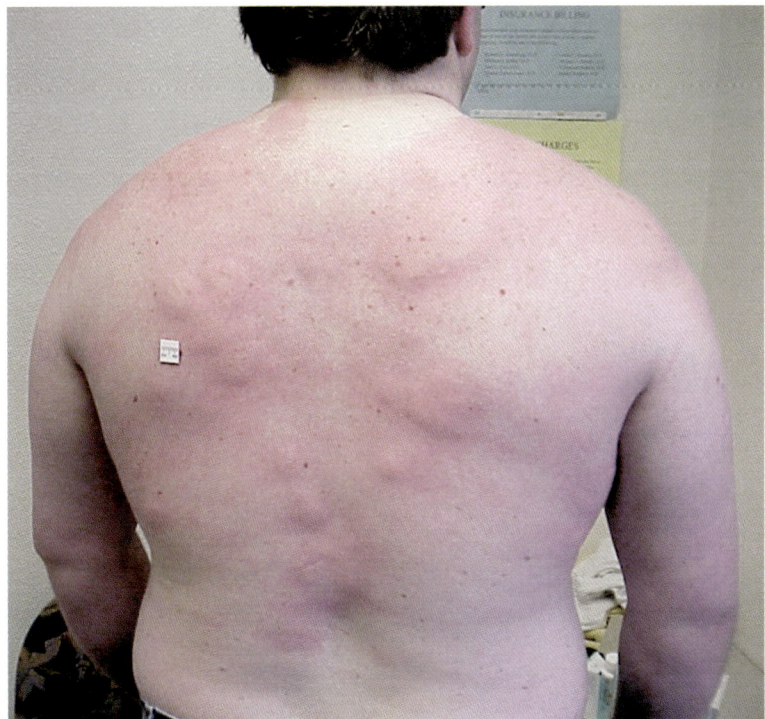

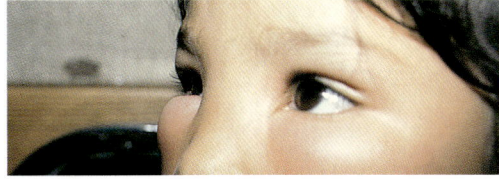

Figure 5-3 Angioedema on the face of a young girl—swelling around the eyes is very notable.

Figure 5-1 Acute urticaria on the extremities and trunk secondary to a sulfa allergy.

III. Etiology

The pathophysiology of angioedema and urticaria can be IgE-mediated, complement-mediated, related to physical stimuli, autoantibody-mediated, or idiopathic. These mechanisms lead to mast cell degranulation, which results in the release of histamine. The histamine and other inflammatory mediators produce the wheals, edema and pruritus.

The following etiologic types exist:

- Immunologic—IgE-mediated, complement-mediated
- Physical urticaria—dermatographism, cold urticaria, cholinergic, pressure, vibratory urticaria
- Urticaria due to mast cell–releasing agents—mastocytosis, urticaria pigmentosa
- Urticaria associated with vascular/connective tissue autoimmune disease

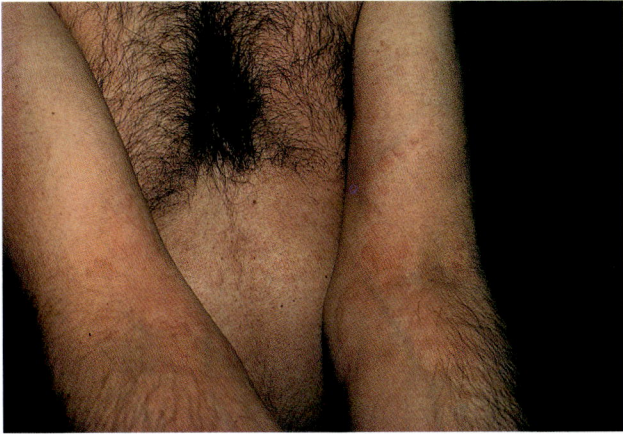

Figure 5-2 Urticaria on the back with angioedema. (Courtesy of Daniel Stulberg, MD.)

- Hereditary angioedema
- Angioedema-urticaria-eosinophilia syndrome
- Urticarial vasculitis

A. Immunologic Urticaria

IgE-mediated urticaria occurs more often in persons with an atopic background. The antigens are most commonly foods or medications. The most common foods include milk, eggs, wheat, shellfish, and nuts.

Complement-mediated urticaria occurs when immune complexes activate complement and release anaphylatoxins, which induce mast cell degranulation.

B. Physical Urticaria

1. *Dermatographism* is also known as "skin writing." It is the most common physical urticaria. Approximately 5% of the population have dermatographism to some degree.[1] Hives occur after rubbing or stroking of the skin (Fig. 5-4). In most cases the cause is unknown, but the hives may be preceded by a viral infection, antibiotic therapy, or psychological distress. Dermatographism occurs most commonly in young people. It may last for weeks to months or even years.
2. *Cold urticaria* usually occurs in children or young adults. The wheals occur in areas exposed to the cold. Most patients have an acquired form, but a rare familial form is inherited as an autosomal dominant disorder. The mean age at onset is 18–25 years, and the condition typically lasts 5–6 years. Patients with cold urticaria often have dermatographism and cholinergic urticaria as well.
3. *Solar urticaria* occurs within minutes after sun exposure. These hives usually disappear in less than 1 hour. This condition is different from a polymorphous light eruption because those lesions are not urticarial.
4. *Cholinergic urticaria* may be provoked by anything that can heat up the body, such as vigorous exercise, heat, or emotional distress (Fig. 5-5). This form of urticaria is characterized by small papular wheals, 2–4 mm in diameter, with an erythematous background. Most cases begin in people between the ages of 10 and 30 years. The wheals typically begin 2–20 minutes after the person becomes overheated. The lesions may last for minutes to hours, with a median duration of 30 minutes.[1]
5. *Pressure urticaria/angioedema* is characterized by swelling that occurs after pressure. Examples include buttock swelling after sitting for an extended period of time, foot swelling after walking, or hand swelling after using a hand tool. Tight-fitting clothing can also bring on this problem. The hands, feet, trunk, buttock, lips, and face are most commonly affected. The painful swelling tends to occur 4–6 hours after the pressure stimulus and lasts 8–72 hours afterward. Various

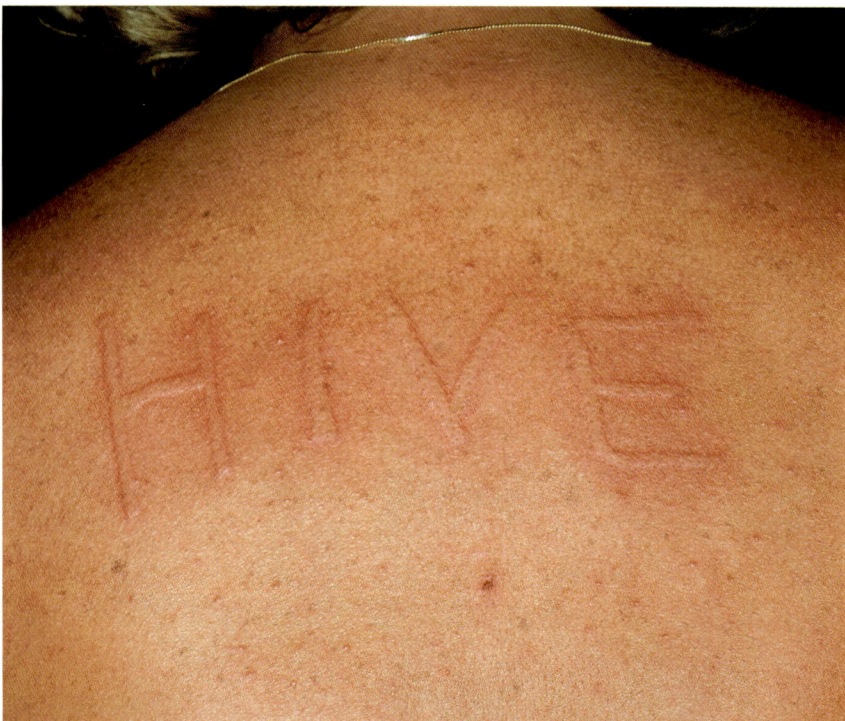

Figure 5-4 Dermatographism is also known as skin writing. (From Habif T: Clinical Dermatology: A Color Guide to Diagnosis and Therapy, 3rd ed. St. Louis: Mosby, 1996. Reproduced with permission.)

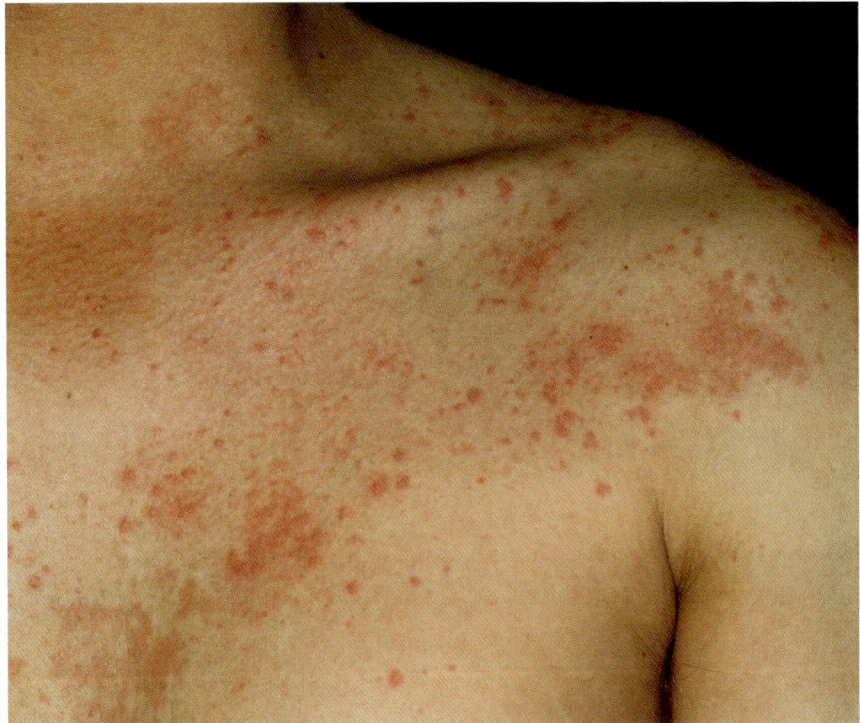

Figure 5-5 Cholinergic urticaria. Round red papules or wheals that occur in response to exercise, heat, or emotional stress. (From Habif T: Clinical Dermatology: A Color Guide to Diagnosis and Therapy, 3rd ed. St. Louis: Mosby, 1996. Reproduced with permission.)

systemic symptoms such as malaise, fever, fatigue, chills, headache, or arthralgia may occur.

6. *Vibratory urticaria/angioedema* occurs after a vibratory stimulus such as the rubbing of a towel back and forth across the skin or working with a jackhammer.

C. Urticaria Due to Mast Cell–Releasing Agents

This form of urticaria occurs when there are too many mast cells in the skin. These mast cells release histamine stored in granules. One example is *cutaneous mastocytosis,* also known as *urticaria pigmentosa.* The cause is unknown.

Most cases of urticaria pigmentosa occur before age 2. These cases gradually improve, usually clearing by puberty. Urticaria pigmentosa that begins after age 10 usually persists and may be associated with systemic disease. Cutaneous mastocytosis manifests with red-brown, slightly elevated plaques averaging 0.5–1.5 cm in diameter. The plaques occur in small groups on the trunk but can occur in other areas as well.

D. Hereditary Angioedema

Hereditary angioedema is a potentially life-threatening disorder that is inherited in an autosomal dominant manner (Fig. 5-6). This disorder usually involves angioedema of the face and extremities, larynx, and bowel wall. Usually there are no wheals seen with this condition. The abnor-

malities are found in the complement system. These abnormalities include:

1. Decreased levels of C1 esterase inhibitor (85%)
2. Dysfunctional C1 esterase inhibitor (15%)
3. Low C4 levels in the presence of normal C1 and C3 levels

E. Angioedema-Urticaria-Eosinophilia Syndrome

This rare syndrome is characterized by severe angioedema involving the face, neck, extremities, and trunk that lasts for 7–10 days. Occasionally it is also accompanied by pruritic urticaria. The patient is febrile, and there is a large amount of fluid retention, causing a 10%–18% increase in normal weight.[2] This is not an inherited abnormality, and the patient will report no family history of this condition. A complete blood cell (CBC) count with differential will show a markedly elevated WBC count of 20,000–70,000/cu mm with 60%–80% eosinophils. Fortunately, the prognosis for resolution is good.

F. Urticarial Vasculitis

Urticarial vasculitis is a type of urticaria associated with vascular/connective tissue autoimmune disease. These urticarial skin lesions persist longer than 12–24 hours and can be associated with purpura (Fig. 5-7). There may be some residual pigmentation due to hemosiderin deposits after involution of the urticaria. Urticarial vasculitis may

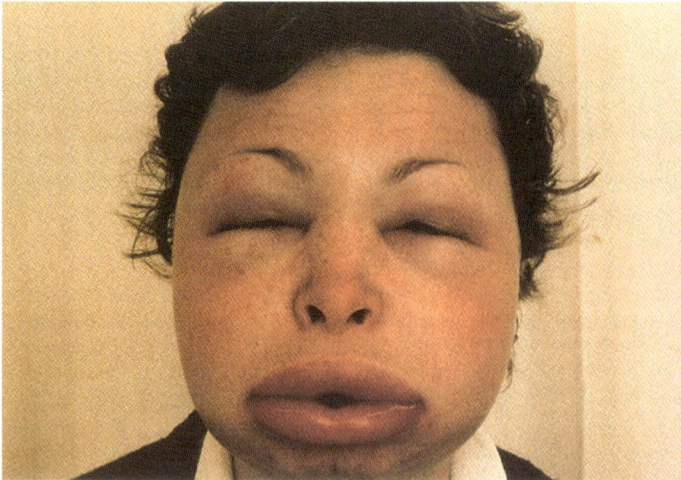

A

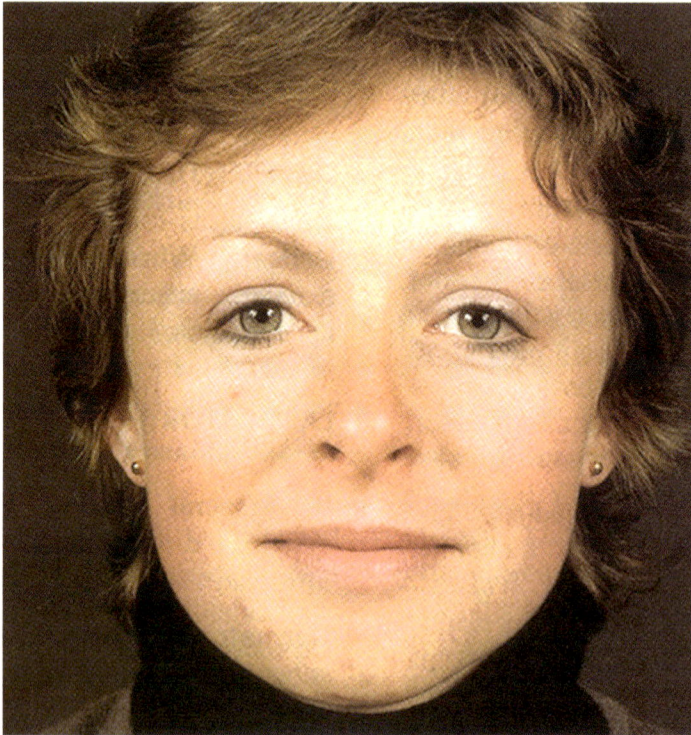

B

Figure 5-6 **A**, Hereditary angioedema. **B**, The same woman from (**A**) after the angioedema resolves. (From Fitzpatrick BF, Johnson RA, Wolff K, Suurmond D: Color Atlas and Synopsis of Clinical Dermatology, 4th ed. New York: McGraw-Hill, 2001. Reproduced with permission.)

be associated with systemic lupus erythematosis (SLE), Sjögren's syndrome, hypocomplementemia, or renal disease.

IV. Clinical Manifestations

A. Itching, Wheals

Patients with hives complain of itching but may also experience burning or stinging. The wheals may vary in size from the small, 2-mm papules of cholinergic urticaria (see Fig. 5-5) to giant hives, in which a single wheal may cover an extremity or part of the abdomen (Fig. 5-8). The wheal may be all red or white, or the border may be red, with the remainder of the surface white. Wheals may be surrounded by a red halo. The larger lesions, >5 mm, are referred to as plaques. In patients with darker skin, the wheals may be skin-colored only, with no visible erythema (Fig. 5-9).

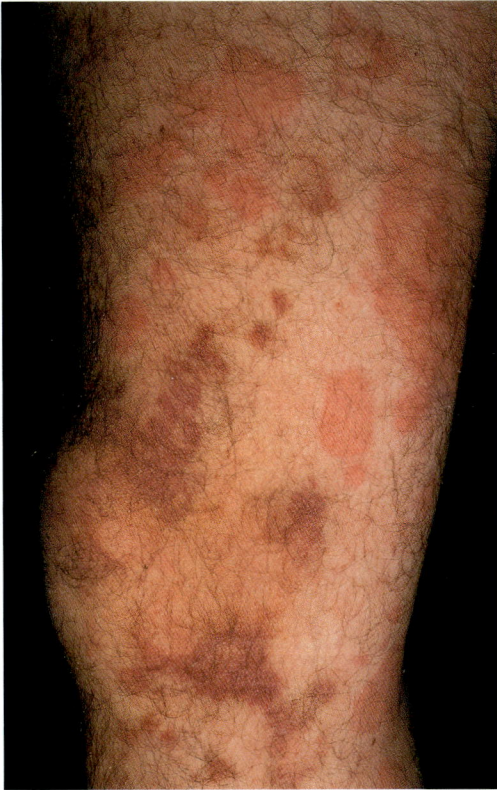

Figure 5-7 Urticarial vasculitis. Purpura occurs as the hive resolves. (From Habif T: Clinical Dermatology: A Color Guide to Diagnosis and Therapy, 3rd ed. St. Louis: Mosby, 1996. Reproduced with permission.)

B. Time Course

Acute urticaria and/or angioedema may present rapidly or gradually. The time course (onset and resolution) of the wheals varies according to the etiology, and even varies from person to person within the same etiologic group. The time to resolution of the wheals is longer in urticarial vasculitis.

C. Angioedema

Angioedema is deeper than a wheal and is caused by transudation of fluid into the dermis and subcutaneous tissue. The lips, tongue, eyelids, and ears may become swollen (Fig. 5-10). Sometimes angioedema occurs on the genitals or the trunk.

D. Dermatographism

If dermatographism is present, there is an exaggerated triple response of Lewis (local reddening, edema, and surrounding flare) that allows one to write on the skin and see the resulting words or shapes (see Fig. 5-4).

E. Unknown Etiology

The etiology is unknown in approximately 80% of cases of chronic urticaria. Emotional stress often seems to be an exacerbating factor and may in fact be a cause of the chronic urticaria.

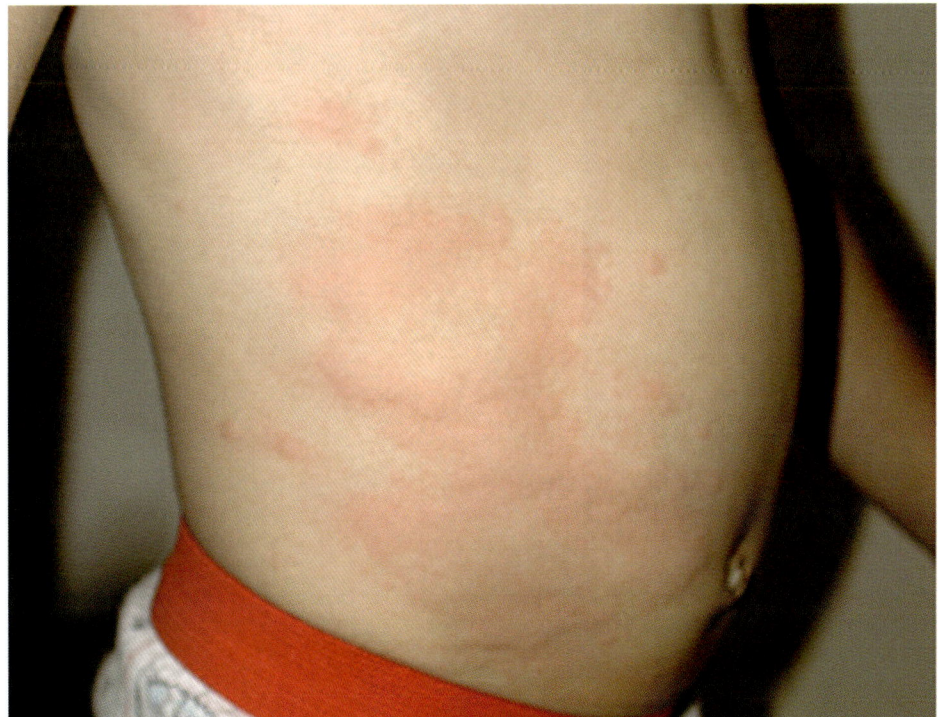

Figure 5-8 Large urticarial plaques on the trunk of a young boy.

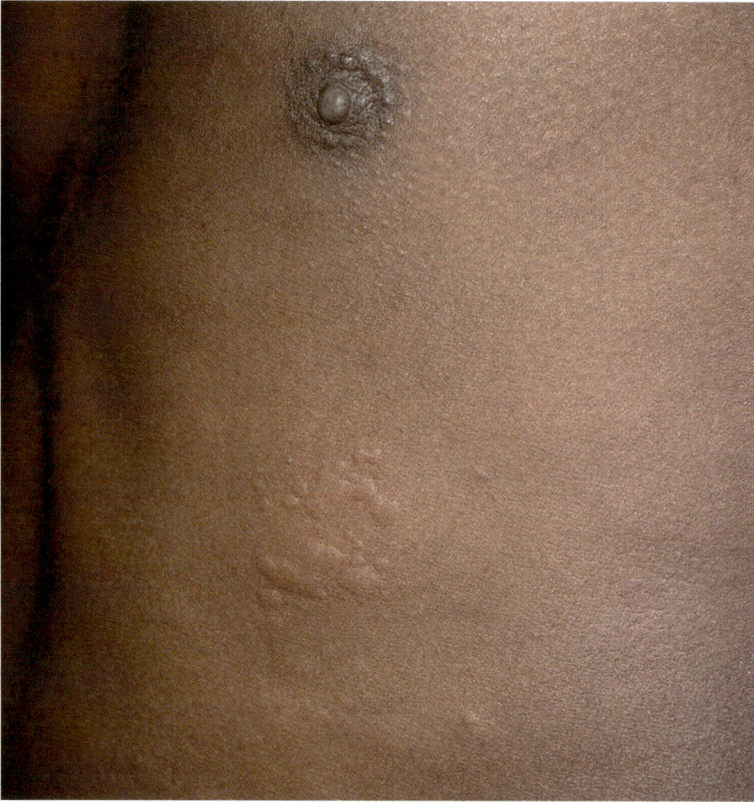

Figure 5-9 Urticaria in a young African-American boy. No erythema is visible but the wheals are otherwise typical.

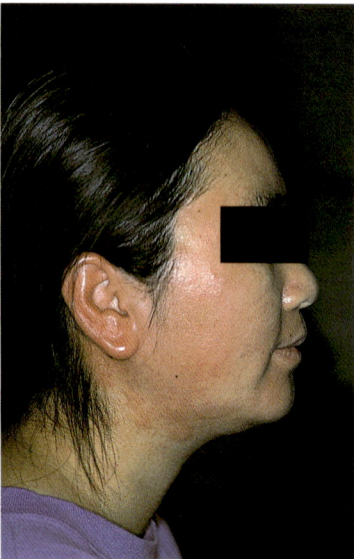

A

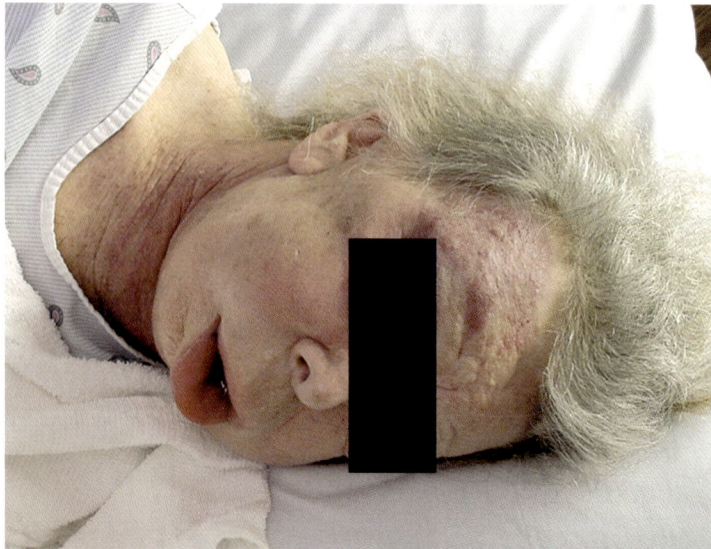

B

Figure 5-10 A, Angioedema on the face of a young woman. Ear involvement is notable. **B**, Severe angioedema on the face of an older woman in the hospital with marked lip involvement. (**B**, Courtesy of Adrian Casillas, MD.)

V. Differential Diagnosis

The differential diagnosis of urticaria includes insect bites, erythema multiforme, bullous pemphigoid, dermatitis herpetiformis, urticarial contact dermatitis, exercise-induced anaphylaxis, pruritic urticarial papules and plaques of pregnancy (PUPPP), mast cell releasability syndromes, and urticarial vasculitis.

A. Insect Bites

A good history and physical examination should help distinguish between insect bites and urticaria. Look for the site where the bite occurred within the swollen red area of the skin (Fig. 5-11).

B. Erythema Multiforme

Like urticaria, erythema multiforme can occur as part of an allergic/immunologic reaction to medications, infections, and neoplasms. The classic lesion of erythema multiforme is the target lesion (Fig. 5-12). If the patient develops erythema multiforme major (Stevens-Johnson syndrome), the patient will have more systemic symptoms, including fever and malaise. Stevens-Johnson syndrome causes mucosal lesions and can be life-threatening.

C. Bullous Pemphigoid and Dermatitis Herpetiformis

The early lesions of bullous pemphigoid and dermatitis herpetiformis (see Fig. 3-21, p. 51) may resemble the papular form of cholinergic urticaria. As bullous pemphigoid progresses to typical bullae, it should become distinguishable from urticaria. Dermatitis herpetiformis is more symmetric, and this differs from the asymmetry of urticaria.

D. Urticarial Vasculitis

The lestions of urticarial vascultis typically last longer than 24 hours. The lesions are found more commonly on the lower extremities, and when they heal they often leave a hyperpigmented area (see Fig. 5-7). Additionally,

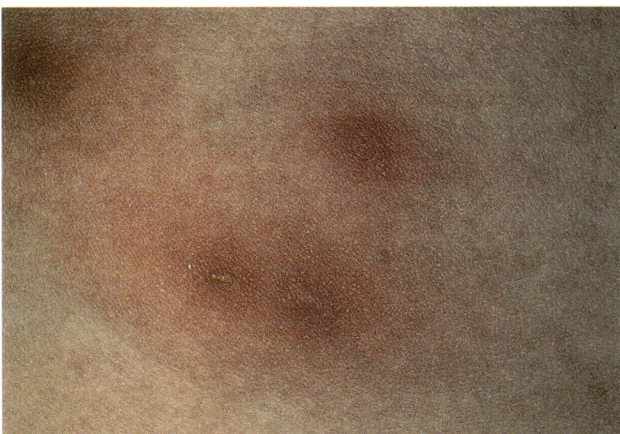

Figure 5-12 This target lesion is the classic lesion of erythema multiforme.

purpura, bruising, livedo reticularis, and petechiae may be present. Patients may also have more burning and pain rather than actual pruritus. Systemic symptoms such as fever, arthralgia/arthritis, gastrointestinal (GI) symptoms, myalgias, malaise, or weight loss may help to distinguish this condition from a more benign urticarial process. One example of this is Henoch-Schönlein purpura (Fig. 5-13).

E. Mast Cell Releasability Syndromes

In these syndromes there are too many mast cells in the skin or other organs of the body. These syndromes include:

1. Cutaneous mastocytosis—i.e., urticaria pigmentosa (Fig. 5-14), solitary mastocytoma, and diffuse cutaneous mastocytosis (without urticaria pigmentosa)
2. Systemic mastocytosis with or without skin involvement
3. Mastocytosis in association with hematologic disorders (e.g., leukemia)
4. Lymphadenopathic mastocytosis with eosinophilia
5. Mast cell leukemia. Flushing, hives, itching, bruising, and tingling are common cutaneous symptoms. Systemic symptoms occur as well.[5]

When angioedema occurs without urticaria, hereditary or acquired C1 esterase inhibitor deficiency should be considered. Isolated angioedema in the upper extremities could be due to the superior vena cava syndrome.

F. Exercise-Induced Anaphylaxis

Patients may develop urticaria, respiratory distress, and hypotension after exercise. Symptoms may progress to laryngeal edema, angioedema, and bronchospasm. This could actually cause upper airway distress and shock. This is most often reported with jogging but can occur with other kinds of exercise. Exercise causes the mast cell degranulation and elevated serum histamine levels. This is different from cholinergic urticaria in that the wheals

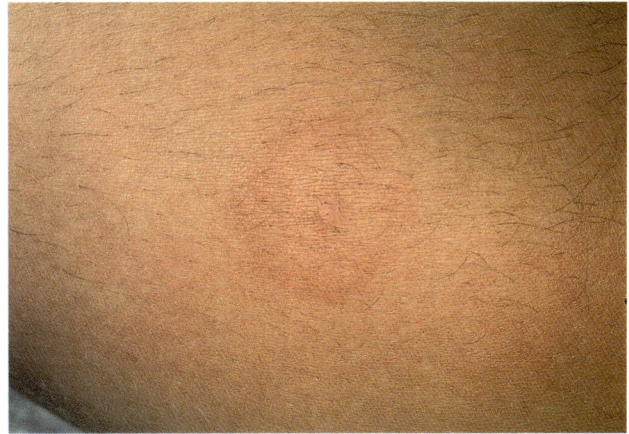

Figure 5-11 Insect bites.

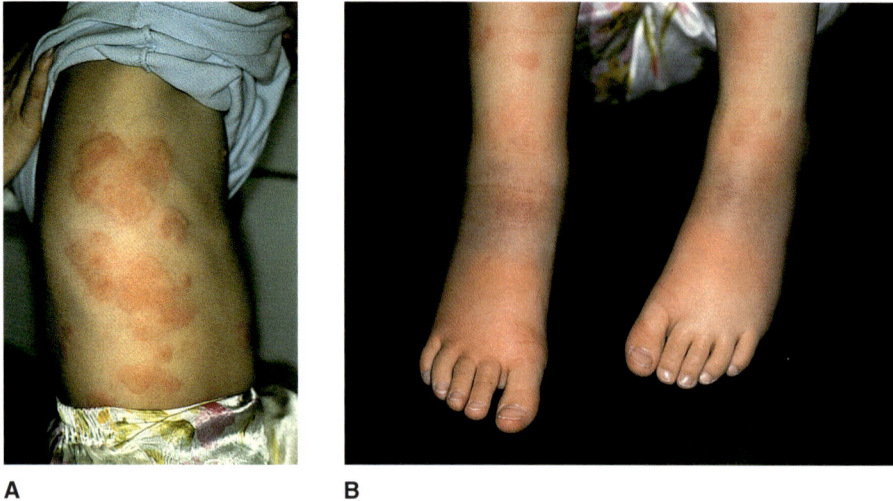

A   **B**

Figure 5-13 Henoch-Schönlein purpura in a young girl that started after she began taking a sulfa antibiotic. **A**, This figure resembles urticaria. **B**, The purpura is seen best in the area of the ankle swelling.

are larger and are not produced by hot showers, heat, or anxiety. It can be differentiated from cholinergic urticaria by a hot water immersion test. Exercise-induced anaphylaxis may occur only after ingestion of certain foods, such as wheat or shellfish.[1]

G. Pruritic Urticarial Papules and Plaques of Pregnancy

PUPPP is the most common pregnancy-related skin disorder and has an incidence of approximately 1 in 160 pregnancies. It is seen most frequently during the first pregnancy and begins late in the third trimester. The papules and plaques appear suddenly and usually appear first on the abdomen (Fig. 5-15). The lesions may spread to involve the buttocks and arms (Fig. 5-16). The face is spared. PUPPP can be differentiated from urticaria because the eruption remains fixed and increases in intensity. In most cases the lesions clear spontaneously before or within 1 week after delivery.

VI. History and Physical Examination

The wheals are usually pruritic and transient. The distribution may be localized, regional, or generalized. The wheals may be as small as 1- to 2-mm papules or as large as 8-cm edematous plaques. The wheals have various shapes as well as sizes. Typical shapes include round, oval, arciform, annular, and serpiginous. The edema in angioedema can cause transient enlargement of portions of the face and extremities. Eyelids, lips, and tongue are often involved and can become massively enlarged (see Figs. 5-6 and 5-10).

If the cause and type of urticaria are obvious from the history, and the physical examination confirms the diagnosis, the following physical examination maneuvers

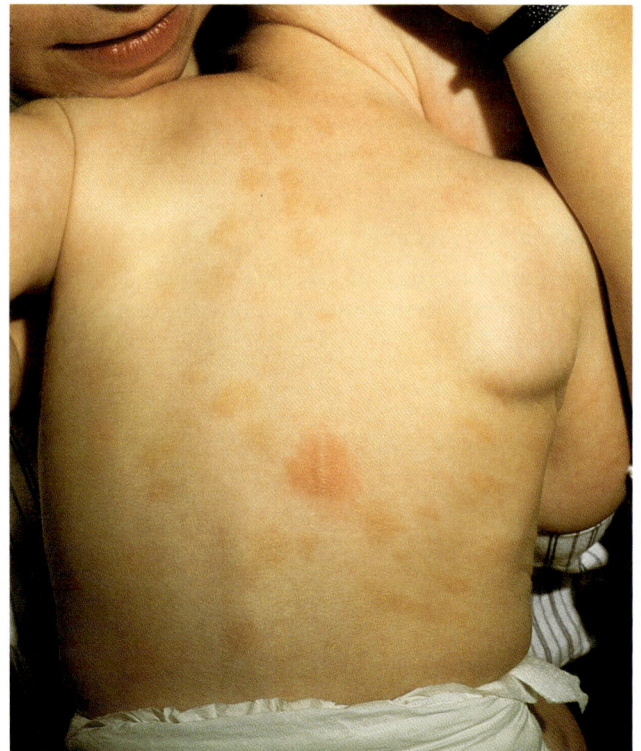

Figure 5-14 Urticaria pigmentosa (cutaneous mastocytosis). Red-brown, slightly elevated plaques averaging 0.5–3.5 cm in diameter typically occur in small groups on the trunk. One lesion turned red after being stroked. (From Habif T: Clinical Dermatology: A Color Guide to Diagnosis and Therapy, 3rd ed. St. Louis: Mosby, 1996. Reproduced with permission.)

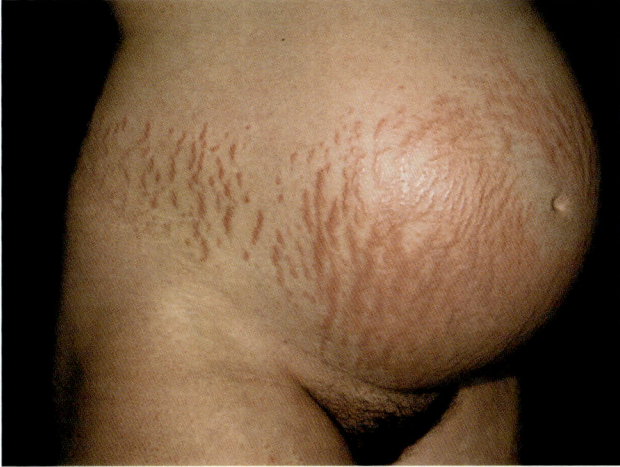

A

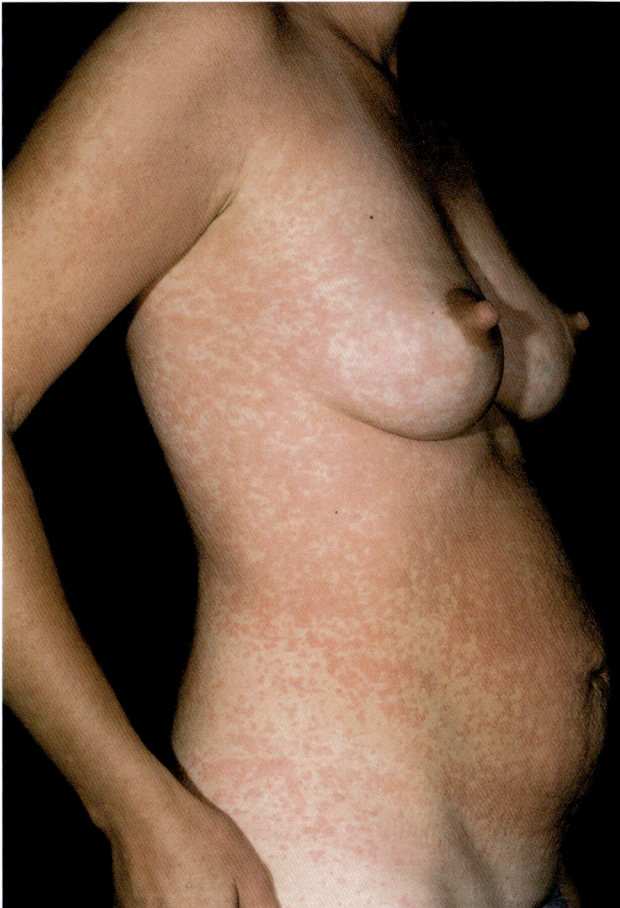

B

Figure 5-15 Pruritic urticarial papules and plaques of pregnancy (PUPPP). **A,** The initial lesions may be limited to the striae. **B,** Fully evolved eruptions. (From Habif T: Clinical Dermatology: A Color Guide to Diagnosis and Therapy, 3rd ed. St. Louis: Mosby, 1996. Reproduced with permission.)

probably will not be needed. If the cause and type of urticaria/angioedema are not obvious, a focused physical examination may yield the information needed to determine the etiology.

In most cases of acute urticaria the history will be most helpful in determining the etiology. In chronic urticaria, careful collection of historical, physical examination, and laboratory evidence may be needed to determine the etiology in the approximately 20% of cases in which the etiology can be discerned.

Carefully examine the patient for these clues:

1. Look for signs of insect bites where the insect pierced the skin.
2. Small papular hives after exercise or heat exposure suggest a possible cholinergic process (see Fig. 5-5).
3. Look to see if the distribution of wheals follows a pattern. In physical urticaria, there is a predilection for sites of pressure. In solar and cold urticaria, there is a predilection for exposed areas.
4. Look for signs of active infection or a recent viral infection.
5. Look for jaundice or icterus, because hepatitis can lead to urticaria. Examine the patient for liver or gallbladder tenderness.
6. Look for sinus or dental infections.
7. Examine the thyroid for signs of enlargement or tenderness.
8. Look for signs of a connective tissue disease.
9. Consider a vaginal or prostate examination for signs of infection or malignancy.
10. Check for dermatographism by stroking the flexor surface of the forearm with a tongue blade (Fig. 5-17)
11. Check for cold urticaria with an ice cube (Fig. 5-18).

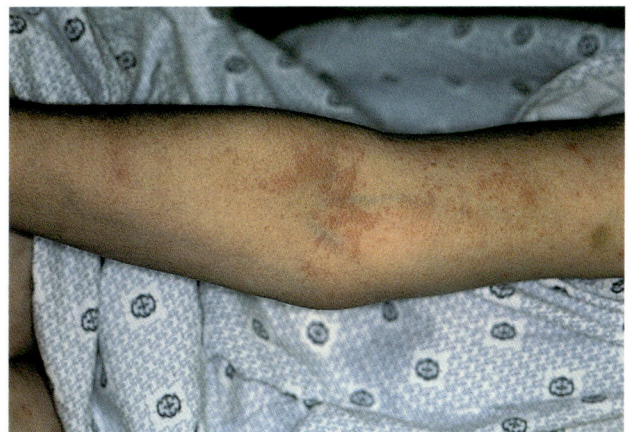

Figure 5-16 PUPPP on the arm of a pregnant woman.

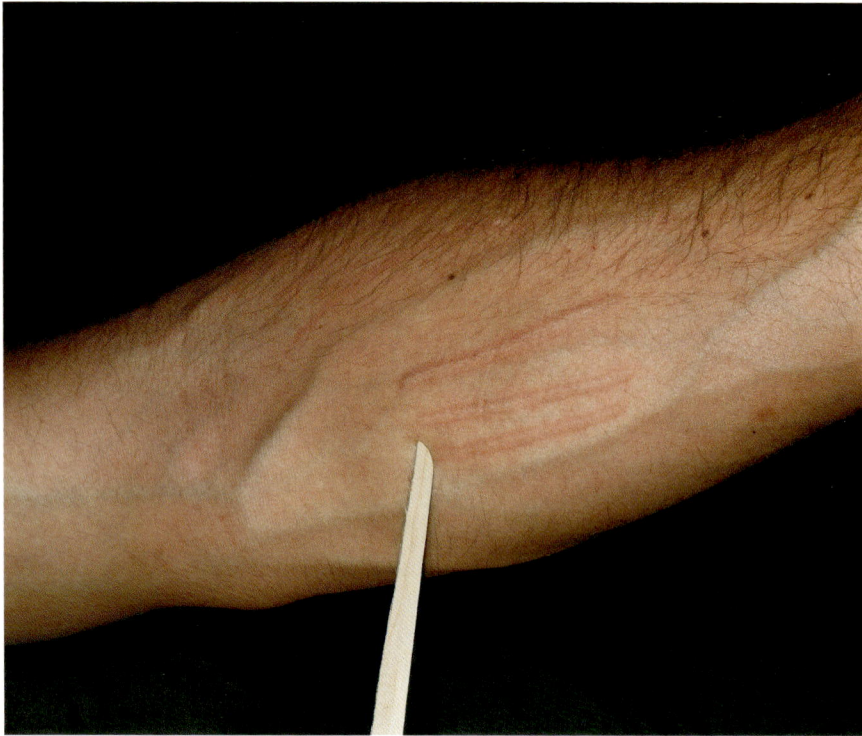

Figure 5-17 Test for dermatographism. The tongue blade drawn firmly across the arm elicits urticaria in susceptible individuals. This simple test should be considered for any patient with acute or chronic urticaria. (From Habif T: Clinical Dermatology: A Color Guide to Diagnosis and Therapy, 3rd ed. St. Louis: Mosby, 1996. Reproduced with permission.)

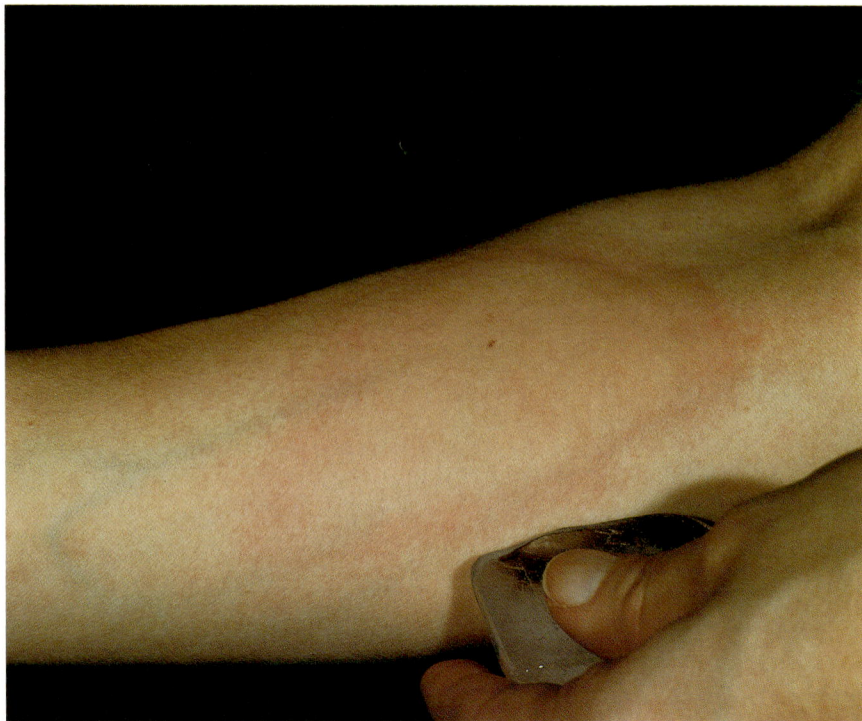

Figure 5-18 Cold urticaria. The wheals occurred within minutes of holding an ice cube against the skin. (From Habif T: Clinical Dermatology: A Color Guide to Diagnosis and Therapy, 3rd ed. St. Louis: Mosby, 1996. Reproduced with permission.)

12. If you suspect urticaria pigmentosa, try stroking a lesion with the wooden end of a cotton-tipped applicator. This will induce intense erythema of the entire plaque, and the wheal is usually confined to the stroke site. This is called Darier's sign.

Warning: If the patient has hypotension, airway obstruction, or GI distress along with the urticaria, the patient may be in the midst of an anaphylactic process, which requires immediate treatment with epinephrine and further intervention. Chapter 6 covers this topic in greater detail.

VII. Laboratory Tests

Laboratory tests are rarely needed in acute urticaria. If laboratory tests are needed, a shotgun approach should not be used. Instead, specific clues from the history and physical examination are used to select those tests with the highest yield.

When urticaria persists, a workup to rule out systemic disease is indicated. Unfortunately, because 80% of cases of chronic urticaria are idiopathic, these workups are rarely productive.

Tests to consider in a workup include:
1. Urinalysis to look for a urinary tract infection.
2. CBC with differential count to rule out hematologic diseases and to look for eosinophilia. Eosinophilia may be seen with reactions to parasites, foods, and drugs. High levels of eosinophilia are seen in the angioedema-urticaria-eosinophilia syndrome.
3. Consider sinus and dental films.
4. Consider a thyroid microsomal antibody test.
5. Consider an antinuclear antibody (ANA) assay if SLE is in the differential diagnosis.
6. Consider hepatitis serologies.
7. The erythrocyte sedimentation rate (ESR) is often elevated in urticarial vasculitis.
8. Obtain a stool specimen to check for ova and parasites.
9. If acute mononucleosis is suspected, consider a mono spot test or Epstein-Barr virus serologies.
10. Specific complement studies (C_3, C_4, CH_{50} quantitative and qualitative C1 esteraste inhibitor levels) to exclude hereditary or acquired C1 esterase inhibitor deficiency may be indicated in patients with recurrent episodes of acute angioedema of the face, tongue, or lips without urticaria and associated with severe abdominal pain.
11. Allergen skin testing and/or in vitro tests for detection of specific IgE antibody to inhalants (e.g., animal danders, pollens, molds) may be useful when the history reveals that urticaria/angioedema occurs after direct contact with a suspected allergen such as animals, weeds, or grass (see Chapters 12 and 13).

12. The physical findings of weight loss, lymphadenopathy, and visceromegaly warrant further medical evaluation to exclude an underlying lymphoreticular malignancy.
13. A punch biopsy (3–4 mm) of an urticarial plaque may help to determine if urticarial vasculitis or mastocytosis is the cause of chronic idiopathic urticaria. (A Giemsa stain is needed for detection of increased numbers of mast cells.)

VIII. Approach to Diagnosis

The duration of the condition determines whether the condition is acute or chronic urticaria. Chronic urticaria is defined as lesions that continue to come and go over 6 or more weeks.

A. If the lesions are recent in onset, determine whether the patient has urticaria or insect bites. Also, be sure that the skin lesions are not the target lesions of erythema multiforme.

B. Determine whether the urticaria is due to a physical cause. Many of these causes can be determined from the history and confirmed on physical examination. Dermatographism can be reproduced in the office.

1. Ask whether physical stimuli such as pressure, exercise, sun, cold, heat, vibration, or water bring on the hives.
2. Ask about food ingestion such as fish, shellfish, nuts, eggs, chocolate, strawberries, tomatoes, pork, cow's milk, cheese, wheat, and yeast (Fig. 5-19).
3. Ask about medication use, especially antibiotics and aspirin. Don't just ask about prescription medications; inquire into the use of over-the-counter (OTC) medicines and supplements.
4. Ask about the use of morphine, codeine, and quinine. These medicines are known to cause an immunologic release of histamine and can cause urticaria and an anaphylactoid reaction.
5. Ask about infections:
   a. Bacterial infections that are chronic—sinusitis, dental infections, pulmonary or urinary tract infections, cholecystitis
   b. Viral infections—hepatitis B, mononucleosis, coxsackievirus
   c. Parasitic infections—especially roundworms, amebiasis, malaria (usually related to travel to or recent immigration from a developing country)
   d. Fungal infections—tinea or *Candida*
6. Ask about a history of atopic conditions such as allergic rhinitis, atopic dermatitis, asthma, and allergic conjunctivitis.

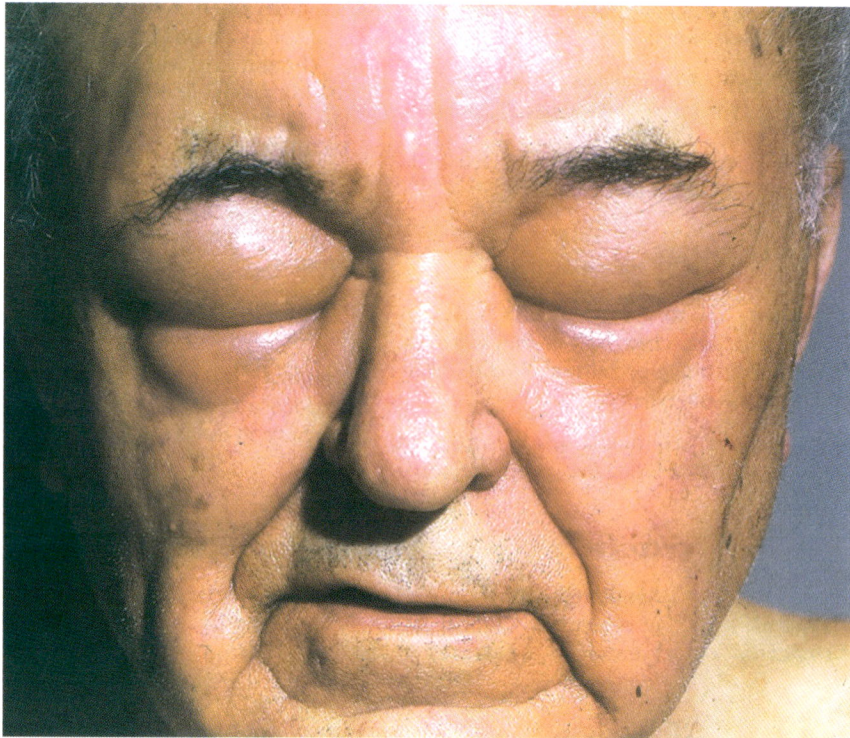

Figure 5-19 Acute urticaria and angioedema after patient ate shellfish. (From Fitzpatrick BF, Johnson RA, Wolff K, Suurmond D: Color Atlas and Synopsis of Clinical Dermatology, 4th ed. New York: McGraw-Hill, 2001. Reproduced with permission.)

7. Ask about exposures to various inhalants, including pollens, mold, spores, animal dander, house dust, aerosols, and chemicals.
8. Ask about previous systemic diseases, including SLE, hyperthyroidism, and cancers.
9. Ask about contact with plants such as nettles, animals such as jellyfish and caterpillars, and the use of DMSO. A linear local wheal pattern raises the suspicion of a contact allergen as the cause of the urticaria (Fig. 5-20).
10. Ask about previous skin diseases. Rare diseases such as dermatitis herpetiformis, pemphigoid, and urticaria pigmentosa can lead to urticaria.
11. Ask about pregnancy or premenstrual syndrome. If the patient is pregnant, she may have PUPPP. Premenstrual symptoms can be related to progesterone levels.
12. Very rare genetic autosomal dominant conditions can cause urticaria and/or angioedema. These are hereditary angioedema, cholinergic urticaria with progressive nerve deafness, amyloidosis of the kidney, familial cold urticaria, and vibratory urticaria.

C. An elimination diet may be tried when there is a suspicious potential food precipitant. While this might be

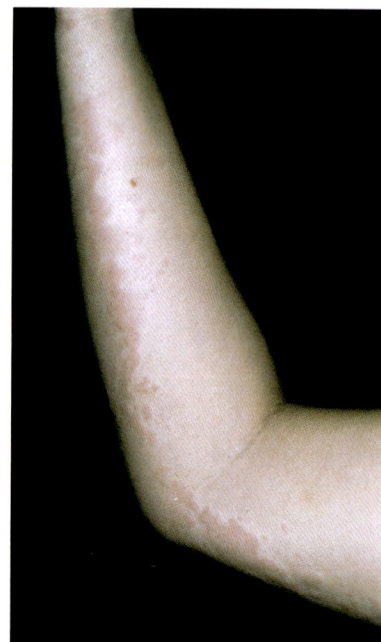

Figure 5-20 Urticaria in a linear pattern may suggest a contact allergen was the provoking agent.

useful in acute urticaria, it is rare to find a food cause of chronic urticaria (see Appendix 6).

IX. Therapy and Management

Determining the cause or type of urticaria can be very helpful in treating the urticaria. This goal is easier to achieve when the urticaria is acute. Urticaria that persists beyond 6 weeks and has not responded to initial therapy is more difficult to treat.

A. Nonpharmacologic Therapy

When a causative agent, stimulus, or antigen is found, the first step is avoidance of the precipitant. This may require elimination diets when a food substance is suspected. Stopping a suspicious medication may also be effective. If a patient has physical urticaria, he or she should try to avoid the specific precipitant when possible.

In chronic urticaria, patients may benefit from avoidance of potential urticarial precipitants such as aspirin, NSAIDs, opiates, and alcohol. Stop all unnecessary OTC medications, supplements, and vitamins.

1. **Stress Management**
   Reassure the patient with chronic urticaria that you understand that this is a very frustrating condition. Reassure patients that there are many medicines available to control the disease, especially when urticaria does not respond to initial therapy.

   It is helpful if patients accept that stress exacerbates urticaria and make an effort to work on stress management techniques (e.g., meditation, yoga, counseling). Sometimes vacations from home and work environments can be helpful.

2. **Restricted Diets and Avoidance**
   In severe refractory chronic idiopathic urticaria, patients may be told to avoid all food additives, tobacco use, vitamins, salicylates, laxatives, antacids, toothpaste, cosmetics and other toiletries, chewing gum, household cleaning solutions, and aerosols. Severe restrictive diets, which may include cessation of eating fruits, tomatoes, nuts, shellfish, chocolate, alcohol, milk, cheese, bread, diet drinks, and junk food, are occassionally recommended by allergists. Most primary care physicians should refer patients to a specialist before instituting such drastic diets or lifestyle changes (see Appendix 6).

B. Pharmacologic Therapy

The H_1 antihistamines are the first line of therapy for urticaria. These antihistamines are H_1-receptor antagonists.

1. **First-Generation Antihistamines**
   First-generation antihistamines such as diphenhydramine, chlorpheniramine, and hydroxyzine can be very effective, especially in acute urticaria (see Appendix 5, Table A5-2, for dose ranges). Diphenhydramine and chlorpheniramine are available OTC and are relatively inexpensive. Hydroxyzine requires a prescription and is more potent than diphenhydramine and chlorpheniramine. These first-generation antihistamines can be sedating. Sedation may be a benefit in reducing pruritus but can pose a danger to persons who drive or operate machinery. Risk-benefit profiles need to be determined for each individual based on their response to the medicine. When urticaria does not resolve quickly, these agents may be limited by their adverse effects, especially daytime sedation and cholinergic-induced dry mouth.

2. **Second-Generation Antihistamines**
   Second-generation H_1 antihistamines, such as fexofenadine, loratadine, desloratadine, and cetirizine are nonsedating and better tolerated for daytime chronic use. Although these medications are more expensive, they play a large role in the management of chronic urticaria.
   a. A systematic review of patients with chronic urticaria demonstrated that nonsedating antihistamines are as effective as sedating antihistamines. The author concluded that "in patients with acute urticaria, effectiveness of antihistamines has not been established with clinical trials, but may be warranted based on clinical experience and experimental evidence. It is reasonable to substitute nonsedating for sedating antihistamines based on conclusions derived from trials in chronic urticaria and experimental urticaria."[6]
   b. To balance the benefits and risks of the different antihistamines it is recommended that clinicians prescribe a first-generation sedating antihistamine at night and a second-generation nonsedating antihistamine during the day. Although this regimen is more complex, it maximizes antihistamine therapeutic effects while minimizing side effects and costs.

3. **Combination Therapy**
   The H_2 antihistamines, such as cimetidine, famotidine, and ranitidine, may be useful in combination with H_1 antihistamines when the urticaria does not respond to the H_1 antihistamines alone. Lin and colleagues showed improved outcomes in patients with acute allergic syndromes, including urticaria, who were treated with both H_1 and H_2 antagonists.[7] However, not all studies have shown an improved outcome when H_2 antihistamines were added to H_1 antihistamines.

4. **Doxepin**
   Doxepin is an antidepressant and an H_1-receptor antagonist as well. Habif states that doxepin is approximately 775 times more potent as an H_1-blocker than diphenhydramine and approximately 56 times more

potent than hydroxyzine.[1] The use of doxepin is limited by the side effects of sedation, lethargy, dry mouth, and constipation. It is best to start doxepin in the evening with a small 10-mg dose. The patient should be warned that he or she will likely feel a bit hung over the first morning. Fortunately, the lethargy and dry mouth decrease rapidly with each daily use. The doxepin dosage can be increased to 25–75 mg before bed. While some sources suggest doses of 10–25 mg three times a day, this schedule is best reserved for patients with severe urticaria who are not working or driving.

5. **Combination Therapy**
Combinations of various antihistamines may be useful in suppressing symptoms. A nonsedating H_1 antihistamine taken during the day can be combined with a sedating H_1 antihistamine and doxepin at night. An H_2 antihistamine can be added to this regimen as well. Occasionally in refractory urticaria, it is necessary to use 2–3 antihistamines simutaneously.

6. **Corticosteroids**
Oral corticosteroids such as prednisone are the most effective medicine for refractory urticaria. Corticosteroids stabilize mast cell membranes and inhibit further histamine release. They also reduce the inflammatory effect of histamine and other mediators. The use of corticosteroids in acute urticaria remains somewhat controversial. Their use generally is limited to more severe, refractory cases. Prednisone is very effective in the treatment of urticaria, but patients need to understand that it has a significant adverse side effect profile.

It may be worth attempting a short course of prednisone, 40 mg/day for 5 days. This can be taken as a single 40-mg dose in the morning with breakfast or as 20 mg bid with meals. While this schedule may control the urticaria temporarily, some patients will experience rebound symptoms once the prednisone is stopped. Physicians and patients will need to discuss the benefits and risks of prednisone. Ideally, prednisone should be tapered and stopped within 2 weeks. On very rare occasions, a punch biopsy may be necessary to identify or verify a disease process that is recalcitrant to therapy.

7. **Epinephrine**
Epinephrine is valuable in treating severe acute urticaria or angioedema, especially if there is a suspicion of airway compromise or anaphylaxis. Subcutaneous epinephrine will result in vasoconstriction of the superficial cutaneous vessels and directly oppose the vasodilatory effect of histamine. Epinephrine has no effect on pruritus but can be lifesaving if there is bronchospasm or airway compromise. An injection of epinephrine solution subcutaneously (SC) or intramuscularly (IM) has a rapid onset of action. The standard adult dose is 0.3–0.5 mL of the 1 : 1000 solution.

Oropharyngeal edema can be treated with a local spray of 2% solution of ephedrine.

8. **Leukotriene Receptor Antagonists**
Leukotriene receptor antagonists are being studied for the treatment of chronic urticaria. Pacor and colleagues performed a double-blind, placebo-controlled comparison of treatment with montelukast and cetirizine in patients with chronic urticaria. These patients had an intolerance to food additives and/or acetylsalicylic acid. They found some benefit with the leukotriene receptor antagonist.[8]

9. **Other Agents**
Other agents that have been used in the treatment of severe refractory urticaria or urticarial vasculitis include methotrexate, colchicine, dapsone, and hydroxychloroquine. In 40% of patients with chronic urticaria, an anti-FRI autoantibody has been identified. These autoantibodies may explain why plasmapheresis, intravenous immune globulins, and cyclosporine may induce remission of disease activity in these patients.[2]

Most primary care physicians should refer patients with severe cases of urticaria or angioedema to a specialist before using these medications. These medications can cause severe side effects. Patients should be made aware of recent data on these less proven therapies.

X. Treatment of Specific Urticarial Syndromes

A. Angioedema

Acute attacks are treated with epinephrine injections, antihistamines, and corticosteroids. IM administration of epinephrine in children results in a faster response than SC administration.[9] Other treatment modalities include parenteral H_1 and/or H_2 antihistamine antagonists and parenteral corticosteroids. Close monitoring of vital signs and oxygen measurements (e.g., pulse oximetry; arterial blood gases) may be necessary. Patients with hereditary or acquired C1 esterase inhibitor deficiency may actually require intubation to overcome a compromised airway. Several EpiPens or Ana-Kits should be prescribed to patients who experience severe anaphylactic reactions so that they have immediate access to epinephrine.

B. Dermatographism

Antihistamines can reduce dermatographism.

C. Pressure Urticaria

Antihistamines may not be helpful but should be tried first. Oral corticosteroids (prednisone) may be the only effective treatment for severe disabling pressure urticaria.

D. Cholinergic Urticaria

Patients with this condition should avoid strenuous exercise when possible. Hydroxyzine, 10–50 mg taken 1 hour before exercise, can diminish the urticaria. If hydroxyzine causes too much sedation, nonsedating H_1 antihistamines may be tried. Showering with hot water may temporarily deplete histamine stores and create a 24-hour refractory period.[1]

E. Cold Urticaria

Avoidance of cold weather and cold water is helpful whenever possible. Severe reactions can occur when patients swim in cold water. The massive transudation of fluid into the skin can lead to hypotension, fainting, shock, and possibly death. Doxepin and cyproheptadine (Periactin) can be effective in suppressing cold urticaria. Cyproheptadine can be used in an oral dose as low as 2 mg once or twice a day.

F. Solar Urticaria

Antihistamines, sunscreens, and graded exposure to increasing amounts of light may be effective therapy.[1]

G. Exercise-Induced Anaphylaxis

Acute treatment of exercise-induced anaphylaxis includes epinephrine injections, antihistamines, airway maintenance, and cardiovascular support as needed. Preventive treatment with H_1 antihistamine before exercise is recommended. Inhaled cromolyn may be used as a mast-cell stabilizer. Avoidance of exercise may not be acceptable. Precipitating foods or medications should be avoided, especially before or after exercise. Tolerance may be induced through regular exercise.[1] Patients should be advised to carry an EpiPen or Ana-Kit at all times, especially while exercising.

H. Pruritic Urticarial Papules and Plaques of Pregnancy

Pruritis can be treated with low-potency topical steroids, H_1 antihistamines (chlorpheniramine, tripelennamine, loratadine, and cetirizine have FDA category B ratings), cool wet compresses, and oatmeal baths. If the itching is intolerable, a short course of prednisone, 40 mg/day, may be considered.

I. Urticarial Vasculitis

After a biopsy diagnosis of urticarial vasculitis is made, the most effective treatment is prednisone, 40–60 mg/day. Other medications reported to be effective are indomethacin (25 mg tid to 50 mg qid), colchicine (0.6 mg two to three times per day), dapsone (up to 200 mg/day), low-dose oral methotrexate, and antimalarial drugs.[1]

J. Urticaria Pigmentosa

The diagnosis and treatment of mastocytosis are complex. If you suspect a patient has cutaneous or systemic mastocytosis, he or she should be referred to a specialist for management.

XI. When to Obtain Consultation

Consultation with or referral to a dermatologist, allergist, immunologist, or rheumatologist may be needed in cases of recurrent angioedema or complicated, recurrent, refractory, severe chronic urticaria.

XII. Practice Guideline

www.jcaai.org/Param/Urticaria.htm
Algorithm from the Joint Task Force on Practice Parameters, published on the web site of the Joint Council on Allergy, Asthma and Immunology

XIII. Internet Resources

www.emedicine.com/emerg/topic628.htm
A chapter on urticaria in the online e-medicine textbook.

dermis.net
An extensive Dermatology Information System (DermIs) from two universities in Germany.

fm.mednet.ucla.edu/derm
An interactive dermatology atlas with over a thousand images that can be searched by many different parameters. This site includes interactive cases and a quiz mode. It was developed by Drs. Usatine and Madden at UCLA.

XIV. ICD-9 Codes

Urticaria	708.9
Allergic	708.0
Non-Allergic	708.1
Idiopathic	708.1
Caused by cold and heat	708.2
Dermatographia	708.3
Vibratory	708.4
Cholinergic	708.5
Chronic	708.8
Angioedema	995.1
Heriditary	277.6

XV. Diagnosis and Management Algorithms

See Figures 5-21, Management of Urticaria and Angioedema, and 5-22, Diagnosis of Angioedema.

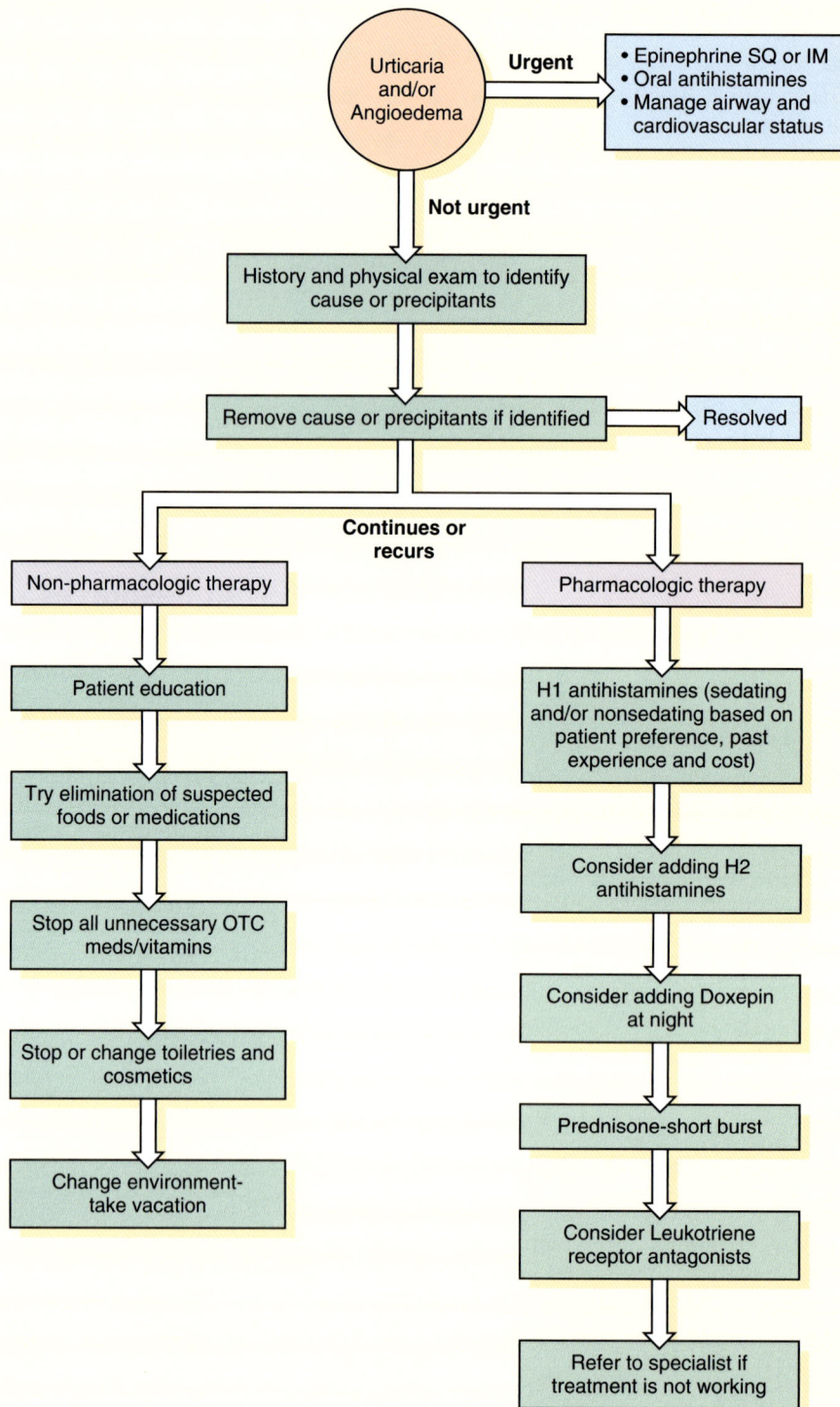

Figure 5-21 Management of urticaria and angioedema.

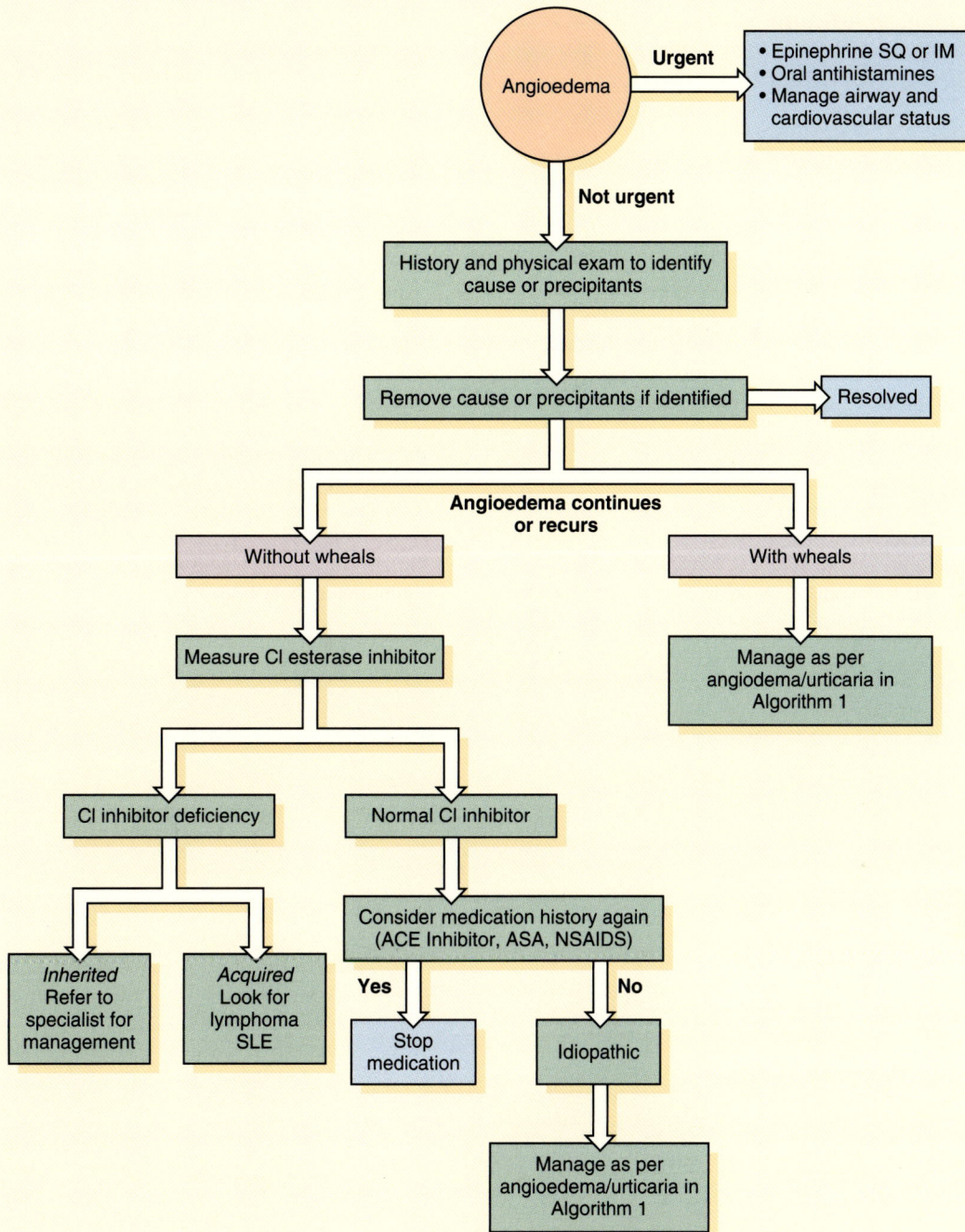

Figure 5-22 Diagnosis of angioedema.

XVI. Patient Education

allergy.mcg.edu/advice/urtic.html
Patient education on urticaria: what can trigger it, types and identification, and treatment from the American College of Allergy, Asthma and Immunology.

www.aad.org/pamphlets/Urticaria.html
Patient education from the American Academy of Dermatology.

Refer to patient education CD, which is provided with this text, for additional patient education information. It has been formatted to provide readily accessible, easy-to-understand handouts for adult patients and the parents of pediatric patients. These handouts can be easily modified to fit specific practice requirements.

REFERENCES

1. Habif T: Clinical Dermatology: A Color Guide to Diagnosis and Therapy, 3rd ed. St. Louis: Mosby, 1996.
2. Fitzpatrick BF, Johnson RA, Wolff K, Suurmond D: Color Atlas and Synopsis of Clinical Dermatology, 4th ed. New York: McGraw-Hill, 2001.
3. Humphreys F, Hunter JA: The characteristics of urticaria in 390 patients. Br J Dermatol 1998;138:635–663.
4. Negro-Alvarez JM, Miralles-Lopez JC: Chronic idiopathic urticaria treatment. Allergol Immunopathol (Madr) 2001;29:129–132.
5. Metcalfe DD: Classification and diagnosis of mastocytosis: Current status. J Invest Dermatol 1991;96:2S–4S.
6. Alper BS: SOAP: Solutions to often asked problems. Choice of antihistamines for urticaria. Arch Fam Med 2000;9: 748–751.
7. Lin RY, Curry A, Pesola GR, et al: Improved outcomes in patients with acute allergic syndromes who are treated with combined H1 and H2 antagonists. Ann Emerg Med 2000;36: 462–468.
8. Pacor ML, Di Lorenzo G, Corrocher R: Efficacy of leukotriene receptor antagonist in chronic urticaria: A double-blind, placebo-controlled comparison of treatment with montelukast and cetirizine in patients with chronic urticaria with intolerance to food additive and/or acetylsalicylic acid. Clin Exp Allergy 2001;31:1607–1614.
9. Simons FE, Roberts JR, Gu X, Simons KJ: Epinephrine absorption in children with a history of anaphylaxis. J Allergy Clin Immunol 1998;101:33–37.

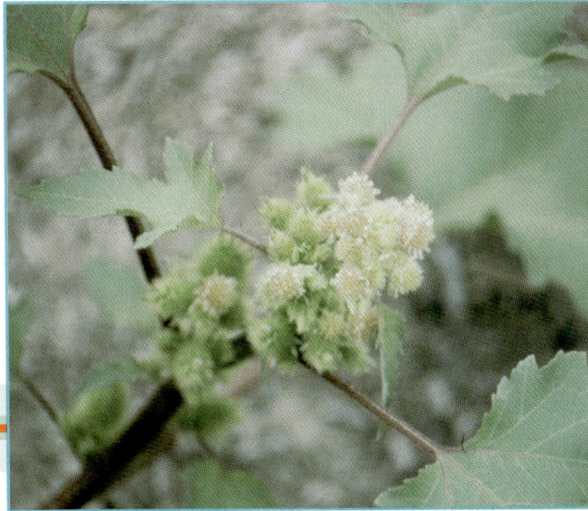

CHAPTER 6
Anaphylaxis

Joe Belleau and Phillip L. Lieberman

I. Introduction

The term *anaphylaxis* refers to a systemic, immediate hypersensitivity reaction resulting from IgE-mediated mast cell or basophil degranulation. This degranulation releases chemicals responsible for the clinical event. The term *anaphylactoid reaction* refers to a clinically similar occurrence not mediated by IgE. In the vast majority of instances the diagnostic approach to and treatment of both disorders are identical, and therefore the terms will be used synonymously in this chapter.

II. Etiology

An etiologic and pathophysiologic classification of anaphylaxis is shown in Box 6-1. This classification lists the most common causes of anaphylaxis and separates them according to the pathophysiologic mechanism of action. The same etiologic agent can cause anaphylaxis through separate pathophysiologic pathways. For example, drugs can cause IgE-mediated anaphylaxis as well as anaphylactoid reactions due to the direct release of mediators from mast cells and basophils without the participation of IgE.

The most common cause of anaphylaxis is food. The most common anaphylasis-provoking food in adults is shellfish; in children it is probably peanuts.

Drugs are the next most common cause of anaphylaxis. Antibiotics are probably the most common drug to produce anaphylactic episodes. Of the drugs, the β-lactam derivatives are the most frequent anaphylaxis culprits. Nonsteroidal anti-inflammatory agents (NSAIDs) are the second most common class of drugs to produce anaphylaxis.

Anaphylaxis can also be caused by physical factors, including exercise and, rarely, cold and sunlight.

Anaphylactic reactions to latex are on the rise because of the increased use of latex gloves in the wake of the AIDS epidemic.

Insect stings and bites have long been a prominent cause of anaphylaxis. Their incidence has probably remained steady over the past five decades, and they still probably account for a small number of deaths annually in the United States. Their importance is accentuated, however, since there is excellent preventive therapy.

In many cases the cause of an anaphylactic event cannot be determined. Often these episodes of unknown

Etiologic and Pathophysiologic Classification of Anaphylaxis and Anaphylactoid Reactions

Anaphylaxis—IgE-mediated reaction
  Food
  Drugs
  Insect bites and stings
  Latex
  Perhaps in some cases, exercise
Anaphylactoid
  Disturbances in arachidonic acid metabolism
    Aspirin
    Nonsteroidal anti-inflammatory drugs
  Immune aggregates
    Gamma globulin
    IgG—anti-IgA
    Possibly protamine, dextran, and albumin
  Direct release of mediators from mast cells and basophils
    Drugs
    Idiopathic
    Exercise
    Physical factors such as cold or sunlight
Miscellaneous and multimediator activity
  Non-antigen-antibody-mediated complement activation
    Radiocontrast material
    Possibly some cases of protamine reactions
    Dialysis membranes
  Activation of contact system
    Dialysis membranes
    Radiocontrast material

etiology are recurrent, and therefore the term *recurrent idiopathic anaphylaxis* has been coined to describe such reactions. In a series of patients presenting to allergists for evaluation after anaphylactic episodes, the incidence of recurrent idiopathic anaphylaxis ranged from 33% to 46%.[1] Thus, idiopathic episodes represent a significant number of anaphylactic events.

III. Epidemiology

The exact incidence of anaphylaxis is unknown. Several studies have attempted to assess the frequency of events. In Ontario, one survey revealed four cases per 10 million population, with two fatalities.[2] It has also been estimated that idiopathic episodes may account for as many as 47,000 cases per year in the United States.[3] A more recent study of cases in Olmstead County, Minnesota, found that the annual incidence rate of anaphylaxis was 21 per 100,000 person-years, with a hospitalization rate of 7% and only one fatality.[4] Regardless of the incidence, since these events are potentially fatal, they represent a significant health problem worldwide.

A. Several factors can affect the incidence. These are noted in Box 6-2.

1. *Atopy*
   For unknown reasons, atopy is a clear risk for anaphylaxis. This is especially true when antigen is administered orally. This risk even extends to those subjects with recurrent idiopathic anaphylaxis.
2. *Sex*
   In most series, female sex is also a risk factor. In some instances this may be due to increased exposure (e.g., nurses with latex anaphylaxis), but in other instances the reason for the preponderance of females in series of anaphylaxis is unknown.
3. *Age*
   Anaphylactic events occur more often in adults than in children. This probably is a function of both increased exposure and maturity of the IgE-mediated realm of the immune response.

B. Both the route and constancy of administration of antigen play a role in the frequency of events. This is of clinical importance.

1. Anaphylaxis has occurred following all routes of administration, including oral, subcutaneous, intramuscular, intravenous, intranasal, intraocular, cutaneous, intravaginal, intrarectal, and intratracheal.
2. However, attacks appear to be more frequent and severe when the agent is injected than when it is ingested. This is of clinical relevance in the prevention of anaphylactic episodes.
3. The constancy of administration of antigen is also important. For example, in most patients with insulin allergy, the anaphylactic reaction does not occur as long as there is uninterrupted administration of the drug. Sensitivity is enhanced when administration becomes intermittent, as, for example, in recurrent glucose intolerance limited to pregnancy.

C. The time elapsing between the original episode and the readministration of antigen plays a role in the frequency of recurrence. The likelihood of a second episode

Factors Affecting the Incidence of Anaphylaxis

Atopy
Sex
Age
Route and constancy of administration of antigen
Time since last reaction

decreases as the time interval between the original event and readministration increases. This is probably due to the catabolism and decreased synthesis of IgE after cessation of antigen exposure.

IV. Clinical Manifestations

The clinical manifestations of anaphylaxis are listed in order of frequency of occurrence in Box 6-3.

A. Time of Symptom Appearance

Symptoms usually begin within 5–30 minutes after the injection of antigen. After oral administration, symptoms usually occur within the first 2 hours, and sometimes within the first 30 minutes. However, there can be a delay of up to 4–6 hours after oral ingestion of antigen. There appears to be a direct relationship between the time of onset of symptoms after the administration of antigen and their severity. That is, the more rapid the onset, the more severe the episode.

B. Signs and Symptoms

1. *Cutaneous*

   Cutaneous signs and symptoms are by far the most frequent manifestations. Urticaria and angioedema, along with pruritus and flush, occur in almost every event. In fact, the absence of cutaneous symptoms suggests a diagnosis other than anaphylaxis. However, on rare occasions, cardiovascular collapse and shock can occur immediately and without any cutaneous or respiratory event.

2. *Respiratory*

   The next most common findings are related to the respiratory tract and consist of shortness of breath and wheezing. Upper airway edema can be responsible for some of these symptoms. Manifestations secondary to hypotension follow respiratory tract symptoms. They include dizziness, syncope, and hypotension.

3. *Gastrointestinal*

   The next most common signs and symptoms occur in the GI system, and include nausea, vomiting, diarrhea, cramping and abdominal pain. GI problems are more frequent when the antigen has been ingested.

4. *Cardiac*

   Cardiac manifestations are varied and can be profound.

   a. Characteristically, anaphylaxis is associated with a compensatory tachycardia that occurs in response to decreased effective vascular volume. This has often been used as a sign to differentiate the anaphylactic episode from a vasodepressor reaction. However, bradycardia, presumably caused by increased vagal activity, can also occur.

   b. Myocardial depression with decreased cardiac output as a result of contractile depression can occur and can persist for several days. This is thought to be due to hypoxemia. In addition, coronary artery vasospasm can occur. This has been documented with coronary angiography. Such vasospasm can result in myocardial infarction, even in the absence of arteriosclerosis.

   c. Shock can be profound. Much of the data regarding the mechanism of production of shock have been obtained through the evaluation of patients experiencing anaphylaxis during cardiac catheterization or anesthesia. During these episodes, hemodynamic measurements have been taken. They have revealed that the major factors causing cardiovascular abnormalities are universal and are due to an initial loss of intravascular fluid and vasodilation, which can be followed shortly by vasoconstriction and then myocardial depression.

   d. Increased vascular permeability can produce a marked and extremely rapid loss of fluid from the vascular space. Fluid shifted to the extravascular space can result in a 50% loss of vascular volume within 10 minutes. The loss of blood volume activates compensatory mechanisms, including the secretion of catecholamines and the conversion of angiotensin I to angiotensin II. This compensatory response is of clinical importance in the patient's recovery, since it can be

---

BOX 6-3

Clinical Manifestations of Anaphylaxis Listed in Order of Frequency of Occurrence

Cutaneous manifestation
    Urticaria
    Angioedema
    Flush
    Pruritus
    Sensation of heat
Dyspnea, wheeze
Dizziness, syncope, hypotension
Gastrointestinal manifestations
    Nausea
    Vomiting
    Diarrhea
    Cramping abdominal pain
Upper airway edema
Headache
Rhinitis
Substernal pain
Seizure

inhibited by β-blockers, angiotensin-converting enzyme (ACE) inhibitors, and angiotensin blockers.

5. Other manifestations include headache, rhinitis, and substernal chest pain. Seizure activity can occur, presumably due to hypotension.

C. Symptom Recurrence

An important clinical feature is the recurrence of symptoms after a relatively asymptomatic period. An episode can abate and then recur several hours after the onset of the original symptoms. Such episodes have been termed *biphasic*. In addition, attacks can be protracted, exhibiting multiple minor remissions followed by recurrent symptoms. Occasionally these recurrent symptoms are crescendo in nature and last several hours. Protracted shock and adult respiratory tract distress syndrome can occur in spite of appropriate therapy, and death can occur at any time during the course of such events.

All of these pathophysiologic events are caused by the release of mast cell and basophil mediators. Some knowledge of these mediators and their activities is important in developing a rational therapy. They are therefore summarized in Table 6-1.

Histamine is perhaps the most important mediator. It exerts its effect by acting both through H_1 and H_2 receptors. This is also of clinical importance, since hypotension, flush, headaches, and excess mucous gland secretion are best treated by a combination of H_1 and H_2 antagonists. The activities of histamine through these receptors are summarized in Box 6-4.

TABLE 6-1

Mast Cell and Basophil Mediators That May Play a Role in Anaphylaxis and Anaphylactoid Reactions

Mediator	Pathophysiologic Event	Possible Clinical Manifestations
Histamine	Acts through H_1, H_2 receptors Increases vascular permeability Vasodilation Contraction of smooth muscle Exocrine gland secretion Sensory nerve stimulation	Flush, urticaria, angioedema, wheeze, hypotension, abdominal cramps, diarrhea
Arachidonic acid metabolites		
Lipoxygenase pathway		
LTB_4	Chemotaxis	Possible role in late-phase response
LTC_4	Contraction of airway smooth muscle	Possible production of wheeze and hypotension
LTD_4	Increased vascular permeability	
Cyclooxygenase pathway	Goblet and mucosal gland secretion	
PGD_2		Flush, hypotension
PGF_2		Possible production of wheeze, myocardial ischemia
Thromboxane A_2	Peripheral vasodilatation Contraction airway smooth muscle Coronary vasoconstriction Goblet, submucosal gland secretion	
Prostaglandin-generating factor of anaphylaxis	Formation of arachidonic acid metabolites of both cyclooxygenase and lipoxygenase pathways	Same as arachidonic acid metabolites above
Platelet-activating factor	Contraction airway smooth muscle Vascular permeability	Wheeze, hypotension
Eosinophil and neutrophil chemotactic factors	Infiltration of and activation of eosinophils and neutrophils	Unclear; theoretically could prolong and intensify reaction, producing late-phase reaction
Tryptase	May activate complement by cleavage of C3 to C3a Cleaves fibrinogen Possibly has kallikrein activity	Unclear; may recruit other pathways of inflammation

Involvement of Histamine Receptors in Anaphylaxis and Anaphylactoid Reactions

H₁ receptor–mediated effects

Vascular permeability
Smooth muscle contraction
Vasodilation
    Endothelial cell relaxing factor (nitric oxide)
    Direct effect
Cardiac effects
    Increased rate of depolarization of sinoatrial node
    Coronary artery vasospasm
Stimulation of nerve endings
    Neuropeptide release
    Pruritus
    Vagal irritant receptors
Increased mucous gland secretion (viscosity)

H₂ receptor–mediated effects

Cardiac effects
    Positive inotropic effects
    Positive chronotropic effects
    Decreased fibrillation threshold
Vasodilation
Mucus glycoprotein secretion from goblet cells and bronchial glands

Require both H₁ and H₂ receptors for maximum effect

Vasodilation
    Hypotension
    Flush
    Headache
Increased mucous gland secretion (amount)

V. Differential Diagnosis

The differential diagnosis of anaphylaxis is summarized in Box 6-5. Clinicians are faced with the differential diagnosis in two settings. The first setting occurs when patients present after the fact. In this instance it must be determined (retrospectively) whether the episode was the result of anaphylaxis or another cause. In the second setting, patients present during an event. In this instance the distinction between anaphylaxis and other causes of shock must be made immediately.

A. Vasodepressor Reaction

The vasodepressor reaction is probably the most common syndrome to mimic anaphylaxis.

1. Vasodepressor reactions are characterized by pallor, weakness, sweating, hypotension, nausea, and occasionally vomiting. They are almost always accompanied by bradycardia (≤60 beats/min). This is one of the most useful differential diagnostic features distinguishing a vasodepressor reaction from an anaphylactic reaction. However, as previously

noted, bradycardia can occasionally during an anaphylactic event.

2. The other important distinguishing feature is the absence of cutaneous symptoms (urticaria, flush, pruritus, angioedema) during a vasodepressor reaction. In vasodepressor reactions the skin is usually pale and there is a cold sweat.

B. Other Forms of Shock

Other forms of shock (hemorrhagic, cardiogenic, and endotoxic) usually present no diagnostic difficulty in that cutaneous symptoms are absent, and accompanying manifestations usually allow clinicians to easily make the distinction between anaphylaxis and these events.

C. Restaurant Syndromes

A number of different events have been grouped under the heading "restaurant syndromes." These reactions can

Differential Diagnosis of Anaphylaxis

Vasodepressor reactions

Other forms of shock
    Hemorrhagic
    Cardiogenic
    Endotoxic

"Restaurant syndromes"

Monosodium glutamate
Scombroidosis
Sulfites

Flush syndromes

Niacin-induced
Carcinoid
Postmenopausal
Chlorpropamide/alcohol
Medullary carcinoma thyroid
Autonomic epilepsy
Idiopathic

Excess endogenous production of histamine syndromes

Systemic mastocytosis
Urticaria pigmentosa
Basophilic leukemia
Acute promyelocytic leukemia (tretinoin treatment)
Hydatid cyst

Nonorganic disease

Panic attacks
Munchausen's stridor
Vocal chord dysfunction syndrome
Globus hystericus

Miscellaneous conditions

Hereditary angioedema
"Red man syndrome" (from vancomycin)

mimic anaphylaxis. They include reactions due to the ingestion of monosodium glutamate (MSG), those due to the ingestion of large amounts of histamine via the ingestion of spoiled fish (scombroidosis), and those due to the ingestion of sulfites.

1. The ingestion of MSG can produce flushing, chest pain, burning of the skin and face, dizziness, sweating, paresthesias, nausea and vomiting, headaches, and palpitations. These symptoms have been referred to as the *Chinese restaurant syndrome*.
   a. The mechanism of production is presumably due to a transient acetylcholinosis secondary to a parasympathetic discharge. Apparently about 14%–20% of the population is susceptible to these events.
   b. The onset of the reactions is no later than 1 hour after the ingestion in most instances, but on occasion reactions can occur up to 14 hours after a meal. It can usually be distinguished from anaphylactic events because there is no urticaria or angioedema.
2. Spoiled fish often contains large amounts of histamine. The histamine is produced by bacterial decarboxylation of histidine during the decay process.
   a. Several bacteria have been incriminated, including *Klebsiella pneumoniae* and *Proteus morgani*.
   b. Symptoms may be identical to those occurring in a true anaphylactic event and consist of flushing, urticaria, angioedema, pruritus, headache, nausea, and vomiting. Anyone eating sufficient quantities of the fish will experience the reaction. Thus, several people eating a meal may be affected. This observation allows the distinction between an anaphylactic event and scombroidosis. Isoniazid appears to make individuals more susceptible to these events.
3. The importance of sulfites as the cause of anaphylactic-like episodes has diminished with the reduction of the use of these agents to preserve foods on salad bars. However, sulfites are still found in high concentration in certain foods, such as pickles, gelatin, wine, fruit juices, sausages, dried fruits, and shellfish. Susceptible individuals will experience flushing, bronchospasm, and occasionally hypotension. Once again, however, there is no urticaria or angioedema.

D. Flushing Syndromes

The flushing syndromes can mimic anaphylaxis. Entities that produce flush should be considered in the differential diagnosis. These include carcinoid syndrome, postmenopausal flush, chlorpropamide-alcohol-induced flush, flush associated with medullary carcinoma of the thyroid, and, rarely, autonomic epilepsy. In most instances, however, the cause of the flush cannot be determined. In such instances the flush is often termed *recurrent idiopathic flush reaction*.

1. One of the entities listed under flush syndrome has become increasingly more frequent with the incorporation of niacin into self-prescribed or physician-prescribed treatment programs.
   a. Niacin can produce a flush accompanied by a sensation of heat and prickling of the skin that can be described by patients as burning and itching.
   b. The niacin flush can occur within minutes or up to hours after the ingestion of a niacin-containing preparation, depending on the pharmacokinetic properties of the tablet, specifically its timed-release or immediate-release features. The diagnosis is established at the time of history and is confirmed by the cessation of events after discontinuation of the niacin ingestion.
2. It is not surprising that the carcinoid syndrome can produce anaphylactic-like symptoms, since carcinoid tumors (as well as medullary carcinoma of the thyroid) can secrete histamine, kallikrein, neuropeptides, and prostaglandins. Patients with carcinoid syndrome have flushing, diarrhea, abdominal pain, wheezing, and cardiovascular distress.
3. Up to 50% of patients with postmenopausal flush experience the flush over the face, neck, upper chest, and breasts. It usually lasts 3–5 minutes and can reoccur several times daily. It is aggravated by alcohol and stress. There is no pruritus and no other manifestation of anaphylaxis.
4. Sulfonylurea agents, especially chlorpropamide, can produce a flush when ingested with alcohol. This can be associated with hypoglycemia and all of its accompanying symptoms. The reaction usually begins about 3–5 minutes after the ingestion of alcohol and peaks within 15 minutes. There is no pruritus, urticaria, or fall in blood pressure.
5. Autonomic epilepsy is a rare disease thought to be due to paroxysmal autonomic discharges. There can be a fall in blood pressure, tachycardia, flush, and syncope.

E. Excess Production of Histamine

Several diseases are associated with the excess endogenous production of histamine. These include systemic mastocytosis, urticaria pigmentosa, basophilic leukemia, acute promyelocytic leukemia treated with tretinoin, and hydatid cysts that rupture. The manifestations of all of these are identical to those of anaphylaxis since the mediators are identical.

F. Nonorganic Syndromes

Nonorganic syndromes are an important component of the differential diagnosis. Panic attacks, Munchausen's stridor, vocal cord dysfunction, and globus hystericus have all been confused with anaphylaxis in the past. There are case reports describing each of these in that context.

1. *Undifferentiated somatoform anaphylaxis* is a term used to describe this group of patients who present with these disorders. Such episodes can be involuntary, as with panic attacks and the vocal cord dysfunction syndrome, or they can be consciously self-induced, as with Munchausen's stridor.
2. Panic attacks are accompanied by tachycardia, flushing, shortness of breath, and GI symptoms.
3. Vocal cord dysfunction syndrome and Munchausen's stridor have similar presentations. The former is due to an involuntary adduction of the vocal cords, occluding the glottic opening. The latter is due to an intentional adduction of the cords. In both instances there is obstruction of respiration on both inspiration and expiration, with accentuation on inspiration. In the former, patients are unaware of the process.

G. Hereditary Angioedema

Episodes of hereditary angioedema, or "red man syndrome," may rarely be confused with anaphylaxis produced by the administration of vancomycin. In hereditary angioedema there is no urticaria, but some individuals with this disorder can exhibit an accompanying evanescent serpiginous erythema that lasts for the first 24 hours of the event. However, there is no pruritus, and the skin lesions usually are not elevated above the skin surface. Red man syndrome can result from histamine release and therefore can mimic anaphylaxis, but there is usually no pruritus or urticaria. It is more closely related to the flush syndromes.

VI. Physical Examination

The physical examination of a patient with anaphylaxis is not challenging. Clinicians should first assess the airways and then the blood pressure and pulse. Of course, cutaneous manifestations are easily seen. However, the degree of urticaria, angioedema, or flush may not correlate with the severity of the reaction. Note should be taken of any arrhythmia, and the vital signs should be monitored frequently during therapy. There are no particularly distinguishing features other than those previously noted.

VII. Laboratory Evaluation

A. Mediators

The differential diagnosis can be assisted via measurement of mediators. If carcinoid syndrome is suspected, serum serotonin and urinary 5-hydroxyindole acetic acid (5-HIAA) should be measured. If a patient is seen shortly after an anaphylactic episode, plasma and urinary histamine or histamine metabolites and serum tryptase determinations may be helpful. Plasma histamine levels begin to rise between 5 and 10 minutes and remain elevated up to 60 minutes. They are of little help if the patient is seen an hour after the event. However, urinary histamine and its metabolites can be elevated for a longer duration and thus might be useful. Serum tryptase levels peak 1 to $1^{1}/_{2}$ hours after the onset of symptoms and persist longer than plasma histamine levels. Elevated tryptase levels may be found as long as 5 hours after the onset of symptoms. Therefore, serum tryptase may be extremely useful in establishing the diagnosis. The best time to measure serum tryptase is between 1 and 2 hours after the onset of symptoms. It is usually of no benefit if measured after 6 hours. The best time to measure plasma histamine is 10 minutes to 1 hour after the onset of symptoms. There may be a disjunction between the histamine and tryptase levels, with some patients exhibiting an elevation of only one of these mediators. It can also be beneficial to obtain serum to identify specific IgE against suspected agents (see Chapter 13, RAST).

B. ECG Abnormalities

A number of different electrocardiographic (ECG) abnormalities can occur. Such ECG abnormalities include S-T segment elevation, flattening and inversion of T waves, and arrhythmias. Transient elevation of cardiac enzymes can also occur.

C. Blood Gas Measurement

Pulse oximetry can reveal desaturation, and blood gases can show a fall in PO_2 and PCO_2 early in the course. If severe respiratory difficulty supervenes, hypoxia worsens and elevation of PCO_2 can occur. The pH will vary with CO_2 retention and with the later onset of metabolic acidosis should cardiovascular failure occur.

D. Allergy Testing

Allergy skin testing and/or in vitro testing can be helpful in determining the etiologic agent in some instances. This is especially true in atopic individuals. Chapters 12 and 13 cover this topic in greater detail.

VIII. Approach to Diagnosis

In the absence of confirmatory elevations of histamine or tryptase, the diagnosis of anaphylaxis is established purely on the basis of the clinical impression. The diagnosis is easily established by history and physical examination, with the laboratory studies noted previously being confirmatory. Rarely, the entities noted previously, especially vasodepressor reactions or flush syndromes, present the clinician with a diagnostic dilemma.

IX. Therapy and Management

Therapy and management can be divided into prevention of anaphylactic events and treatment of acute events. In addition, the measures used to prevent anaphylactic episodes can be divided into general and patient-specific measures. The preventive measures are listed in Box 6-6.

Many of the procedures used to prevent anaphylactic episodes are self-evident. A thorough history should be taken to identify any form of drug allergy, which also requires knowledge of immunologic and biochemical cross-reactivity between drugs. All medications should be checked for proper labeling because individuals presenting with anaphylactic events may have mistakenly taken an incorrect drug. In such instances clinicians should ask patients to bring all drugs to the office to check containers for proper contents.

A. Drugs should be administered orally rather than parenterally if possible. As noted, anaphylaxis is more frequent and more severe with parenteral administration. When parenteral administration is necessary, patients should be kept in the office for 20–30 minutes after injection.

B. Certain patients are at risk for anaphylactic episodes. These patients include hymenoptera-sensitive subjects, latex-sensitive subjects, and subjects with recurrent, idiopathic anaphylaxis. These individuals should wear an identifying Medic-Alert bracelet or necklace (Medic-Alert, 2323 Colorado Ave., Turlock, CA 95382) and should keep identification cards listing their allergies in their wallet or purse. All such patients should keep a self-injection kit of epinephrine on their person. Such kits are available in two forms: Ana-Kit, where patients must learn to inject the medication, and EpiPen, which has an automatic injector mechanism triggered by pressure. Some patients should be given more than one kit because they either need more than one injection or because they have a tendency to forget to carry the kit. Kits should be placed in strategic areas such as automobiles, homes, and offices. It is essential that trained personnel, either clinicians or a designated substitute, teach the injection of epinephrine to the patient. Each epinephrine injection kit comes with specific instructions, and use of the kit should be demonstrated in person.

C. Patients at risk for anaphylaxis should avoid drugs that would enhance a reaction, increase its severity, or complicate its therapy. These agents include β-adrenergic blockers, ACE inhibitors, angiotensin-blocking agents, monoamine oxidase inhibitors (MAOIs), and certain tricyclic antidepressants.

1. β-adrenergic blocking agents inhibit the activity of epinephrine and can enhance hypotension due to blockade of the compensatory mechanism of endogenous catechol release. ACE inhibitors and angiotensin-blocking agents also prevent the compensatory response.
2. There is an endogenous conversion of angiotensin I to angiotensin II during an anaphylactic event. This conversion is an important mechanism to maintain blood pressure. Both MAOIs and tricyclic antidepressants can increase a patient's sensitivity to epinephrine therapy and produce an exaggerated hypertensive response. This can be dangerous, especially in an elderly patient with arteriosclerotic vascular disease. MAOIs prevent the catabolism of epinephrine, and tricyclic antidepressants prevent the reuptake of catechols into peripheral nerve endings.

D. Occasionally, patients must undergo a procedure or receive a medication that places them at risk. The classic example is a patient who has had a previous reaction to radiocontrast media and must receive this agent again for diagnostic purposes. A standard pretreatment protocol exists for such circumstances (Box 6-7). This protocol has been successfully used to prevent reactions during plasma

---

BOX 6-6

Measures to Reduce the Risk of Anaphylactic Episodes

General

Obtain thorough history to identify drug allergy.

Avoid drugs that have immunologic or biochemical cross-reactivity with any agents to which the patient is sensitive.

Check all drugs for proper labeling.

Administer drugs orally rather than parenterally when possible.

When parenteral administration is necessary, keep patients in the office 20–30 minutes after injections.

For patients at risk

Have patients wear Medic-Alert bracelet or necklace and carry identification card.

Teach self-injection of epinephrine and advise patients to keep epinephrine kits with them.

Avoid prescribing β-adrenergic-blocking agents, ACE inhibitors, angiotensin blockers, MAO inhibitors, and tricyclic antidepressants.

Use preventive techniques, including pretreatment, provocation challenge, and desensitization, when patients are required to undergo a procedure or receive an agent that places them at risk (see text).

ACE = angiotensin converting enzyme; MAO = monoamine oxidase

BOX 6-7

Prevention of Anaphylactic Reactions to Radiocontrast and Other Agents

Document the need for the study.

Obtain informed consent.

Pretreat with:

Prednisone, 50 mg orally, 13, 7, and 1 hour before procedure.

Diphenhydramine, 50 mg intramuscularly, 1 hour before procedure.

Ephedrine sulfate (when not contraindicated because of cardiovascular disease), 25 mg orally, 1 hour before procedure.

Use a low-osmolar radiocontrast agent in cases of radiocontrast readministration.

Discontinue, if possible, β-adrenergic-blocking agents, ACE inhibitors, angiotensin blockers, MAO inhibitors, and tricyclic antidepressants.

Use an H_2 antagonist (cimetidine, 300 mg, or ranitidine, 300 mg, orally) 2–3 hours before the procedure (optional).

ACE = angiotensin converting enzyme; MAO = monoamine oxidase

---

exchange, fluorescein administration, and in patients with cold urticaria who must undergo coronary bypass surgery. However, it has not been effective in preventing perioperative anaphylaxis in patients with latex allergy.

E. Individuals experiencing anaphylaxis to hymenoptera stings should be evaluated by an allergist and in appropriate instances should receive desensitization with hymenoptera venom. Chapter 9 covers this topic in greater detail.

F. The treatment of an *acute episode* is summarized in Box 6-8.

Therapy can be divided into those actions that are taken immediately and those that are initiated after evaluation. An important principle in managing an acute episode is rapid recognition.

1. After recognition, the immediate events are carried out rapidly. They consist of checking the airway, a rapid evaluation of the level of consciousness, and an evaluation of vital signs.

2. Once the diagnosis is established, epinephrine is administered without further hesitation, and the patient is placed in the supine position with the legs elevated unless the patient is having difficulty breathing or is wheezing severely. Oxygen should be administered simultaneously with these actions.

3. Some authorities recommend placing a tourniquet proximal to the injection site if the antigen was administered by injection. If this is done, the tourniquet should be released every 5–10 minutes to ensure blood flow.

4. Other authorities recommend injecting a small dose of epinephrine (0.1–0.2 mL of 1:1000 preparation) at the site of injection of antigen.

   a. Epinephrine is the drug of choice for all cases of anaphylaxis, and as noted, must be administered immediately. The adult dose is 0.3–0.5 mL (0.3–0.5 mg of a 1:1000 aqueous solution), and the pediatric dose is 0.01 mL/kg of the same 1:1000 solution.

   b. All injections should be injected intramuscularly (IM). This route is superior to subcutaneous (SC) administration.[5]

   c. Intravenous (IV) administration should be avoided whenever possible. It is indicated only for life-threatening reactions not responding to the IM route. For IV administration, 1 mL of the 1:1000 solution is diluted in 10 mL of saline to obtain a 1:10,000 concentration. Doses of 0.1–0.2 mL can be given by IV bolus every 5–20 minutes, depending on the patient's response.

G. *Cardiovascular collapse* is the second most frequent cause of death, after airway obstruction. Therefore, if hypotension is still present after the administration of epinephrine, attention should be given to the administration of IV fluids.

1. Hypotension can be severe and resistant to therapy, especially in patients who have been taking β-blockers. As previously discussed, hypotension is due

BOX 6-8

Treatment of Anaphylaxis

Immediate action

Assessment

Check airway and secure if needed.

Rapidly assess level of consciousness.

Assess vital signs.

Treatment

Give epinephrine.

Place patient in the supine position with legs elevated.

Give oxygen.

If the antigen (or other causal agent) has been injected, place a tourniquet proximal to the injection site.

Evaluation-dependent options

Peripheral intravenous fluids

H_1 and H_2 antagonist

Vasopressors

Corticosteroids

Glucagon or atropine

Electrocardiographic monitoring

Hospitalization

to a shift of fluid from the intravascular to the extravascular space. This event appears to be more significant than vasodilation in causing hypotension.

    a. Fluids are necessary to restore intravascular volume in hypotensive patients not responding to epinephrine. This is best accomplished by rapid administration of large volumes of colloid- or crystalloid-containing fluids.

    b. The most important aspect of fluid therapy is the volume administered. Large volumes of lactated Ringer's solution or normal saline should be given rapidly at a rate of 5–10 mL/kg in an adult in the first 5 minutes. Children should receive up to 30 mL/kg of crystalloid solution in the first hour.

  2. An alternative to crystalloid therapy is the colloid, hydroxyethyl starch.

H. Greater volumes may be necessary in patients who have been taking a β-adrenergic agent.

I. Vasopressors can be administered simultaneously. The drug of choice is dopamine, which should be administered at a rate of 2–20 μg/kg/min and titrated according to the recorded blood pressure.

J. In patients taking β-adrenergic-blocking agents, both the blood pressure and pulse may be resistant to epinephrine and vasopressor therapy. These patients can experience refractory hypotension and bradycardia. In such instances atropine can be used for the bradycardia and glucagon can be used to stimulate chronotropic and inotropic cardiac activity. Atropine sulfate can be injected IM in a dose of 0.3–0.5 mg every 10 minutes, to a maximum of 2 mg. The cardiac activity of glucagon is not dependent on the β-receptor. The dose of glucagon is 1–5 mg IV as a bolus, followed by an infusion of 5–15 μg/min, titrated according to the clinical response.

K. Antihistamines control cutaneous symptoms and can be helpful in the treatment of hypotension as well. The combined use of an H_1 and an H_2 antagonist is superior to use of an H_1 antagonist alone for the treatment of headache, hypotension, flush, and urticaria. Diphenhydramine, 25–50 mg, can be given IM or IV, and ranitidine, 1 mg/kg, or cimetidine, 4 mg/kg, can be given IV.

L. Corticosteroids do not exert an immediate effect; however, they may be indicated for two reasons. They increase the availability of β-receptors, and they ameliorate the events that occur in the late-phase or recurrent response.

M. Wheezing that is refractory to epinephrine can be treated with inhaled albuterol.

The patient should be transferred to a hospital when fluids or IV vasopressors are needed.

There is no standard observation period after an anaphylaxis event. It would seem reasonable that patients should be observed for 2 hours after a mild event and up to 24 hours after a severe event. Although there is no established definition of mild or severe, an event can be considered mild if there is an immediate response to epinephrine without hypotension. An observation period is required because of the possibility of a biphasic reaction or a protracted reaction, as previously described.

X. Special Considerations in Patient Subsets

Exercise-Induced Anaphylaxis

Exercise-induced anaphylaxis is rare. Patients are usually well-trained athletes who experience symptoms with vigorous exercise. Symptoms do not always occur each time they exercise, and the same duration and level of physical exertion may not always reproduce the same reaction.

  1. The first signs are fatigue, diffuse warmth, pruritus, and urticaria. Without treatment, patients may develop angioedema, laryngeal edema, nausea, vomiting, and vascular collapse.

  2. The exact cause has not yet been determined, although in a subset of these individuals consumption of a food prior to exercising is a contributing factor.

  3. Patients with exercise-induced anaphylaxis can be categorized as having either food-dependent or food-independent reactions.

  4. Patients who suffer from this condition can exercise without any apparent reaction as long as they refrain from food for several hours prior to exercise.

  5. Persons with food-dependent exercise-induced anaphylaxis are more likely to have a personal and family history of atopic disease and are skin prick test positive to the provoking item. However, they are usually asymptomatic when ingesting the food without exercise, or vice versa.

  6. Unlike individuals with cholinergic urticaria, patients with exercise-induced anaphylaxis do not experience symptoms under stress, during a hot shower, or with an increase in body temperature.

  7. Prophylactic medications have not been shown to be useful in controlling symptoms in this disorder. Therefore, general guidelines suggest that exercise should be discontinued at the first indication of symptoms. Affected individuals should refrain from eating 4–6 hours prior to exercise, always carry a self-injectable epinephrine preparation, and exercise with a partner.

XI. When to Obtain Consultation

Any patient who has experienced an episode of anaphylaxis of unknown etiology should be referred for an allergy evaluation.

XII. Practice Guidelines

Practice guidelines for therapy and management can be found in the Joint Task Force on Practice Parameters (www.jcaai.org/param/anaphylaxis.htm). There is variability on what in-office equipment should be required for proper treatment of anaphylaxis; position papers have been published but there is still no general consensus on this issue.[6-9] Box 6-9 provides a compilation list of equipment based on these statements. The Joint Task Force is the most consistent statement to date.[9]

BOX 6-9

Equipment and Medication to Treat Anaphylaxis in Office

Primary
Tourniquet
1-mL and 5-mL disposable syringes
Oxygen tank and mask/nasal prongs
Epinephrine solution (aqueous) 1:1000 (1-mL ampules and multidose vials)
Epinephrine solution (aqueous) 1:10,000 (commercially available preloaded intrinsic asthma syringe)
Diphenhydramine injectable
Ranitidine or cimetidine injectable
Injectable corticosteroids
Ambu-bag, oral airway, laryngoscope, endotracheal tube, No. 12 needle
Intravenous setup with large-bore catheter
IV fluids: 2000 mL crystalloid, 1000 mL hydroxyethyl starch
Aerosol β_2 bronchodilator and compressor nebulizer
Glucagon
Electrocardiogram
Normal saline, 10-mL vial, for epinephrine dilution

Supporting
Suction apparatus
Dopamine
Sodium bicarbonate
Aminophylline
Atropine
IV setup with needles, tape, and tubing
Nonlatex gloves

Optional
Defibrillator
Calcium gluconate
Neuroleptics for seizures
Lidocaine

XIII. Internet Resources

www.aafa.org
Asthma and Allergy Foundation of America

www.aaai.org
American Academy of Allergy, Asthma and Immunology

allergy.mcg.edu
American College of Allergy, Asthma and Immunology

www.vivra.com
Vivra Asthma and Allergy Group

foodallergy.org
Food Allergy Network

www.immune.com/allergy/allabc.html
Allergy Internet Resources

www.national-jewish.org
Allergy Internet National Jewish Medical and Research Center

XIV. ICD-9 Code

995.0   Anaphylaxis

XV. Diagnosis and Management Algorithm *(Fig. 6-1)*

XVI. Patient Education Materials and Handouts

Anaphylaxis is a generalized allergic response to a substance that has entered the body. The most common route of entry is ingestion, but anaphylaxis can occur after injections, eyedrops, suppositories, or even creams or ointments placed on abraded skin.

Symptoms occur shortly (usually within minutes) after the substance enters the body. The most common symptoms are:

- Flushing and a sensation of heat; itching; and the appearance of welts (hives) or swelling (angioedema) on the lips, eyes, hands, or feet
- Wheezing, coughing, and shortness of breath
- A sensation of dizziness or loss of consciousness
- Nausea, vomiting, and diarrhea

The most common causes of anaphylaxis are foods and drugs. In adults, the most common food to produce an anaphylactic reaction is shellfish, and the most common food in children is peanuts. However, anaphylaxis can occur in response to any food. Other common offenders are milk, eggs, and tree nuts.

The most common drugs to cause anaphylaxis are antibiotics. The next most common are nonsteroidal antiinflammatory drugs (NSAIDs). These drugs are taken to

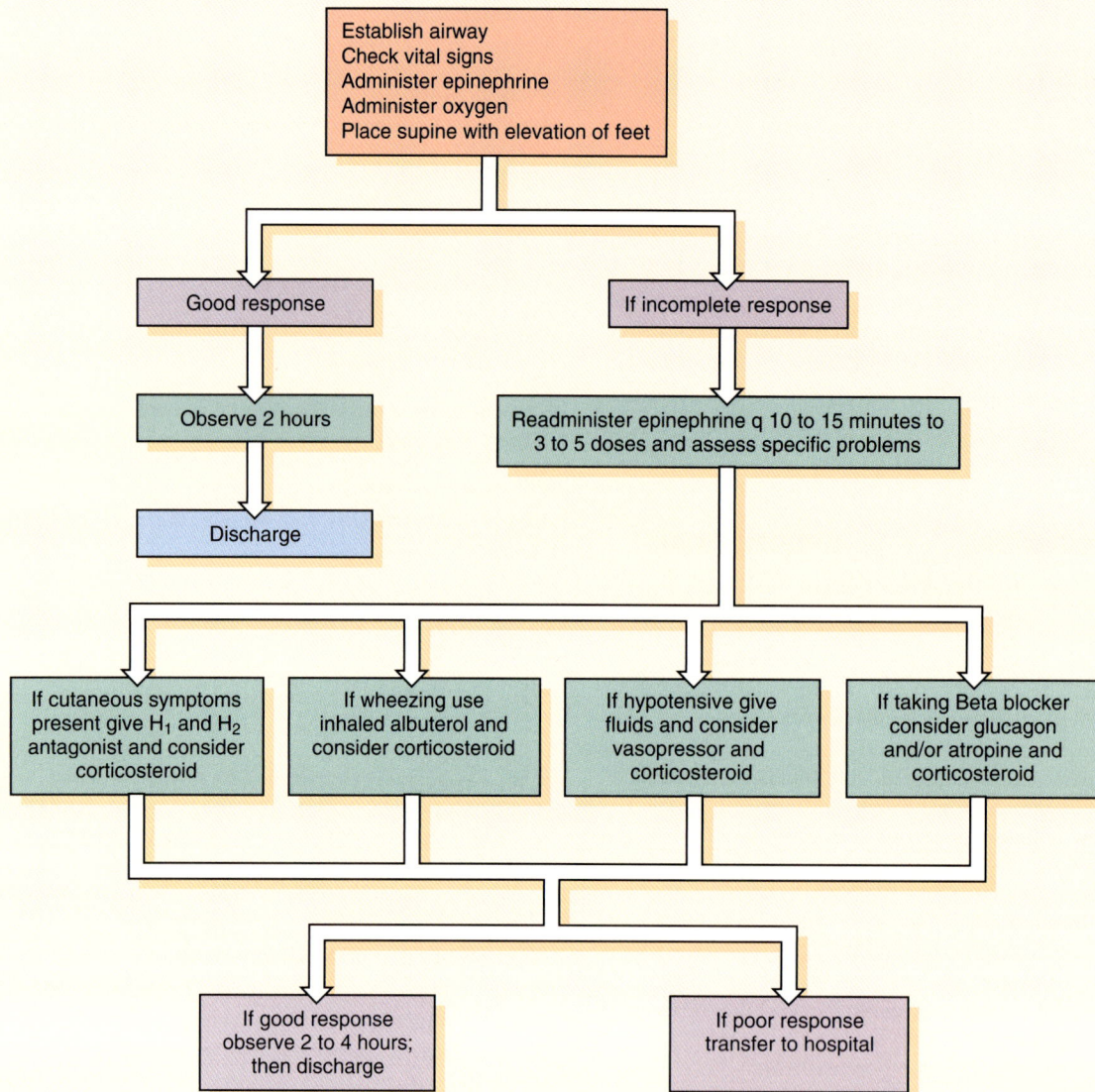

Figure 6-1 Algorithm for management of anaphylaxis in the office: Immediate actions.

treat pain or inflammation such as occurs in arthritis. They include aspirin, ibuprofen (Advil), Nuprin, naproxen (Naprosyn), and many others.

Other common causes of anaphylaxis are insect stings and bites, and latex (rubber).

Individuals who are subject to anaphylactic reactions should always keep epinephrine with them. Epinephrine can be prescribed by your clinician in a kit that can be easily self-administered. Your clinician and assigned personnel can instruct you in the use of such a kit. Common

names for such kits are EpiPen and Ana-Kit. There are others available as well.

In addition, patients subject to anaphylactic episodes should wear a Medic-Alert bracelet or necklace and carry an identification card in their wallet or purse listing their allergies. You can write for a Medic-Alert bracelet or necklace to: Medic-Alert, 2323 Colorado Ave., Turlock, CA 95382.

Also, patients subject to such events should in many instances avoid drugs that might further predispose them to an episode or make such an episode more difficult to treat. Drug classes that might do this are:

- β-blockers
- Angiotensin-converting enzyme inhibitors (ACE inhibitors)
- ACE blockers
- Monoamine oxidase inhibitors (MAOIs) and tricyclic antidepressants

Your physician can assist you in identifying drugs that might increase your risk of an event.

Refer to patient education CD, which is provided with this text, for additional patient education information. It has been formatted to provide readily accessible, easy-to-understand handouts for adult patients and the parents of pediatric patients. These handouts can be easily modified to fit specific practice requirements.

REFERENCES

1. Lieberman P: Anaphylaxis. In Kaliner M (ed): Current Review of Allergic Diseases, vol I, pp 133–141. Philadelphia: Blackwell Science/Current Medicine, 1999.
2. Orange RP, Donsky GJ: Anaphylaxis. In Middleton E Jr, Reed CE, Ellis EF (eds): Allergy: Principles and Practice, p 564. St. Louis: Mosby, 1978.
3. Patterson R, Hogan M, Yarnold P: Idiopathic anaphylaxis. Arch Intern Med 1995;155:869–871.
4. Yocum MW, Butterfield J, Klein J, et al: Epidemiology of anaphylaxis in Olmstead County: A population-based study. J Allergy Clin Immunol 1999;104:452–456.
5. Gu X, Simons FER, MacNair KR: Epinephrine absorption after different routes of administration (abstract). J Allergy Clin Immunol 1999;103:S554.
6. American Academy of Pediatrics Committee on Drugs: Anaphylaxis. Pediatrics 1973;51:136–140.
7. Journal of Allergy and Clinical Immunology: Position statement. J Allergy Clin Immunol 1986;77:271–273.
8. Journal of Allergy and Clinical Immunology: Position statement: Guidelines to minimize the risk from systemic reactions caused by immunotherapy with allergen extracts. J Allergy Clin Immunol 1994;93:811–812.
9. Joint Task Force on Practice Parameters: The diagnosis and treatment of anaphylaxis. Allergy Clin Immunol 1998;S428–S465.

OTHER SUGGESTED READING

Lieberman P: Anaphylaxis: How to quickly narrow the differential diagnosis. J Respir Dis 1999;20:221–231.
Lieberman P: Anaphylaxis: Tips on prevention and management. J Respir Dis 1999;20:309–316.
Lieberman P: Anaphylaxis and anaphylactoid events. In Middleton E Jr, Reed CE, Ellis EF, Adkinson F Jr., Yunginger JW, and Busse W. (eds): Allergy: Principles and Practice, 5th ed, vol II, pp 1079–1092. St. Louis: Mosby, 1998.
Lieberman P: Anaphylaxis. In Allergic Diseases: Diagnosis and Treatment, pp 47–64. Humana Press, 1997.
Lieberman P: Specific and idiopathic anaphylaxis: Pathophysiology and treatment. In Bierman W, Pearlman D, Shapiro G, Busse W (eds): Allergy, Asthma and Immunology from Infancy to Adulthood, 3rd ed, pp 297–320. Philadelphia: WB Saunders, 1996.

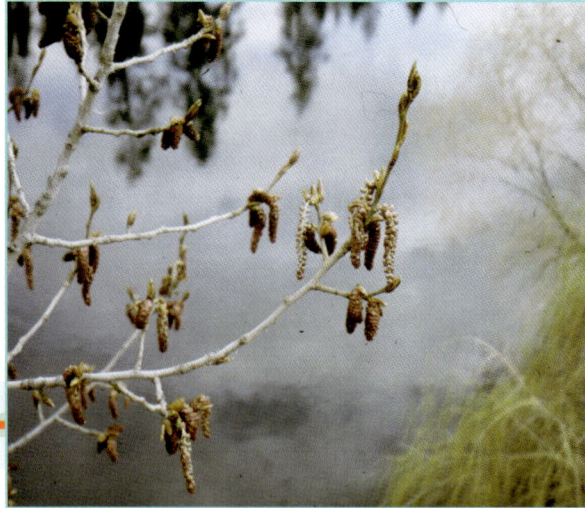

Common Cottonwood Courtesy of Hollister-Stier Laboratory

CHAPTER 7
Food Allergy

Ricardo A. Tan

I. Introduction

Technology and progress have made available to the ordinary consumer foods from all over the world. As people are exposed to new foods, additives, and preservatives, an increasing number of symptoms and conditions with unclear causes are being attributed to food. The term *food allergy* is frequently used by laypeople as well as health care practitioners to refer to a wide range of adverse experiences perceived to be induced by food. This often leads to confusion or misconceptions about the nature of and approach to food-related symptoms. The European Academy of Allergy and Clinical Immunology classification recommends the term *adverse food reaction* to refer to any adverse experience associated with food ingestion.[1] An adverse reaction is *nontoxic* if only certain individuals are susceptible to it and *toxic* if it occurs in all exposed individuals. A food allergy or hypersensitivity is a nontoxic reaction with an *immunologic* mechanism. A food intolerance is also nontoxic but has a *nonimmunologic* mechanism. Food intolerance probably accounts for the majority of cases of food-related complaints (Box 7-1). Food allergy can have an IgE-mediated, non-IgE-mediated, or mixed mechanism. Also known as immediate-type hypersensitivity, IgE-mediated

reactions are the type of food allergy most patients seek treatment for.

II. Etiology

Every growing infant or child has the ability to develop oral tolerance or immunologic unresponsiveness to each new food antigen that he or she ingests orally. This is essential to prevent the immune system from reacting adversely every time one eats.

A. Mechanism

The mechanism is not completely understood but involves both the T- and B-cell systems and may involve clonal anergy, clonal deletion, and active suppression by CD8+ T-cells.[2]

1. Oral tolerance, in certain individuals, does not develop to a food antigen. Instead, the infant or child could become sensitized, develop food-specific IgE, and later exhibit allergic responses on subsequent reexposure to the specific food.[2]

2. The development of IgG, IgM, and IgA antibodies is part of the normal response to food antigens and does not indicate food allergy.[3]

BOX 7-1

Classification of Adverse Food Reactions

1. Toxic (e.g., *Salmonella* toxin, tuna scombroid poisoning)
2. Nontoxic
   Food intolerance (nonimmunologic mechanism) (e.g., caffeine, lactose intolerance)
   Food allergy or hypersensitivity (immunologic mechanism)
   IgE-mediated (e.g., peanut allergy, shrimp allergy)
   Mixed IgE- and non-IgE-mediated (e.g., allergic eosinophilic gastroenteritis)
   Non-IgE-mediated (e.g., dietary protein enterocolitis)

3. Important factors influencing the appearance of food allergy include a personal or family history of atopy, the integrity of the intestinal barrier, and the timing of exposure to foods.[4]
4. Breast-feeding: Several studies have suggested that breast-feeding can help prevent food allergy and enhance oral tolerance by lowering early exposure to foreign proteins and strengthening the infant's intestinal barrier and immune system with maternal IgA and other soluble factors in breast milk.[5,6]

B. IgE-Mediated

Sensitization to or prduction of IgE directed to a specific food occurs when a predisposed individual is first exposed to that food allergen. Specific IgE then attaches primarily to the surface of mast cells, basophils, and macrophages in the skin, respiratory tract, and gastrointestinal (GI) tract. Reexposure to the food allergen will cause cross-linking of IgE molecules on the mast cell surface and lead to release of histamine and other inflammatory mediators, which produce symptoms ranging from urticaria and sneezing to bronchospasm and anaphylaxis. IgE-mediated reactions are also referred to as immediate or type I hypersensitivity reactions.

C. Mixed and Non-IgE-Mediated Reactions

These are rare conditions that most commonly involve infiltration of the walls of the GI tract with eosinophils, lymphocytes, and other inflammatory cells. Type II to IV hypersensitivity may also be involved. Abdominal cramps, vomiting, and nausea are common symptoms. Results of serum and skin testing for food-specific IgE are usually negative. These disorders include *food-induced enterocolitis* and *proctocolitis,* which occur in infants; and *allergic eosinophilic gastroenteritis* and *celiac disease* (*gluten-sensitive enteropathy*), which may occur later.[7–10]

D. Cross-Reactivity with Other Allergens

Cross-reactivity between foods and pollen is most likely due to shared or homologous proteins.[11] Examples of this phenomenon include mugwort pollen cross-reacting with kiwi, apple, and celery,[12] and birch pollen cross-reacting with carrot, potato, and celery.[13] Latex has also been found to cross-react with avocado, banana, chestnut, and kiwi.[12]

E. Food Allergy and Atopic Dermatitis

Food allergies can be present and be a contributing factor in approximately one-third of cases of atopic dermatitis in children.[14] In up to 90% of younger children under 2 years of age with atopic dermatitis, food allergy can be an important trigger.[15] In adults, food allergy is usually not a major trigger or aggravating factor for atopic dermatitis.

III. Epidemiology

Approximately 2% of adolescents and adults and 2%–5% of children in the United States are estimated to have food allergies.[2] Infants have the highest prevalence of food allergy at 7%–8%.[16] The majority of food allergies start in childhood. Most children lose or "outgrow" their food hypersensitivity by 3 years of age.[17] Most food allergies can resolve with at least 2 years of strict avoidance except for allergies to peanuts, tree nuts, fish, and shellfish, which tend to persist into adulthood.[18,19] New-onset food allergies in adulthood are rare.

The most common causes of food allergens in children are milk, soy, egg, wheat, and peanuts. The most common causes of food allergens in adults are peanuts, tree nuts, fish, and shellfish. These foods account for the majority of food allergies practitioners will encounter.

IV. Clinical Manifestations

A. Signs and Symptoms

1. ***IgE-Mediated***
   IgE-mediated symptoms and signs of food allergy usually manifest within an hour of ingesting the offending food. Symptoms are often primarily in the skin, respiratory tract, and GI tract. Itching, urticaria, angioedema, sneezing, nasal congestion, abdominal pain, nausea, and vomiting are often seen. With more severe reactions, patients may have laryngeal edema or bronchospasm leading to respiratory distress. Anaphylaxis with hypotension and shock can occur, occasionally resulting in death.
2. ***Non-IgE-Mediated***
   Non-IgE-mediated food allergy or hypersensitivity encompasses a spectrum of conditions that have primarily GI manifestations. Varying degrees of

food-induced nausea, vomiting, diarrhea, steatorrhea, abdominal discomfort, weight loss, and blood in the stool are seen. In infants and small children, dehydration and failure to thrive frequently occur.

3. ***Time of Appearance***

The temporal relationship between the food intake and the onset of symptoms should be established. A thorough review of all the patient's meals in the last 24 hours should be done. A food diary may be helpful if symptoms have been recurrent for an extended period of time. Spices and additives can be responsible for missed or "hidden" food allergies.[20] If patients have eaten a certain food without problems many times, it is unlikely that the food is responsible for new symptoms. Multiple food allergies to four or more allergens is unusual. Concurrent illnesses involving the skin, respiratory tract, and GI tract that may produce symptoms similar to allergy or anaphylaxis should be identified.

B. Oral Allergy Syndrome

This syndrome is characterized by itching and swelling limited to the mouth and throat, most commonly in response to fruits and vegetables. Patients with this syndrome often have an allergy to the pollen, with cross-reactivity to the allergenic fruit or vegetable. This syndrome is believed to be a form of contact urticaria (see Chapter 12 for details on evaluation of syndrome).[21]

C. Exercise-Induced Food Anaphylaxis

Some patients will have allergic reactions to specific foods only when they undergo exertion or exercise after consuming the food.[22,23] No reaction is observed if the patient does not exercise after eating. This condition has been called exercise-induced food anaphylaxis. The mechanism for this condition is unclear. Skin testing is usually positive to the suspected food (see Chapters 6, 12, and 13).

D. Migraine

A subset of patients with migraine and other vascular headaches have symptoms induced by intake of alcohol, caffeine, tyramine, and other substances that affect cerebral blood flow. Food-induced migraine is most likely a food intolerance rather than a true food allergy.[24]

E. Conditions Not Proved to Be Related to Food Allergy

Studies have not provided evidence that food allergy is a cause of seizure disorders, autism, attention deficit disorder, memory loss, rheumatoid arthritis, osteoarthritis, or chronic fatigue syndrome.[25–27]

V. Differential Diagnosis

Food allergy is only one type of reaction in a spectrum of adverse food reactions. Since eating is a daily activity, patients often mistakenly perceive associations between their symptoms and food intake, especially if the symptoms are nonspecific. Therefore, it is important to rule out underlying skin, pulmonary, GI, and other systemic disorders that may be present. Patients who claim to be allergic to numerous foods, including foods they have previously eaten without problems, should be investigated for conditions other than food allergy (Box 7-2).

A. Toxic Food Reactions

Toxic food reactions are frequently referred to as "food poisoning" and are due to ingestion of spoiled or

---

BOX 7-2

Differential Diagnosis of Food-Induced Symptoms

1. Toxic food reactions
   Ciguatera poisoning (snapper, grouper, barracuda)
   Scombroid poisoning (tuna, skipjack, mackerel)
   Fungal toxins
   Mold contamination
   Bacterial toxins (*Salmonella, Botulinum*)

2. Food intolerance (nonimmunologic food reactions)
   Caffeine
   Alcohol
   Tyramine
   Tryptamine
   Antibiotics
   Serotonin
   Pesticides
   Dyes
   Sulfites
   Nitrates
   Monosodium glutamate (MSG)
   Enzyme deficiencies
       Lactose and other carbohydrate intolerance
       Phenylketonuria

3. Gastrointestinal disorders
   Peptic ulcer disease
   Crohn's disease
   Ulcerative colitis
   Cancer
   Pancreatic insufficiency
   Irritable bowel syndrome
   Dumping syndrome
   Hiatal hernia
   Congenital structural abnormalities
       Pyloric stenosis
       Hirschsprung's disease

4. Psychiatric disorders
   Eating disorders (anorexia nervosa, bulimia)
   Anxiety disorders

5. Chronic idiopathic urticaria

contaminated food. Ciguatera poisoning from snapper, scombroid poisoning from tuna, and fungal contamination with aflatoxin are toxic food reactions. Almost all persons who consume the food will be affected.

B. Food Intolerance

Enzyme deficiencies (lactase deficiency), pharmacologic effects (caffeine, alcohol, tyramine in cheese, tryptamine in fruits and vegetables), and additives and preservatives (dyes, sulfites, nitrates, monosodium glutamate) are all causes of food intolerance. Muscarinic receptor-associated rhinorrhea induced by spicy foods is termed *gustatory rhinitis.*[28]

C. Gastrointestinal Disorders

Peptic ulcer disease, Crohn's disease, ulcerative colitis, cancer, pancreatic insufficiency, irritable bowel syndrome, dumping syndrome, hiatal hernia, and structural abnormalities will all have symptoms associated with eating and can be ruled out based on their other clinical manifestations.

D. Psychiatric Disorders

Eating disorders such an anorexia nervosa and bulimia as well as anxiety disorders have food-related symptoms and should be ruled out.

E. Chronic Urticaria

Urticaria lasting for 6 weeks or longer with no apparent cause is termed chronic idiopathic urticaria. Many patients with chronic urticaria believe they have multiple food allergies. However, no consistent pattern of food-induced reactions is seen. Elimination diets are rarely effective, since studies have shown that chronic urticaria is rarely associated with food allergy.[29] The pathophysiology of chronic urticaria has not been established, but an autoimmune mechanism involving antibodies to the IgE receptor is thought to be present.[30]

VI. Physical Examination

Patients experiencing IgE-mediated food allergy often have localized or generalized urticaria or angioedema.[23] Nasal congestion, rhinorrhea, conjunctival congestion, and tongue swelling may be seen. Dyspnea and loss of voice or hoarseness are signs of laryngeal edema. Wheezing, intercostal retractions, nasal flare, and dyspnea indicate bronchospasm. Loss of consciousness and hypotension are signs of anaphylactic shock. Cyanosis may result from laryngeal obstruction or respiratory failure. Abdominal tenderness and increased bowel sounds may be present in both IgE-mediated and non-IgE-mediated food allergy reactions.

VII. Laboratory Evaluation

A. Serum-Specific IgE

RAST (radioallergosorbent test) testing of food antigen-specific IgE can be performed if skin testing cannot be performed (due to extensive skin disease, recent ingestion of antihistamines, refusal of the patient, or some other reason). Serum testing is considered to correlate less well with clinical reactivity than skin testing.[31] Chapter 13 covers this topic in greater detail.

B. Serum-Specific IgG

Testing for food antigen-specific IgG has not been shown to be of any value in evaluating clinical food allergy (see Chapter 21).[32]

VIII. Diagnosis

The diagnosis of food allergy is made following diagnostic testing.

Diagnostic testing should be guided by the patient's history. During the initial evaluation, suspected foods can be tested for individually or a screening panel of common food allergens can be utilized for skin and serum testing. All positive skin and serum testing results should be correlated with clinical symptoms before a diagnosis is made. The need for diagnostic elimination diets and food challenges should be based on the history, initial laboratory test results, and suggestive positive results on skin testing (see Fig. 7-1 for diagnosis and management algorithm). There is no scientific basis for intradermal skin testing with food antigens.

A. Skin Testing

Skin testing is the first procedure that should be done to screen for or confirm suspected food allergy. Chapter 12 covers this topic in greater detail.

1. *Prick* or *puncture skin testing* consists of placing a droplet of food antigen on the skin and pricking the skin through the droplet with a needle device, usually made of plastic.[33,34] Up to 80 foods can be evaluated by skin testing. Testing for more foods has not been shown to improve yield. Most food extracts for skin testing are commercially available. Patients generally have to refrain from taking antihistamines for 3–10 days prior to skin testing. A negative food skin test is more accurate in ruling out a specific food allergy than a positive food skin test is in ruling in a specific food allergy.

2. *Intradermal testing,* which is done for inhaled antigens, is not routinely performed for food allergens due to a high rate of false-positive reactions and a higher risk of a systemic allergic reaction.[34]

B. Elimination Diets

Most patients will have tried removing certain suspected foods from their diet even before they see their clinician. It is very important that any elimination diet be done with supervision to avoid malnutrition and other harmful outcomes. In the clinical setting, diagnostic elimination of a food from the diet is prescribed based on the history and results of skin or serum testing. Improvement or resolution of symptoms after a food is eliminated confirms the food allergy.[35] A medically supervised limited diet consisting primarily of lamb and rice (considered among the least allergenic of foods) may be indicated if the patient or clinician continues to suspect food-induced symptoms despite negative diagnostic testing.[36] If symptoms improve, foods should be reintroduced one at a time in a systematic fashion until a culprit is identified. Various regimens have been recommended, and practitioners should choose one based on the severity of the patient's symptoms and the patient's tolerance for restricted diets (see Appendix 6).

C. Food Challenge

The double-blind, placebo-controlled food challenge (DBPCFC) is considered the gold standard for the diagnosis of food allergy.[37,38] It is indicated if the history and laboratory testing are not adequate to confirm the presence or absence of a food allergy. It is often performed by a clinician to dissuade a patient from a persistent belief that a certain food item is responsible for his or her symptoms. The DBPCFC avoids patient or clinician bias in reporting of symptoms. It should be performed in the practitioner's office. Emergency resuscitation equipment should be available, especially if patients have experienced serious or life-threatening reactions. Having patients eat the suspected food in regular quantities in the practitioner's office should be done to further confirm a negative DBPCFC result. Box 7-3 shows a suggested DBPCFC regimen.

D. Unproven Diagnostic Techniques

A sublingual or subcutaneous provocative food challenge with patients reporting subjective symptoms has not been shown to be a valid diagnostic procedure.

Cytotoxic testing, which involves observing the effect of adding a food allergen to the white blood cells in a blood sample, has no scientific basis (see Chapter 21).[39]

IX. Therapy and Management

A. Avoidance

1. Removal of the food from the diet is the primary treatment for food allergy. This may be easier said than done, since small quantities of a food allergen can be easily missed among the multiple ingredients in today's manufactured foods. Patients should check the ingredient lists on the labels of store-bought products.

BOX 7-3

DBPCFC for Suspected IgE-Mediated Food Allergy

1. The patient should be in a fasting state.
2. The suspected food should have been avoided for at least 1 week prior to challenge.
3. Withhold all antihistamines for at least 3 days.
4. Prepare food in dry or powdered form and insert into blinded capsules. Food may be added to formulas, juices, or soft foods for children. All contents should be prepared by and known only to a third person who is not the clinician.
5. The challenge should start with 25–500 mg of the food. The dose may be doubled every 15–60 minutes if there is no reaction.
6. Placebo challenges may be given before the patient receives the test food.
7. The challenge is stopped if the patient reports or the clinician observes any reaction, or when 10 g has been ingested without incident for at least 2 hours.
8. If the challenge is negative, the food is then given openly to the patient in meal-sized amounts to confirm the result.

From Sampson HA: Food allergy: Part 2. Diagnosis and management. J Allergy Clin Immunol 1999;103:981–989. Reproduced with permission.

---

2. Clinicians should assist persons with allergies to common foods (e.g., milk, egg, soy) in designing food allergen-free diets. Guidance from a nutritionist may be necessary to maintain good nutrition (see Appendix 6).
3. When eating in restaurants, the person with a food allergy should make sure a food allergen is not part of salads or sauces. Egg, soy, fish, or shellfish may be inadvertently eaten in salads.
4. Infants and children with cow's milk allergy commonly react to goat's milk as well.[29]
5. Milk-allergic persons should watch for and avoid casein- and whey-containing foods.
6. Egg-allergic persons should avoid foods containing ovalbumin, ovomucoid, and ovotransferin. Most egg-allergic persons can tolerate chicken meat.[29]
7. The American Academy of Pediatrics Committee on Infectious Diseases currently has the following recommendations (summarized here from the 2000 Red Book) regarding giving vaccines grown in egg-related culture media to egg-allergic individuals.[40]
   a. Children with egg allergy are at low risk for anaphylactic reactions, and current measles and mumps vaccines do not contain significant amounts of egg cross-reacting proteins. Therefore, children with egg allergy routinely may be given MMR, measles, or mumps vaccine without prior skin testing.

b. Persons with a history of anaphylactic reactions to egg should be skin-tested with yellow fever vaccine. Those with a history of local or less severe reactions to egg may receive the vaccine without skin testing.

c. Persons with a history of anaphylactic reactions to egg generally should not receive influenza vaccine because of the risk of reaction, the need for yearly vaccination, and the availability of prophylactic medications against influenza. Those with a history of local or less severe reactions may receive the vaccine without skin testing.

d. If skin testing to vaccine is negative, it may be given. If the skin test is positive, the vaccine may still be given if the need is great, by using a desensitization protocol. (Clinicians facing an ambivalent situation are advised to consult the 2000 Red Book from the American Academy of Pediatrics.)

8. Peanut is a legume and does not need to be avoided by persons with a tree nut allergy. Peanut allergic persons do not have to avoid all legumes but should be tested for allergies to other legumes to delineate individual sensitivities.[41,42]

9. The Food Allergy Network, a nonprofit organization (www.foodallergy.org), regularly releases alert bulletins regarding "hidden" allergens in commercial products.

B. Medications

1. Mild urticaria, itching, or GI symptoms may be treated with first-generation antihistamines such as oral diphenhydramine, 25–50 mg every 4–6 hours, or hydroxyzine, 25–50 mg every 4–6 hours as needed. Cetirizine, 10 mg once daily, may be effective. Antihistamine therapy is usually given for at least 3 days to prevent recurrence of symptoms.

2. Patients with extensive urticaria, respiratory difficulty from throat swelling or bronchospasm, significant nausea and vomiting, hypotension, and other signs of anaphylaxis should be treated and observed in an emergency room.[43] Intramuscular or subcutaneous epinephrine (1 : 1000 solution) at a dose of 0.2–0.5 mL (0.2–0.5 mg) in adults, or 0.01 mg/kg to a maximum of 0.5 mg (0.5 mL) in children, should be given immediately. This dose may be repeated in 15 minutes for a total of two doses, and then every 4 hours as needed. Albuterol or other β-agonist therapy should be given through nebulization if wheezing or dyspnea persists after epinephrine. Intramuscular corticosteroids such as Depo-medrol, 40–60 mg, may be given, followed by a course of oral steroids (prednisone, 1 mg/kg/day × 4 days) to prevent recurrence of symptoms. Oxygen support and intravenous fluids should be started if symptoms are severe (see Chapter 6).

3. Patients with a history of serious or life-threatening reactions, including throat swelling and hypotension, should be prescribed a portable epinephrine autoinjector (Epipen) to carry with them at all times for use in emergencies.

4. Anti-IgE monoclonal antibody therapy has shown promising protective benefits against peanut allergy and may become a useful tool in preventing reactions from other foods as well.[44]

C. Immunotherapy

At the present time, immunotherapy or desensitization for food allergies is associated with a high risk of allergic reactions and is not an accepted form of therapy.[3]

X. When to Obtain Consultation

When food-related allergic symptoms are suspected by the primary care provider, it is often recommended to seek consultation with an allergist as soon as the diagnosis is considered. Certain food allergies can cause life-threatening reactions, and it is important to identify these allergens by skin testing as soon as possible. Based on the clinical evaluation and skin testing, the specialist can recommend reasonable and specific measures for avoidance of the implicated food allergens, if indicated. If the patient's symptoms are assessed as *not* due to food allergy, the specialist can also give advice on stopping unnecessary elimination diets that can lead to malnutrition and otherwise affect the patient's health and well-being. For patients with allergies to very common foods (e.g., eggs, wheat, peanuts), the specialist can work with a nutritionist and the primary care provider in designing safe and nutritionally healthy diets.

XI. Practice Guidelines

The Joint Task Force on Practice Parameters of the American Academy of Allergy, Asthma and Immunology and the American College of Allergy, Asthma and Immunology has published practice parameters to guide practitioners on the topics of allergy diagnostic testing[34] and the diagnosis and management of anaphylaxis.[43] Practice parameters for the diagnosis and treatment of food allergy will be available soon (www.jcaai.org/param/anaphylaxis.htm and www.jcaai.org/param/aller.htm).

XII. Internet Resources

www.foodallergy.org
Food Allergy Network

www.aaaai.org
American Academy of Allergy, Asthma and Immunology

www.acaai.org
American College of Allergy, Asthma and Immunology

www.niaid.nih.gov
National Institute of Allergy, Immunology and Infectious Disease

www.aafa.org
Asthma and Allergy Foundation of America

www.eatright.org
American Dietetic Association

XIII. ICD-9 Code

693.1   Food allergy

XIV. Diagnosis and Management (Fig. 7-1)

XV. Patient Education

A. Work closely with patients with chronic nonspecific symptoms to determine which symptoms reflect true food allergy so that unnecessary or harmful food elimination can be avoided or stopped.

B. Educate patients on the difference between food allergy and food intolerance.

C. Prepare a written action plan for patients to follow in the event of an allergic reaction. This plan should include specific medications, doses, instructions for emergencies, and important phone numbers (e.g., clinic, emergency room).

D. Instruct patients with a history of anaphylactic reactions on the use of auto-injectable epinephrine for use in emergencies.

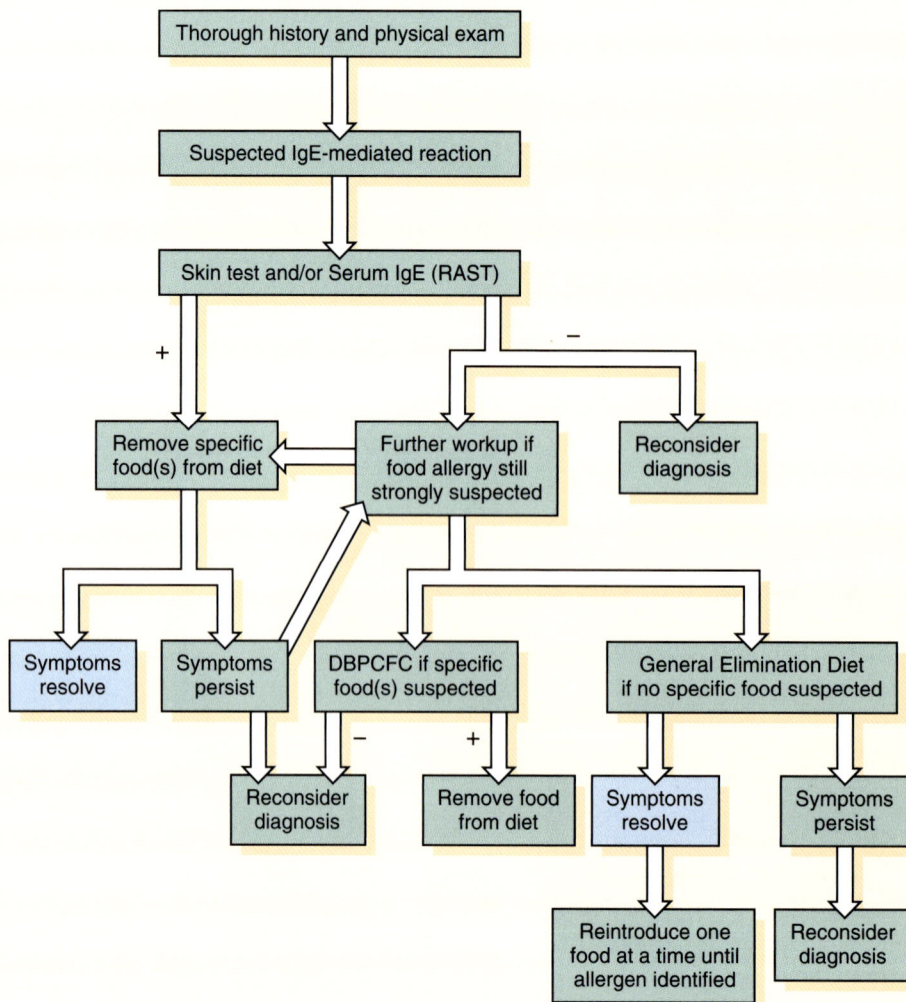

Figure 7-1 Diagnostic algorithm for the evaluation of adverse food reactions.

E. Emphasize to patients that the only treatment for food allergy is avoidance of the offending food.

F. Instruct patients on reading labels on food and beverage products for foods to which they are allergic.

G. Instruct patients to request that specific ingredients be omitted from salads, sauces, and other foods with multiple ingredients when dining in restaurants or other people's homes.

H. Provide support for patients when they are frustrated or discouraged by their allergies.

XVI. Patient Education Materials and Handouts

A. *What is a food allergy?*

Food allergy is susceptibility to developing an adverse reaction to eating specific foods because of an exaggerated response of the immune system. It is important to know whether a reaction is a true food allergy, because while some reactions are mild, others can be fatal.

B. *Are all reactions to food due to food allergy?*

No. Most reactions to food are due to food intolerance, which is not caused by the immune system but by other causes such as enzyme deficiences (e.g., lactose intolerance) or the intrinsic effects of the food (e.g., jitteriness from caffeine, headache from MSG).

C. *What are the symptoms of food allergy?*

Symptoms can include itching, hives, abdominal cramps, or diarrhea, usually appearing within an hour of eating. More serious symptoms include throat swelling, difficulty breathing, shock, and even death.

D. *What tests do I need to have to find out if I have a food allergy?*

The history of a pattern of symptoms related to food is the starting point for diagnosing food allergy. The next step is to check for allergic antibodies (IgE) to foods by skin testing or by a blood test. Both skin and blood testing provide information, but skin testing appears to be more sensitive.

E. *Can my child outgrow his or her food allergy?*

Many children outgrow their food allergies, with the exception of peanut, tree nut, fish, and shellfish allergies, which tend to persist into adulthood.

F. *What is the treatment for a food allergy?*

Avoidance is the only treatment for food allergy at this time. It is important to read labels on store-bought products and to inquire about ingredients when eating in restaurants to avoid accidentally eating something to which you are allergic.

G. *What should I do if I accidentally eat something I'm allergic to and have a reaction?*

An antihistamine such as diphenhydramine (Benadryl) should be taken immediately at the first sign of an allergic reaction. Persons who have had serious allergic reactions, including throat swelling, shortness of breath, or anaphylactic shock, should always carry a self-injectable preparation of epinephrine (EpiPen, Ana-kit) that they can use at the first sign of these symptoms while on the way to the emergency room or calling 911.

H. *Can I get allergy shots to make my food allergy go away?*

At this time, allergy shots like those given for pollen allergy are not acceptable for food allergy because the risk of allergic reactions to the shots is too high.

I. Refer to patient education CD, which is provided with this text, for additional patient education information. It has been formatted to provide readily accessible, easy-to-understand handouts for adult patients and the parents of pediatric patients. These handouts can be easily modified to fit specific practice requirements.

REFERENCES

1. Bruijnzeel-Koomen C, Ortolani C, Aas K, et al: Adverse reactions to food. Allergy 1995;50:623–635.
2. Sampson HA: Food allergy: Part 1. Immunopathogenesis and clinical disorders. J Allergy Clin Immunol 1999;103: 717–728.
3. Sampson HA: Food allergy: Part 2. Diagnosis and management. J Allergy Clin Immunol 1999;103:981–989.
4. Sbothill JF, Stokes CR, Turner MW, et al: Predisposing factors and the development of reaginic allergy in infancy. Clin Allergy 1976;6:305–319.
5. Machtinger S, Moss R: Cow's milk allergy in breast-fed infants: The role of allergen and maternal secretory IgA antibody. J Allergy Clin Immunol 1986;77:341–347.
6. Sigurs N, Hattevig G, Kjellman B: Maternal avoidance of eggs, cow's milk and fish during lactation: Effect on allergic manifestations, skin-prick tests, and specific IgE antibodies in children at age 4 years. Pediatrics 1992;89:735–739.
7. Lee C, Changchien C, Chert P, et al: Eosinophilic gastroenteritis: 10 years experience. Am J Gastroenterol 1993; 88:70–74.
8. Moon A, Kleinman R: Allergic gastroenteropathy in children. Ann Allergy Asthma Immunol 1995;74:5–12.
9. Min KU, Metcalfe D: Eosinophilic gastroenteritis. Immunol Allergy Clin North Am 1991;11:799–813.
10. Sicherer SH, Eigenmann PA, Sampson HA: Clinical features of food protein-induced enterocolitis syndrome. J Pediatr 1998;102:e6.
11. Bircher AJ, Van Melle G, Haller E, Curty B, Frei PC: IgE to food allergens are highly prevalent in patients allergic to pollens with and without symptoms of food allergy. Clin Exp Allergy 1994;24:367–374.

12. Pastorello EA, Incorvaia C, Pravetonni V: New allergens in fruits and vegetables. Allergy 1998;53:48–51.

13. Dreborg S, Foucard T: Allergy to apple, carrot and potato in children with birch-pollen allergy. Allergy 1983;38: 167–172.

14. Sampson HA, Jolie PL: Increased plasma histamine concentrations after food challenges in children with atopic dermatitis. N Engl J Med 1984;311:372–376.

15. Eigenmann PA, Sicherer SH, Borkowski TA, Cohen BD, Sampson HA: Prevalence of IgE-mediated food allergy among children with atopic dermatitis. Pediatrics 1998; 101:e8.

16. Bock SA: Prospective appraisal of complaints of adverse reactions to foods in children during the first three years of life. Pediatrics 1987;79:683–688.

17. Host A, Halken S: A prospective study of cow milk allergy in Danish infants during the first three years of life. Allergy 1990;45:587–596.

18. Bock SA, Atkins FM: The natural history of peanut allergy. J Allergy Clin Immunol 1989;83:900–904.

19. Bock SA: The natural history of food sensitivity. J Allergy Clin Immunol 1982;69:173–177.

20. Steinman HA: "Hidden" allergens in foods. J Allergy Clin Immunol 1996;98:241–250.

21. Amlot PL, Kemeny DM, Zachary C, Parkes P, Lessof MH: Oral allergy syndrome (OAS): Symptoms of IgE-mediated hypersensitivity to foods. Clin Allergy 1987;17:33–42.

22. Horan RF, Sheffer AL: Food-dependent exercise-induced anaphylaxis. Immunol Allergy Clin North Am 1991;11: 757–766.

23. Shimamoto SR, Bock SA: Update on clinical features of food-induced anaphylaxis. Curr Opin Allergy Clin Immunol 2002;2:211–216.

24. Weber RW, Vaughan TR: Food and migraine headache. Immunol Allergy Clin North Am 1991;11:831–841.

25. Warner JO: Food and behavior: Allergy, intolerance or aversion? Pediatr Allergy Immunol 1993;4:112–116.

26. Mahan LK, Chase M, Furukuwa CT, et al: Sugar "allergy" and children's behavior. Ann Allergy 1988;61: 453–458.

27. Panush RS: Food induced ("allergic") arthritis: Clinical and serologic studies. J Rheumatol 1990;17:291–294.

28. Raphael G, Raphael M, Kaliner M: Gustatory rhinitis: A syndrome of food-induced rhinorrhea. J Allergy Clin Immunol 1989;83:110–115.

29. Sampson HA: Adverse reactions to food. In Middleton E, Ellis EF, Yunginger JW, et al (eds): Allergy: Principles and Practice, 5th ed, pp 1162–1182. St. Louis: Mosby, 1998.

30. Kaplan AP: Urticaria and angioedema. In Middleton E, Ellis EF, Yunginger JW, et al (eds): Allergy: Principles and Practice, 5th ed, pp 1104–1122. St. Louis: Mosby, 1998.

31. Sampson HA, Albergo R: Comparison of results of skin tests, RAST, and double-blind, placebo-controlled food challenges in children with atopic dermatitis. J Allergy Clin Immunol 1984;74:26–33.

32. Metcalfe D, Sampson HA: Workshop on experimental methodology for clinical studies of adverse reactions to foods and food additives. J Allergy Clin Immunol 1990; 86:421–442.

33. Bock S, Buckley J, Holst A, May C: Proper use of skin tests with food extracts in diagnosis of food hypersensitivity. Clin Allergy 1978;8:559–564.

34. Joint Task Force on Practice Parameters: Practice parameters for allergy diagnostic testing. Ann Allergy Asthma Immunol 1995;75(Pt 2):585.

35. Pastorello E, Stocchi L, Pravetonni V, et al: Role of the food elimination diet in adults with food allergy. J Allergy Clin Immunol 1989;84:475–483.

36. Condemi J, Metcalfe DD: Food allergy in adults. In Lichtenstein LM, Fauci AS (eds): Current Therapy in Allergy, Immunology and Rheumatology, 5th ed, pp 145–149. St. Louis: Mosby, 1996.

37. Sampson HA: Immunologically mediated food allergy: The importance of food challenge procedures. Ann Allergy 1988;60:262–269.

38. Bock SA, Atkins FM: Patterns of food hypersensitivity during sixteen years of double-blind, placebo-controlled food challenges. J Pediatr 1990;117:561–567.

39. Condemi JJ: Unproved diagnostic and therapeutic techniques. In Metcalfe DD, Sampson HA, Simon RA (eds): Food Allergy: Adverse Reactions to Foods and Food Additives, pp 392–404. Boston: Blackwell Scientific, 1991.

40. Peter G (ed): Report of the Committee on Infectious Diseases—Red Book, pp 35–36. Elk Grove Village, IL: American Academy of Pediatrics, 2000.

41. Sampson HA: Peanut allergy. N Engl J Med 2002;346: 1294–1299.

42. Sicherer SH: Clinical update on peanut allergy. Ann Allergy Asthma Immunol 2002;88:350–361.

43. Joint Task Force on Practice Parameters: Practice parameters for the diagnosis and management of anaphylaxis. Ann Allergy Asthma Immunol 1998;101:S465–S528.

44. Leung DY, Sampson HA, Yunginger JW, et al: Effects of anti-IgE therapy in patients with peanut allergy. N Engl J Med 2003;348:986–993.

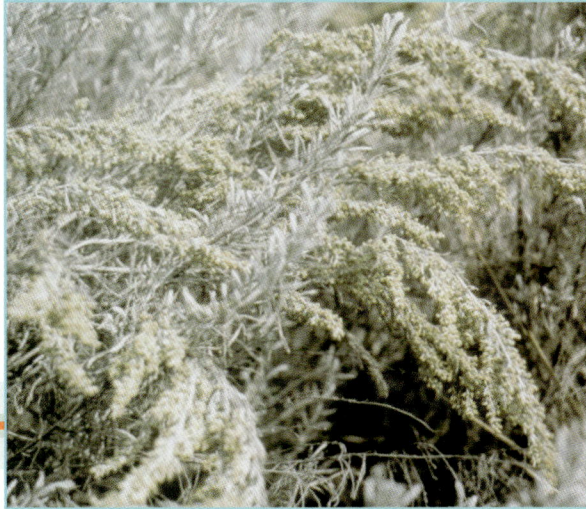
Common Sagebrush *Courtesy of Hollister-Stier Laboratory*

CHAPTER 8
Allergic Disorders of the Eye

George W. Bensch

I. Introduction

The eye as a target organ for allergy is often overlooked in evaluation by both primary care and specialty practitioners. Patients do not report ocular symptoms spontaneously and often self medicate with over-the-counter (OTC) eye drops. Furthermore, patients can be more interested in the cosmetic prospect of having bright nonerythematous eyes and will take OTC eye drops to clear erythema and may ignore important signs and symptoms. It is imperative for practitioners to question patients specifically about eye discomfort and use of eye drops and to heighten their awareness of significant signs and symptoms that may be masked by these OTC medications.

II. Incidence and Epidemiology

Allergic conjunctivitis occurs in approximately 25% of the U.S. population.[1,2] Triggers for allergic eye symptoms are generally similar to those for allergic rhinitis and include airborne allergens such as pollen, dust mites, and environmental pollutants.

A. In a 1991 study by Juniper, itchy eyes associated with head and nose congestion caused poor sleep patterns in

87% of patients, chronic fatigue in 93% of patients, and irritability in greater than 90% of patients experiencing allergy.[3]

B. Pruritis, redness, and tearing can be social impediments, and lead to a poorer quality of life.

III. Etiology

Ocular allergy is based on the classic IgE-mediated histamine response.

A. In the eye, the highest concentration of mast cells is in the limbus, just at the junction of the sclera and cornea. These mast cells, when activated, release histamine in the early phase reaction and kinins, leukotrienes, prostaglandins, and superoxide free radicals in the late phase. The early phase reaction usually occurs within twenty minutes after exposure and produces the classic ocular allergy signs and symptoms of watery eyes, pruritus, and erythema.

B. The late phase reaction occurs four to eight hours after the initial exposure and involves adhesion molecules and other cytokines that promote the influx of inflammatory cells including T-lymphocytes, monocytes, basophils, and eosinophils. These inflammatory cells in turn release numerous other pro-inflammatory mediators such as IL4, ICAM-1, tryptase, and TNF -alpha, which lead to further inflammation of the surrounding tissue.

C. It is interesting to note that mast cells in the quiescent eye are mostly in the substantia propia, but in the allergic state they are found in more superficial layers and are, therefore, easier to activate on exposure to specific antigens.

D. As in asthma and allergic rhinitis, eosinophils are most responsible for damage to epithelial tissue, primarily through the release of major basic proteins and eosinophil cationic proteins.

IV. Clinical Manifestations

There are six basic types of allergic and allergic-like ocular diseases. Each type has different historical presentations, symptoms, and physical findings. These differences are summarized in the differential diagnosis and in Table 8-1.

V. Differential Diagnosis

A. Seasonal Allergic Conjunctivitis

Seasonal allergic conjunctivitis (Fig. 8-1A) is the most common type of allergic conjunctivitis and represents about half of all cases. It is generally associated with rhinitis and results from airborne allergens. Depending on geography, spring and fall are usually the worst seasons of the year due to pollination of many tree and weed species. A history of atopic disease in immediate family members is usually associated with this illness, as well.

1. Signs and symptoms include pruritis, tearing, and erythema that are usually bilateral. A clear, stringy discharge is often seen. Symptoms are usually seasonal but can be present year round, especially if not treated properly and with overlapping seasonal exacerbations (Table 8-2).
2. Laboratory evaluation is not needed for diagnosis. Scraping the conjunctival surface for eosinophils is often negative. When eosinophils are present they are associated with more severe and long-standing ocular allergy and ocular tissue damage. Skin testing is often performed in conjunction with evaluation of allergic rhinitis.

B. Perennial Allergic Conjunctivitis

Perennial allergic conjunctivitis, like perennial rhinitis, is caused by sensitivities to allergens that are present year-round. Symptoms are usually due to animal dander, molds, and dust mites. Clinical findings are the same as those for seasonal allergic conjunctivitis.

C. Giant Papillary Conjunctivitis

Giant papillary conjunctivitis (GPC) is an inflammatory reaction to contact lens and other ocular prostheses but can be mistaken for ocular allergy.

1. Although GPC may be associated with pruritis, in contrast to allergic conjunctivitis, the prominent

---

TABLE 8-1

Distinguishing Characteristics of Ocular Allergic and Allergic-like Diseases

Allergy	*Characteristic*
Allergic conjunctivitis (seasonal and perennial)	Self-limiting, bilateral inflammation; seasonal and/or perennial manifestation. Symptoms include itching, redness, tearing; no threat to vision. IgE-mediated type I hypersensitivity reaction of the conjunctiva.
Atopic keratoconjunctivitis	Bilateral, sight-threatening disease; typically occurs in patients with atopic dermatitis. Serum IgE; cell-mediated immunity. Symptoms include significant redness, eventual fibrosis, keratinization of conjunctiva surface, cataract formation, and lid malposition.
Vernal keratoconjunctivitis	Intensely pruritic, sight-threatening chronic allergic conjunctivitis characterized by large "cobblestone" papillae on the underside of eyelid. Associated findings may include asthma and atopic dermatitis, serum histaminase activity, and levels of nerve growth factor.
Giant papillary conjunctivitis	Generally not considered an allergic condition; may be confused with ocular allergy. Not associated with itching. Giant papillae on underside of eyelid are a distinguishing symptom.
Irritative conjunctivitis	Commonly confused with allergic disease. Signs and symptoms include only conjunctival hyperemia and ocular irritation, caused by environmental pollutants and smoke.

Used with permission of Health Learning Systems.

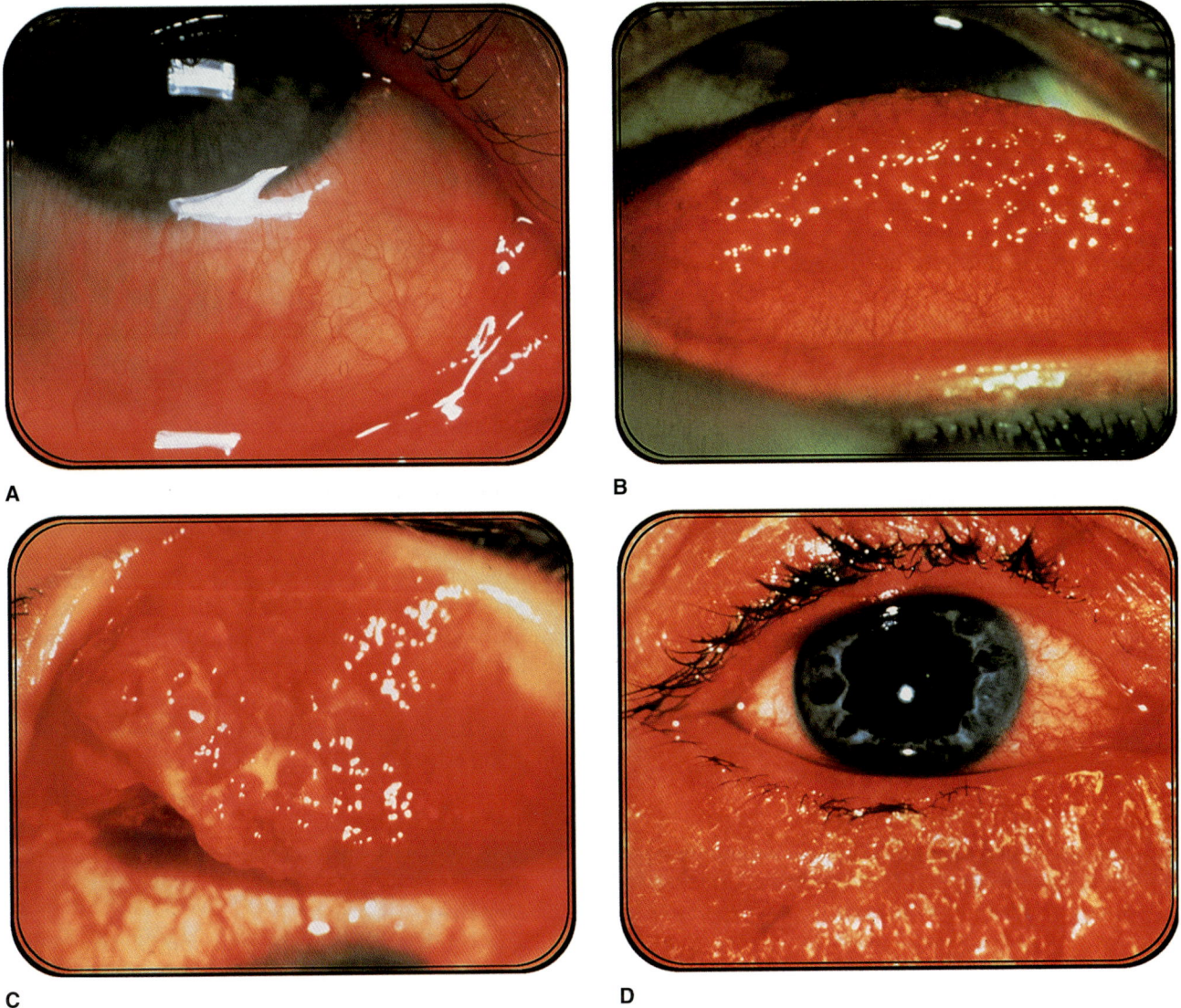

Figure 8-1 Different types of conjunctivitis. **A**, Allergic acute conjunctivitis; **B**, Giant papillary conjunctivitis; **C**, Vernal conjunctivitis; **D**, Atopic keratoconjunctivitis.

symptoms are burning and pain. Coincidently, symptoms may also increase during the spring pollen season. The hallmark of this disease is the presence of giant papillae (cobblestoning) on the underside of the upper eyelid (Fig. 8-1B). Conjunctival redness and swelling, as well as yellowish dots known as Trantas' dots may be seen.

2. The pathophysiology of GPC is still unclear but may involve an immune response to protein deposits on the contact lens surface.

TABLE 8-2

Signs and Symptoms of Allergic Conjunctivitis

Sign	Symptom
Hyperemia	Redness
Chemosis	Itching
Lid edema	Tearing
Mucous discharge	

Used with permission of Health Learning Systems.

D. Vernal Keratoconjunctivitis

Vernal keratoconjunctivitis (Fig. 8-1*C*) is an exceedingly pruritic chronic conjunctivitis that can be sight threatening. It usually is not seen in the United States. It occurs commonly in the early spring in young males in countries close to the equator.

1. Symptoms include tearing and intense pruritus.
2. Sight can be threatened by the development of ulcers on the corneal epithelium.
`3. Physical findings include papillary hypertrophy on the underside of the upper lid, Trantas' dots, conjunctival redness, an extra lower lid crease (Dennie's line), and excessive mucus in the mucosa of the upper lid (Maxwell-Lyons sign).
4. Severe cases can exhibit corneal ulceration with plaque formation.
5. Histamine levels in tears are extremely high in this condition. Eosinophilic granules are common on eye scrapings and can be helpful in differentiating vernal keratoconjunctivitis from seasonal or perennial allergic conjunctivitis.

E. Atopic Keratoconjunctivitis

Atopic keratoconjunctivitis (AKC; Fig. 8-1*D*) is a chronic, usually year-round, severe conjunctivitis associated with atopic dermatitis of the eyelids. Patients usually have a significant history of atopic diseases such as atopic dermatitis or asthma (Box 8-1).

1. AKC is a potentially vision threatening disease, especially when it is associated with secondary infections of the eyelids both from viruses such as herpes and from nasal pathogens transmitted by autoinoculation.
2. This disease usually first appears in the twenty-to-fifty age range and more commonly in women.[4]
3. The major symptoms include pruritus, redness, burning, tearing, blurry vision, and photophobia.
4. On examination, the outer surface of the eyelid shows typical atopic dermatitis signs, which include scaling, dermatitis, erythema, and lichenification. Loss of

---

BOX 8-1

Signs of Atopic Keratoconjunctivitis

- Cicatrizing conjunctivitis (scarring, hypertrophy)
- Swollen, eczematous lids
- Superficial punctate keratitis/ulcers
- Superficial corneal infiltrates
- Keratoconus
- Anterior polar cataracts

Used with permission of Health Learning Systems.

---

eyelashes on the lid margins may be seen in severe, long-standing cases. Papillary hypertrophy may be seen in both upper and lower eyelids. Trantas' dots, Dennie's lines, loss of eyebrows due to rubbing (de Hertoghe's sign) may also be seen.

5. The hallmarks of AKC in severe cases are keratinized or scarred conjunctivae, erythema, and chemosis. Herpetic keratitis occurs in one sixth of these patients, which can lead to vascularization and ulceration of the cornea over time. Anterior cataracts are associated with 10% of cases of AKC, while posterior cataracts are more often seen with corticosteroid overuse.

F. Irritative conjunctivitis is commonly confused with allergic disease.

1. Smoke, environmental pollutants, and dryness all contribute to irritative conjunctivitis, which is generally self-limited and easily treated with artificial tears.
2. These patients typically complain of redness and burning with minimal itching, which differentiates irritative conjunctivitis from true allergic conjunctivitis.

G. Other conditions that should be considered in the differential diagnosis.

1. *Chronic Follicular or Papillary Conjunctivitis*
This condition is associated with infections, toxins, or reactions to various chemicals such as preservatives in eye drops.
2. *Dry Eye*
This condition usually presents with burning rather than itching. A burning, "sandy" feel to the eye, with a dry mouth and stiff hands may be associated with autoimmune disease.
3. *Ocular Rosacea*
This condition is characterized by irritation of the eyes, blepharitis, and recurrent chalazions. It is also associated with facial rosacea changes, which include telangiectasia and enlarged sebaceous cysts. About 20% of patients first present with eye symptoms before skin manifestations appear.
4. *Bacterial Conjunctivitis*
This condition presents with a purulent discharge and lid crusting that is worse in the morning. Cultures are usually unnecessary with a single isolated infection.
5. *Viral Conjunctivitis*
This condition is self-limiting and presents with blurred vision, irritation, and inflammation of the palpebral and/or bulbar conjunctiva. Viral conjunctivitis can be associated with pretragal lymph nodes, chemosis, keratitis, and tarsal plate papillary hypertrophy and lymphoid follicles.

6. ***Chlamydia Infections***
   These eye infections begin with tearing and ocular irritation. Pretragal lymph nodes, urethritis, and a mixed follicular papillary reaction can also be associated with this condition.

7. ***Pemphigoid***
   This condition can decrease vision by corneal scarring. Vesiculated hyperemia and thickening of the eyelid is found in this condition as well.

VI. History and Physical Examination

There are several general principles in the history and physical examination of the eye that can help differentiate allergic eye disease from nonallergic conditions.

A. Allergic eyes itch and only sting after intense rubbing.

B. The same allergens that cause rhinitis also affect the eye, and, therefore, a careful environmental contact history should be obtained.

C. There is usually a history of atopy in the immediate family.

D. Symptoms usually occur in the spring and fall.

E. The physical examination must be preceded by removal of all makeup from the eyes and face to determine eyelid dermatitis and facial rosacea.

F. The conjunctiva will be hyperemic, with increased tearing.

G. Symptoms are bilateral in allergic conjunctivitis. If they are unilateral, they favor the dominant hand.

H. The eye is usually the predominantly affected organ. However, there can be symptoms and signs of allergic rhinitis and even sinusitis, which is often overlooked.

VII. Laboratory Evaluation

Laboratory evaluation is usually not necessary except to isolate the specific antigens responsible for the patient's symptoms.

A. This evaluation is best carried out with traditional skin testing and RAST by clinicians well trained in this area. Chapters 12 and 13 cover this topic in greater detail.

B. Conjunctival smears of the eye for eosinophils are often negative by Hansel's stain. However, this procedure can be a sensitive allergic diagnostic tool even when only a few granules are seen. Eosinophils in large numbers suggest a more chronic condition, such as vernal conjunctivitis. Chapter 14 covers this procedure in greater detail.

C. Serum IgE testing is not recommended because levels of IgE in tears and mucus can be several times higher than serum levels. Serum IgE levels are generally not helpful in diagnosing allergic disease.

VIII. Approach to Final Diagnosis

A careful history linking common antigens such as pollens or animals to allergic conjunctivitis is sufficient to make the diagnosis. This is especially true if upper respiratory symptoms such as paroxysmal sneezing and rhinorrhea are present. Pruritis of the eye is the most salient historical finding.

IX. Therapy and Management

A. Nonpharmacologic Management

1. ***Environmental Control***
   Environmental control should begin in the home. The effects of environmental exposure to pollen, animal dander, dust mites, mold spores, cockroach antigen, and irritants such as smoke and fragrances can be cumulative. Exposure to these allergens is especially intensified during seasons where there is an increase of outdoor allergens. General measures for allergic rhinitis apply to allergic conjunctivitis as well.
   a. Air-conditioning systems using evaporative or swamp coolers are especially deleterious because they can become contaminated with mold spores.
   b. Increased humidity can increase house dust mite concentration, aggravating symptoms.
   c. Animals' access to bedrooms should be discouraged. In homes where animals are removed, it can take five to seven months to reduce animal dander to acceptable levels. Washing of pets to minimize indoor exposure is controversial.
   d. To reduce pollen exposure, patients should be instructed to keep windows closed at home, work, and in moving vehicles. Washing hair and changing out of street clothes after returning home is advised to avoid increasing pollen contamination throughout the house.

2. ***Saline Irrigation***
   Saline eye drops (e.g., Artificial Tears) can provide an inexpensive soothing treatment especially if cooled before administration. They also are effective in moisturizing and flushing aeroallergens and irritants from the eye (Table 8-3).

B. Pharmacologic Management (Table 8-4)

1. ***Antihistamines***
   a. Oral antihistamines are often useful for both eye and nose symptoms, although they are not as

TABLE 8-3

OTC Topical Agents Used to Manage Ocular Allergy

Agent	Dosage	Comments
Artificial Tears (dextran/hydroxypropyl methylcellulose)	As needed	• Help to wash the eye • Inexpensive • Safe • Provide additional comfort • Minimally effective • Require frequent use, sometimes hourly
Preservative-Free Tears Tears Natural Free Genteal	As needed	• Somewhat effective treatment for small children <3 years old
Vasoconstrictor		
Visine L.R. (oxymetazoline HCl)	Up to 4 times daily	• Constricts ocular blood vessels; makes eyes white • Eyes look better for short periods • Does not block allergic process • Has potential for ocular irritation • Potential development of rebound hyperemia and corresponding overuse of drug • Can interact with MAO inhibitors • Contraindicated in patients with narrow angle glaucoma
Antihistamine vasoconstrictors		
Naphcon A, Opcon-A (pheniramine maleate/ naphazoline HCl)	Up to 4 times daily	• Contain both antihistamine and ocular vasoconstrictors • Rapid relief of mild symptoms • Short duration of action • Have potential for rebound hyperemia and corresponding overuse of drug • Interact with MAO inhibitors • Contraindicated in patients with narrow angle glaucoma
Vasocon-A (naphazoline HCl antazoline phosphate)	Up to 4 times daily	

Used with permission of Health Learning Systems.

effective for eye symptoms Nonsedating antihistamines can be helpful but can contribute to eye dryness and may not be completely effective for allergic conjunctivitis.

b. Topical ocular antihistamines are very effective for pruritus and hyperemia. They are more effective when applied prior to known exposure.

Most OTC topical antihistamines are short acting (only 3–4 hours) and require reapplication four times a day for complete relief of symptoms throughout the day. A newer preparation, azelastine 0.05% (Optivar), can be administered one drop every 12 hours as needed. Pediatric safety for these medications has not been established for patients under the age of three. Side effects include eye burning and stinging in about 30% of patients and headaches in about 15% of patients. Topical antihistamines can dry the eyes after prolonged use. Other preparations include emedastine difumarate 0.05% (Emadine) and levocabastine hydrochloride 0.05% (Livostin).

2. **Topical Vasoconstrictors**
   a. Many patients prefer to use vasoconstrictors such as oxymetazoline (Visine) for improved cosmetic results. While they do clear conjunctival erythema, they do not treat either itching or irritation or block the allergic process. Rebound hyperemia can occur with frequent use. These agents are contraindicated in patients with narrow angle glaucoma.
   b. Combination antihistamine-vasoconstrictor preparations are available OTC and include pheniramine maleate 0.3%/naphazoline 0.025% (Naphcon A; Opcon A) and antazoline 0.5%/ naphazoline 0.025% (Vasocon A). These medications can be applied four times a day and provide rapid relief of mild symptoms, especially hyperemia and itching. They are contraindicated in patients with narrow angle

TABLE 8-4

Prescription Agents Used to Manage Ocular Allergy

Agent	Dosage	Comments
Antihistamines		
Emadine (emedastine difumarate)	I drop up to 4 times daily	• Selective H_1-receptor antagonist • Gives effective relief • Safe in patients 3 years of age and older
Livostin (levocabastine HCl)	1 drop 4 times daily	• H_1-receptor antagonist • Gives effective relief • Safe in patients 12 years of age and older • Short duration of action
Mast cell stabilizers		
Alocril (nedocromil sodium)	2 times daily	• Inhibits type I hypersensitivity reaction; prevents release of mast cell mediators • Safe and comfortable • Equivalent to cromolyn for allergic conjunctivitis • Slow onset of action • Dosing twice daily can enhance patient compliance • Provides relief of itching only • Headaches were reported • Long-term use is necessary
Alomide (iodoxamide tromethamine)	4 times daily	• Inhibits type I hypersensitivity reaction; prevents release of mast cell mediators • Effective for all ocular allergic disease with corneal changes • Safe and comfortable • More potent than cromolyn • Slow onset of action • Long-term use necessary since drug is preventive only
Opticrom (cromolyn sodium)	4 to 6 times daily	• Inhibits type I hypersensitivity reaction; prevents release of mast cell mediators • Safe and comfortable • No immediate relief • Long-term use necessary since drug is preventive only
Antihistamine–mast cell stabilizers		
Patanol (olopatadine HCl)	1 drop twice a day	• Single agent with both antihistamine and mast cell stabilization action • Rapid relief of signs and symptoms of allergic conjunctivitis, including itching and redness • Long duration of action • Dosing twice daily can enhance patient compliance • Safe for unlimited length of use • Approved for use in children 3 years of age and older
Zaditor (ketotifen fumarate)	1 drop twice a day	• Histamine antagonist (H_1-receptor) and mast cell stabilizer • Effective in preventing ocular itching associated with allergic conjunctivitis • Rapid onset of action • Mild headaches and rhinitis were reported in 10%–25% of cases
NSAID		
Acular (ketorolac tromethamine)	4 times daily	• Inhibits prostaglandin synthesis • Temporary relief of ocular itching • Stinging/burning experienced by 40% of patients may reduce compliance
Corticosteroids		
Alrex (Ioteprednol)	4 times daily	• Suppress inflammatory response • Recommended for short-term use
Decadron (dexamethasone)	4 times daily	• May cause secondary infection, increase intraocular pressure, glaucoma, cataracts • Contraindicated in patients with herpes simplex or ocular viral,
Vexol (rimexolone)	4 times daily	fungal, or mycobacterial infection • Therapy should be monitored by an ophthalmologist

Used with permission of Health Learning Systems.

glaucoma and should not be used with MAO inhibitors.

3. ***Nonsteroidal Anti-inflammatory Agents***
These agents provide temporary relief of ocular itching through the inhibition of prostaglandin synthesis and can be used every six hours. Available preparations include ketorolac tromethamine 0.5% (Acular) and diclofenac sodium 0.1% (Voltaren). Stinging and burning can occur in 40% of patients, which may reduce compliance.

4. ***Mast Cell Stabilizers***
   a. The general mechanism of this class of medication involves inhibition of IgE-mediated reactions by preventing release of mast cell mediators. Mast cell stabilizers are exceedingly safe but have a slow onset of action, sometimes up to 5–7 days.
   b. Available preparations include nedocromil sodium 2% (Alocril), lodoxamide tromethamine 0.1% (Alomide), cromolyn sodium 4% (Opticrom) and pemirolast 0.1% (Alamast). Except for nedocromil, which can be used twice daily, the other preparations must be applied four times a day for effective relief of symptoms. A second rescue antihistamine eye drop may be needed for immediate relief while waiting for the mast cell stabilization to occur. Reports of immediate relief with mast cell stabilizers are probably due to flushing out the antigens.

5. ***Corticosteroids***
   a. Topical corticosteroids are used in refractory cases to suppress inflammatory responses, such as those seen in vernal keratoconjuctivitis. It is recommended to consult ophthalmologists for patients with atopic keratoconjunctivitis, especially when colonization of the eczematoid lesions of the eyelids with herpes simplex or other pathogens occurs. It is estimated that 40% of these eczematoid lesions harbor herpes simplex. It is also important to note that increased ocular pressure can occur within ten to fourteen days of corticosteroid eye drops usage. Available preparations include loteprednol etabanate 0.2% (Alrex); rimexolone 0.1% (Vexol); dexamethasone 0.1% (Decadron); fluorometholone 0.1%, 0.25%; medrysone 1%; and prednisolone acetate 0.125%, 1%.
   b. Systemic corticosteroids (conventionally used as an oral steroid burst, e.g., Prednisone 40 mg/day [20 mg bid] for 5–7 days) may be used for patients with severe episodes.

6. ***Antihistamine–Mast Cell Stabilizers***
   a. The best control of mild to moderate ocular conjunctivitis can be obtained by using combination antihistamine–mast cell stabilizers. These medications have the ability to provide both immediate relief of pruritis, tearing, and hyperemia and long-term mast cell stabilization.
   b. The available preparations include olopatadine hydrochloride 0.1% (Patanol) and ketotifen fumarate 0.025% (Zaditor), which are both effective at twice daily dosing and approved for children three years of age and older. They are effective immediately and, therefore, circumvent the need for a second rescue eye drop. In a study comparing the two medications, Patanol caused less stinging and headaches than did Zaditor[5] and reduced hyperemia more quickly, as well.[6]

C. Immunotherapy

Immunotherapy has been shown to improve eye symptoms as well as nasal symptoms. It is usually recommended for patients with both rhinitis and conjunctivitis. The indications and dosing are identical to those for allergic rhinitis.[7] Chapter 11 and Appendix 1 cover this topic in greater detail.

X. Special Considerations in Patient Subsets

A. Pruritic eyes will often lead to excessive rubbing and cause recurrent conjunctivitis by repeated autoinoculation.

B. Nasal pathogens typically cause conjunctivitis because the nose and eyes are often manually rubbed without hand washing.

C. Eyelid contact dermatitis can develop from being rubbed by hands with soaps, hand lotions, and even latex gloves.

XI. When to Obtain Consultation

A. Referrals to ophthalmologists should be made if the primary care clinician is uncertain of the diagnosis, if the presence of herpes simplex is suspected, and if prolonged use of intraocular topical steroids is being considered.

B. Referrals to allergists are appropriate for skin testing to help identify the inciting antigen and for initiation of immunotherapy, as well as for other diagnostic and therapeutic dilemmas.

XII. Practice Guidelines

Although practice guidelines are not yet available, the following list of principles is recommended for proper ocular allergy management.

A. There can be no doubt that environmental control is by far the most effective method of treatment.

1. Changing filters in heating and air conditioning systems; removing animals; and control of mites, molds, and cockroach antigens are of primary importance.
2. Closing windows at night to protect against pollen antigens and using dust mite mattress covers can be invaluable.

B. Oral antihistamines and nasal steroids probably contribute little to ocular allergy control.

C. Direct eye drop administration is very important. Refrigerated OTC preservative-free tears can flush and wash eyes effectively and provide significant relief.

D. Vasoconstrictor eye drops, while whitening the eyes, do nothing for itching and can actually dry eyes out.

E. Topical steroids should probably not be prescribed without consulting an ophthalmologist, unless used for short periods of time.

F. The combination of antihistamine–mast cell stabilizers is the safest and most effective therapy for ocular allergy, especially since it can be used for both relief of acute symptoms and/or for chronic anti-inflammatory maintenance therapy.

G. It is crucial for proper ocular allergy management to differentiate allergic eye diseases from nonallergic ocular burning and painful conditions.

XIII. Internet Resources

www.revoptom.com/handbook/SECT2A.HTM
www.familydoctor.org/handouts/678.html
www.contactlenses.co.uk/education/public/
seasonal_allergic_conjunctivitis.htm

XIV. ICD-9 CODES

370.31   Atopic keratoconjuntivitis (e.g., conjunctivitis and eczema)
372.14   Chronic atopic conjunctivitis
372.13   Vernal conjunctivitis
372.05   Atopic conjunctivitis with hay fever

XV. Diagnosis and Management Algorithm (*Fig. 8-2*)

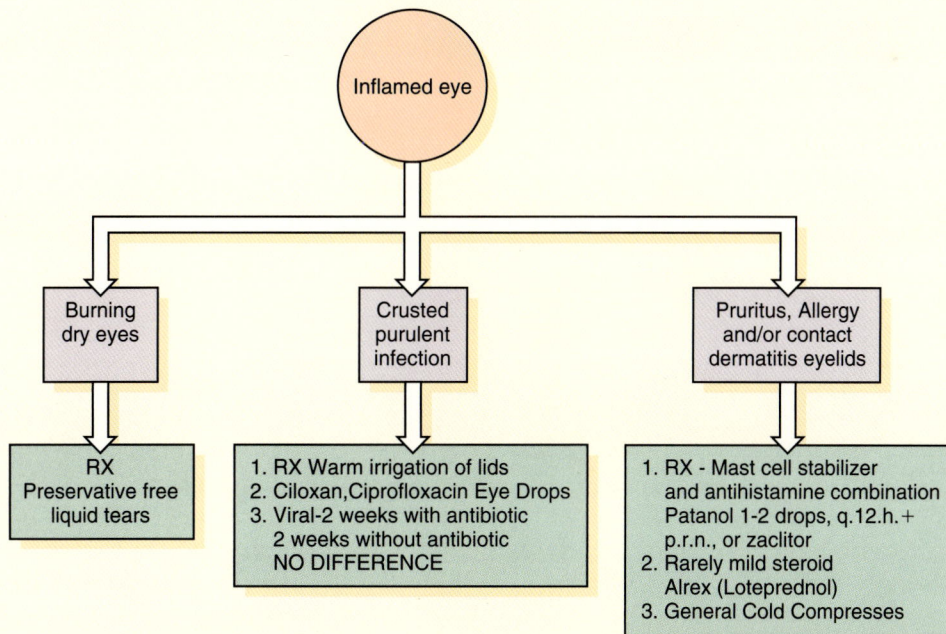

Figure 8-2 Diagnosis and management algorithm.

XVI. Patient Education Materials and Handouts

To alleviate allergic or itchy eyes, patients should:

- Practice environmental control (e.g., close the windows at night and keep animals out of sleep areas).
- Never rub the eyes. Rubbing introduces new antigens into eyes and makes them more sensitive.
- Use Emadine eye drops or a nonstinging equivalent for relief of itching. Use of cold compresses and refrigerated eye drops can help soothe eye discomfort.
- Take a contact lens "vacation" while treating allergic conjunctivitis.
- Avoid eye makeup, which can be rubbed into eyes and exacerbate symptoms.
- See patient education CD, which is provided with this text, for additional patient education information. It has been formatted to provide readily accessible, easy-to-understand handouts for adult patients and the parents of pediatric patients. These handouts can be easily modified to fit specific practice requirements.

REFERENCES

1. Bielory L, Friedlander MH, Fujishima H: Allergic conjunctivitis. Immunology Allergy North America, 1997;17:19–31.
2. Bielory L: Allergic and immunologic disorders of the eye. Part II: ocular allergy. J Allergy Clin Immunol 2000;106:1019–1032.
3. Juniper EF, Guyatt GH: Development and testing of a new measure of health status for clinical trials in rhinoconjunctivitis. Clinical Experimental Allergy 1991;21:77–83.
4. Hogan MJ: Atopic keratonjunctivitis. Am J of Ophthalmology 1953;36:937–947.
5. Aguilar A: Olopatadine Vital Signs: Ketotifen in the Treatment of Allergic Conjunctivitis. Paper presented at: Second International Symposium on Ocular Allergy, Leeds Castle; V. June 1999.
6. Deschenes J, Discepola M, Abelson M: Comparative evaluation of olopatadine ophthamlic solution (0.1%) vs. ketorolac ophthalmic solution (0.5%) using Provocative Antigen Challenge Model. Asta Ophthalmol Scand Suppl 1999;228:47–52.
7. Bielory L, Mongia A: Current opinion of immunotherapy for ocular allergy. Curr Opin Allergy Clin Immunol 2002; 2:447–452.

OTHER SUGGESTED READING

Katelaris CH, Brfemond-Gignac D, Leonardi A, Stahl J: Ocular allergy. Curr Allergy Asthma Rep 2002;2:319–332.

Stahl JL, Cook EB, Graziano FM, Barney NP: Human conjunctival mast cells: Expression of FcRI, cKit, ICAM-1, and IgE. Arch Ophthalmol 1999;117:493–497.

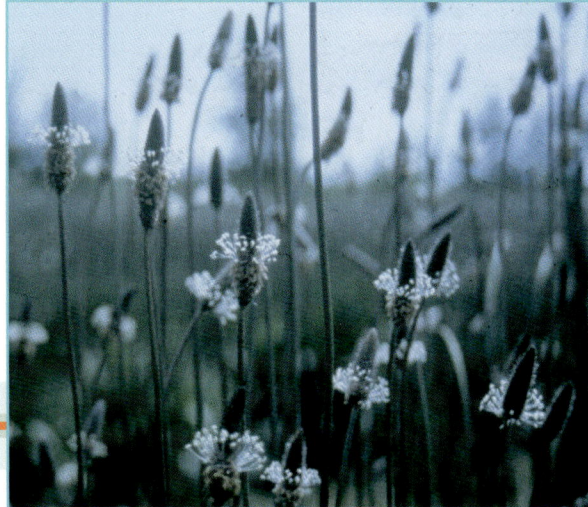

English Plantain Flower *Courtesy of Hollister-Stier Laboratory*

CHAPTER 9
Insect Hypersensitivity

John E. Moffitt and Anne B. Yates

I. Introduction

Anaphylaxis from insect stings causes at least 40 deaths in the United States each year. The stinging insects responsible for these reactions are members of the Hymenoptera family and include yellow jackets, wasps, hornets, honeybees, and fire ants.[1,2] Management of insect sting allergy includes treatment of the acute anaphylactic episode and institution of measures to reduce the patient's risk from subsequent stings. These measures include education of the patient about the self-treatment of anaphylaxis, insect avoidance measures, and evaluation of the patient as a potential candidate for allergen immunotherapy, which is highly effective in reducing the likelihood and severity of a future sting reaction.[1,2]

II. Epidemiology

Insect sting allergy prevalence is probably about 0.5%, although estimates as high as 1.5%–2% have been reported. Persons with insect sting allergy have approximately a 30%–50% risk of reaction with a future sting by the same insect to which they are allergic. Asymptomatic sensitization, the development of measurable venom-specific IgE in the absence of a clinical reaction, occurs in up to 25% of recently stung individuals but is often transient. Sensitized individuals without a history of anaphylaxis appear to have approximately a 17% risk of systemic reaction following subsequent sting.[3,4]

The most common culprit insect in most of the United States is the yellow jacket.[1,2]

The most common culprit insects in the southeastern United States are the imported fire ant and wasp.[5] The domain (Fig. 9-1) of the imported fire ant continues to expand and now extends beyond the southeastern United States.

Other stinging insects include hornets and bees. Figures 9-2 through 9-6 show several types of stinging insects.

III. Etiology

Anaphylactic reactions to insect stings are classic immediate-type hypersensitivity reactions.

A. Mechanism

Reactions occur in previously sensitized individuals when venom-specific IgE molecules attached to mast cells are cross-linked by venom proteins and mast cell mediators are released.

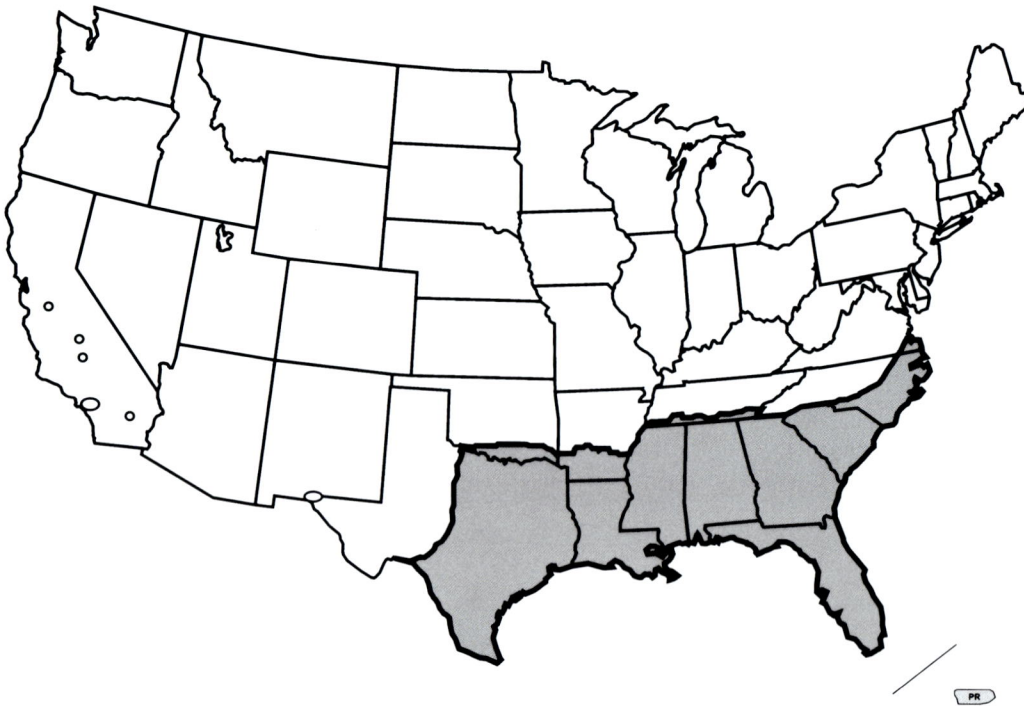

Figure 9-1 Distribution of the imported fire ant in the United States in 1999. (Modified from USDA.)

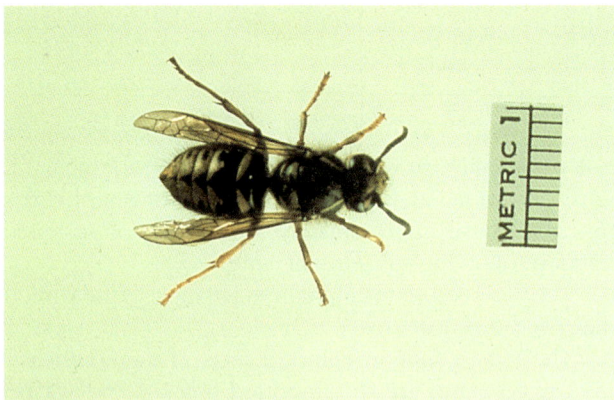

Figure 9-2 Yellow hornet.

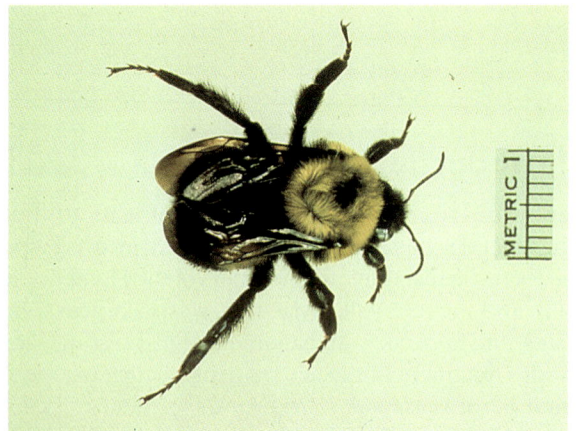

Figure 9-4 Bumblebee.

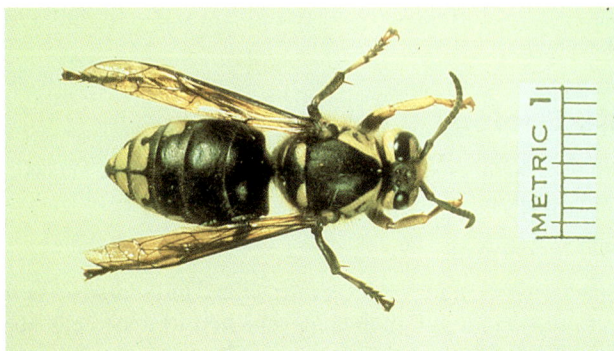

Figure 9-3 White faced hornet.

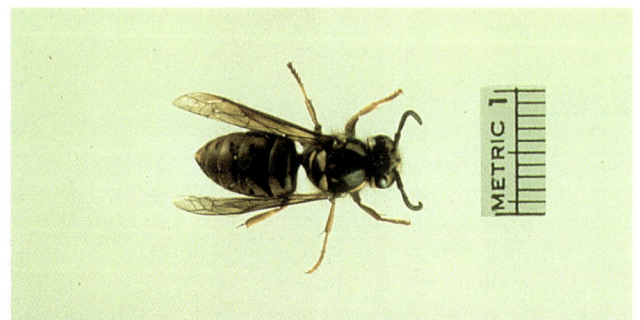

Figure 9-5 Yellow jacket.

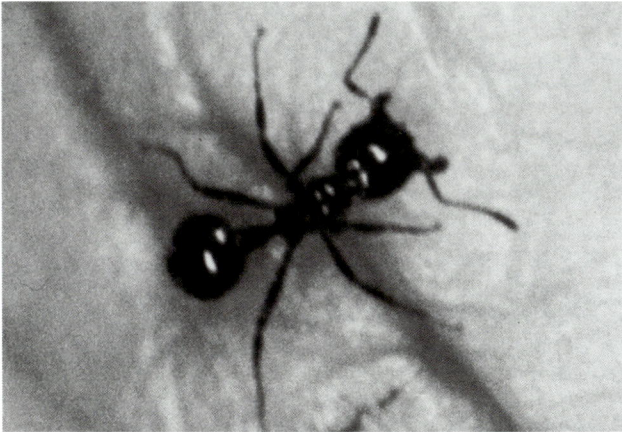

Figure 9-6 Fire ant in the process of stinging. (Courtesy of Dr. James Jarrett, Mississippi Cooperative Extension Service, Mississippi State University.)

B. Sting Reaction

The normal reaction is local; is characterized by pain, erythema, and swelling; and is caused by the direct effects of venom constituents, including histamine, kinin-like substances, enzymes, and other biologically active components.

1. Large local reactions, which appear to be IgE-mediated in most persons, are characterized by more prominent swelling. Patients with large local reactions rarely have systemic reactions to future stings.[1–3]
2. Toxic reactions may occasionally mimic anaphylaxis. They usually occur only after many stings and are due to the direct action of venom constituents, which share physiologic properties with mast cell mediators.[2]

IV. Clinical Manifestations

A. Systemic Allergic Reactions

Systemic allergic reaction to insect stings is similar to anaphylaxis from other causes. Manifestations may be mild, with only flushing, pruritus, angioedema, and urticaria, or the reactions may be life-threatening, usually due to respiratory obstruction with symptoms such as stridor, wheezing, throat tightness, respiratory distress, and shock due to vasodilation or vascular leakage.

B. Normal Sting Reaction

A normal sting reaction consists only of a small area of erythema, local swelling, and pain. The sting of the imported fire ant is unique in that a sterile pustule develops 24 hours after the sting. An imbedded stinger, which usually identifies the culprit insect as a honeybee, may occasionally be seen following stings of other insects.

C. Large Local Reactions

Large local reactions are usually allergic and consist of large areas of local erythema and swelling at the sting site. Swelling of the entire involved extremity may occur, but does not extend beyond that extremity.

D. Toxic Reactions

Toxic reactions occasionally mimic anaphylactic reactions. In these reactions the physiologic effects of venom can cause generalized edema and hypotension. Patients with these reactions usually have received multiple stings. Culprit insects most likely to sting multiple times are the Africanized or "killer" honeybee, the yellow jacket, and the imported fire ant. The "killer" honeybee (Fig. 9-7), which has reached the United States (Fig. 9-8), is more aggressive than native honeybees and may attack in swarms if disturbed. Its venom is nearly identical to that of the native honeybee.

V. Differential Diagnosis

When a patient presents with classic findings of anaphylaxis after a sting, the diagnosis of insect allergy is usually straightforward. However, confirmation of the diagnosis requires demonstration of venom-specific IgE at a later date. At times the diagnosis is not always clear, and the differential diagnosis may be quite extensive.[1–3] Diagnostic considerations may include:

- Anaphylaxis or urticaria from other causes (e.g., food, drug, exercise-induced)
- Coincidental flares of allergic rhinitis or asthma
- Anxiety or hyperventilation reactions
- Vasovagal reactions
- Toxic reactions to insect venom constituents (usually associated with multiple stings)
- Mast cell disorder

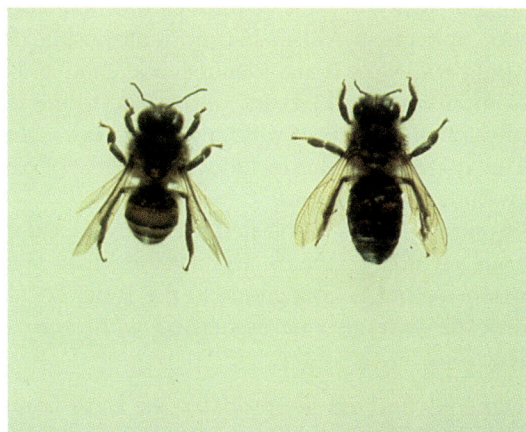

Figure 9-7 Honeybee. (AAAAI. All rights reserved.)

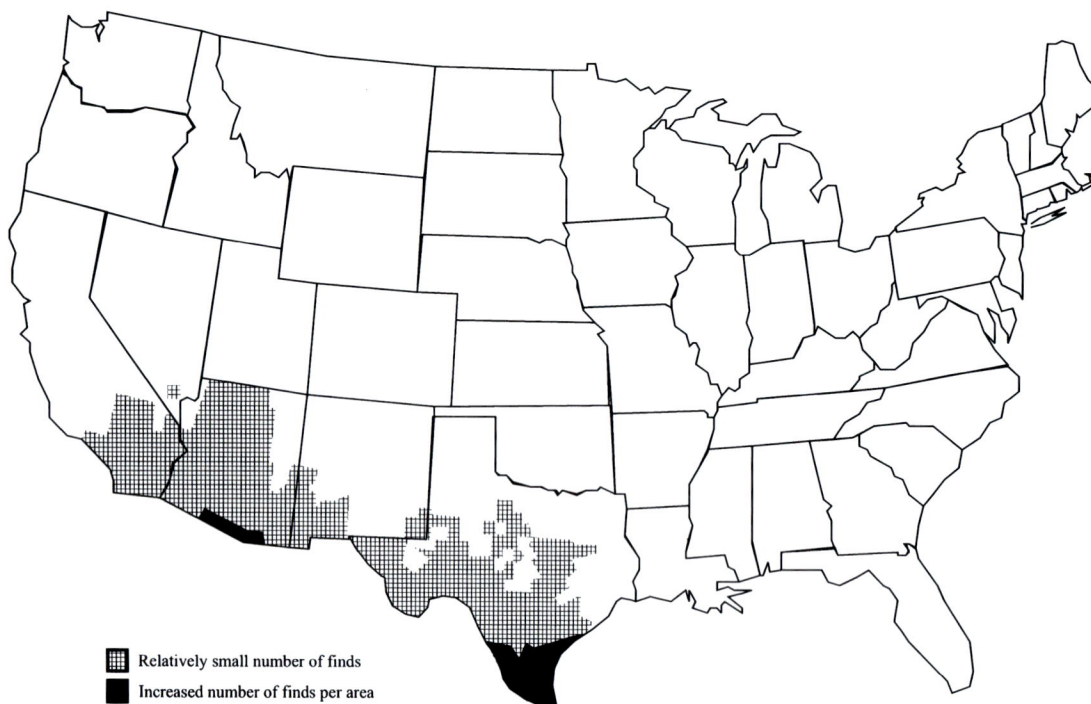

Relatively small number of finds
Increased number of finds per area

Figure 9-8 Distribution of the Africanized honeybee in the United States in 1999. (Modifided from USDA.)

- Other causes of sudden dyspnea or collapse (e.g., seizure, myocardial dysfunction)

VI. Physical Examination

The physical findings of anaphylaxis due to insect allergy are no different from those of anaphylaxis due to other causes, with the exception of the usual presence of one or more sting sites.[1,2]

A. The physical examination should focus initially on findings that indicate a potentially life-threatening condition and that aid in establishing the diagnosis.

1. The physician should examine for presence of a stinger, which usually implicates the honeybee as the culprit insect. A characteristic sterile pustule developing within 24 hours identifies the sting as being from an imported fire ant, and is due to the direct physiologic effects of venom constituents.
2. The "normal" reaction includes a small area of painful swelling and erythema.
3. Physical findings associated with large local reactions include erythema and swelling that may be extensive but is contiguous to the sting. Localized urticaria may also be associated with large local reactions.

B. Cutaneous findings are probably the most common physical findings of anaphylaxis. It is important to document the findings accurately, not only for acute management, but also because the severity of the reaction has bearing on whether or not to start immunotherapy.

1. Findings include urticaria, angioedema, flushing, and/or itching.
2. Patients may also demonstrate rhinorrhea, sneezing and other findings of allergic rhinoconjunctivitis, and vomiting or diarrhea.
3. Myocardial infarctions and spontaneous abortions have also been reported.

C. Deaths from anaphylaxis mainly result from airway obstruction and cardiovascular shock. Usually the large airway is involved, but the lower airway may also be involved (see Chapter 6).[1,2]

1. Signs of airway compromise include stridor, wheezing, and general signs of respiratory distress. Tongue or uvular swelling, hoarseness, voice changes and a sensation of throat tightness may precede more overt signs of airway compromise.
2. Shock is caused by vasodilation and vascular leakage. Physical findings of shock include hypotension and tachycardia, often accompanied by profound edema.

VII. Laboratory Evaluation

In the classic picture of anaphylaxis, laboratory tests are unnecessary. Measurement of tryptase can be useful at

TABLE 9-1

Preventive Management by Reaction Type

Reaction Type	Positive Skin Test (or RAST)	Epinephrine Kit	Insect Avoidance	Immunotherapy
Systemic in adult or child (respiratory/cardiovascular)	Yes	Yes	Yes	Yes
Systemic in adult (dermal only)	Yes	Yes	Yes	Yes
Systemic in child (dermal only)	Yes (if done)	Yes	Yes	Usually no (see text)
Systemic	No	Yes	Yes	No

times because it may remain elevated in some patients for several hours after an anaphylactic episode.

In vitro assays can be used to confirm the presence of venom-specific IgE but are generally less sensitive than immediate hypersensitivity skin testing.

A. Skin Testing Procedures

1. If a flying Hymenoptera is recognized as the culprit insect, patients are usually skin-tested with all five of the available Hymenoptera venoms (yellow jacket, yellow hornet, white-faced hornet, wasp, and honeybee). Most authorities recommend that preliminary prick testing be performed first, and if negative, intradermal skin testing with each venom, starting with a concentration in the range of $0.001\,\mu g/mL$ and increasing by 10-fold increments until the patient develops a positive test to that venom or until a maximum concentration of $1.0\,\mu g/mL$ is reached.
2. For fire ants, if prick tests are negative, then intradermal testing is performed, usually starting with a concentration in the range of $1:1,000,000\,wt/vol$ and increasing by 10-fold increments until a positive reaction develops or a maximum concentration of $1:1000\,wt/vol$ is reached. Patients should be referred to an allergist for this procedure.

VIII. Diagnosis

The diagnosis depends on a history of a reaction consistent with a systemic allergic reaction and demonstration of IgE antibody to a venom.

A. Immediate hypersensitivity skin testing is the method usually employed to demonstrate specific IgE antibody to insect venom because it provides greater sensitivity than in vitro assays.

B. In vitro assays may be used, however, in special circumstances. Also, some patients with negative initial skin tests are later found to have venom-specific IgE. Performance of in vitro testing or repeat skin testing may be

appropriate for patients with more serious reactions if initial skin testing is negative.[6]

1. Skin testing for hypersensitivity should be recommended for patients who would be candidates for venom immunotherapy if positive.
2. Testing to confirm the presence of specific IgE is not necessary in cases where the diagnosis is straightforward and the patient would not meet criteria for institution of venom immunotherapy. However, even in those cases skin testing is an acceptable option for confirmatory purposes. Referral to an allergist is recommended for any patient who may have suffered a systemic reaction and for whom skin testing is indicated.

IX. Therapy and Management

A. Acute Anaphylaxis

1. Treat acute anaphylaxis the same way as for other causes (see Chapter 6, Anaphylaxis, for further discussion of this topic).
2. Remove imbedded stinger by scraping, if present. Do not use forceps, which might inject additional venom from the venom sac into the patient.

B. Preventive (Table 9-1)

1. Prescribe epinephrine kit and educate about use (Table 9-2).

TABLE 9-2

Epinephrine Devices for Self-Administration

Device	Dose	Type
EpiPen	0.3 mg	Spring-loaded autoinjector
EpiPen Jr.	0.15 mg	Spring-loaded autoinjector
Injectable epinephrine (Ana-Kit or Ana-Guard)	Titratable (self-dosed)	Vial

2. Instruct on insect avoidance measures (see Patient Education Material later in this chapter).
3. Consider patient as potential candidate for venom immunotherapy.
   a. Immunotherapy to flying hymenoptera (bees, wasps, hornets, yellow jackets)
      1) Reduces risk of future sting reactions from 30%–50% to 2%–5%.
      2) Indicated for adults and children with systemic allergic reactions involving respiratory and/or cardiovascular symptoms who have venom-specific IgE (by skin test or RAST).
      3) Indicated for adults with systemic cutaneous allergic reactions who have venom-specific IgE.
      4) Children with reactions consisting only of urticaria and/or subcutaneous angioedema are not generally considered candidates for venom immunotherapy because their risk for future systemic allergic reactions is only 10%, and subsequent reactions are also usually limited to urticaria. However, immunotherapy may be considered in select patients and at parental request.
   b. Fire ant immunotherapy
      1) Utilizes whole body extract as opposed to venom product used for flying hymenoptera.[5]
      2) Efficacy is less well defined but appears similar to that of venom immunotherapy used for flying hymenoptera.
      3) Patient selection for fire ant immunotherapy is similar to that for venom immunotherapy. However, it has not been established that children with only dermal allergic reactions are at similarly low risk of severe allergic reactions for subsequent stings. Therefore, immunotherapy is optional for these children.
   c. Duration of immunotherapy
      Usually 3–5 years of therapy is adequate. Recent evidence indicates that the risk of reactions after subsequent stings rises slightly after discontinuation of immunotherapy to around 10%. It may be reasonable to continue immunotherapy for longer periods in cases in which patients have severe reactions (i.e., loss of consciousness).[4]

C. Treatment of Large Local Reactions

These reactions usually require only palliative treatment with analgesics and oral antihistamines. Corticosteroids have not been proven beneficial in controlled trials, but clinical experience suggests they reduce the severity of the swelling. Compartment syndrome occurs rarely and may require fasciotomy. While immunotherapy may reduce the severity of large local reactions, these are not considered an indication for immunotherapy except in the most severe cases.

X. Special Considerations in Patient Subsets

A. Concomitant Medications

Concomitant use of β-blocking medications and possibly angiotension-converting enzyme inhibitors may increase the risk of severe anaphylaxis from stings, immunotherapy reactions, or other causes.

B. Age

Children suffering only mild cutaneous reactions are not usually placed on immunotherapy because they have only a small risk of future severe reactions.

C. Lifestyle

Likelihood of exposure to insect stings may play a role in the decision to institute or discontinue immunotherapy.

XI. When to Obtain Consultation

Consultation with an allergist is indicated when a patient is a candidate for immunotherapy if skin tests prove to be positive. Consultation is appropriate but not mandatory for any patient wth a systematic reaction after an insect sting, even if the patient would not meet criteria for immunotherapy. Consultation is also appropriate when insect sting allergy is suspected but the diagnosis is uncertain.

XII. Practice Guidelines

A. Acute anaphylaxis should be treated similarly to anaphylaxis from other causes (see Chapter 6, Anaphylaxis, for further discussion of this topic and www.jcaai.org/param/anaphylaxis.htm).

B. Patients who have had a systemic reaction to insect stings should:

1. Keep epinephrine for emergency use (see Table 9-2).
2. Be educated about insect avoidance.
3. Consider wearing a medical ID tag.
4. Be considered for skin testing and venom immunotherapy.

C. Venom immunotherapy is indicated for patients with a systemic reaction to insects and venom-specific IgE with the following considerations:

1. Venom immunotherapy is usually not prescribed for children with only cutaneous allergic reactions.

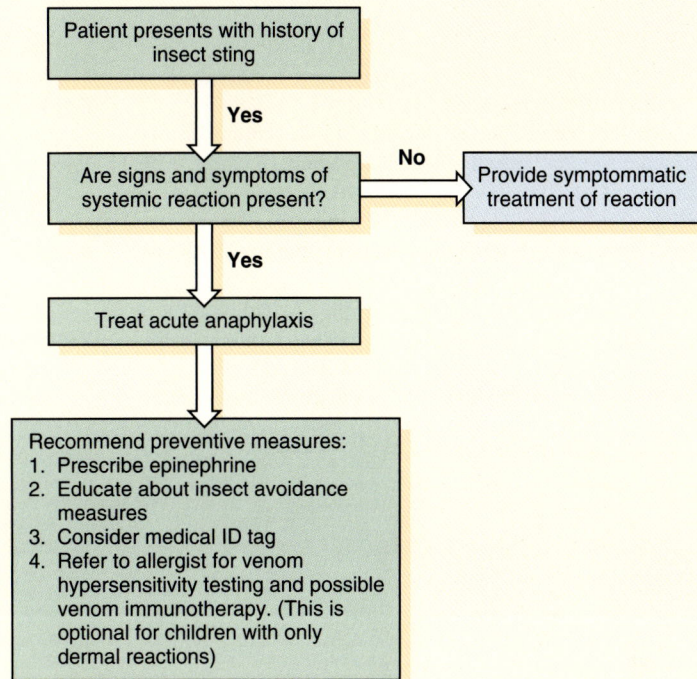

Figure 9-9 Diagnosis and management algorithm.

2. The natural history of cutaneous reactions to fire ant stings in children is not established. Immunotherapy is optional in this group of patients.

XIII. Internet Resources

allergy.mcg.edu
Allergy, Asthma, and Immunology Online—general reference

www.aaaai.org
Web site for American Academy of Allergy, Asthma, and Immunology—general reference

agnews.tamu.edu/bees/stings.htm
Web site for Texas A&M University; emphasis on Africanized honeybee

www.focusonallergies.com
General reference

XIV. ICD-9 Codes

989.5   Anaphylactic shock or reaction following stings
919.4   Insect bite or sting without infection
919.5   Insect bite or sting, infected
E905.3 Modifier to indicate a flying insect

XV. Diagnosis and Management (Fig. 9-9)

XVI. Patient Education Materials and Handouts (Box 9-1)

Refer to patient education CD, which is provided with this text, for additional patient education information. It has been formatted to provide readily accessible, easy-to-understand handouts for adult patients and the parents of pediatric patients. These handouts can be easily modified to fit specific practice requirements.

BOX 9-1
Insect Sting Avoidance Measures

- Avoid close contact with known nests.
- Have nests around the patient's home exterminated professionally.
- Avoid wearing colognes, perfumes, or other fragrances.
- Avoid wearing flowery clothing.
- Wear long-sleeved shirts, long pants, and closed-toe shoes.
- Exercise caution around compost areas, garbage containers, eaves, attics, bushes, picnic areas, and other areas where food or drinks may be served outdoors.

REFERENCES

1. Reisman R: Insect stings. N Engl J Med 1994;331:523-527.
2. Portnoy J, Moffitt JE, Golden DBK, et al: Stinging insect hypersensitivity: A practice parameter. J Allergy Clin Immunol 1999;103:963–980.
3. Golden DB, Marsh DG, Feidhoff LR, et al: Natural history of Hymenoptera venom sensitivity in adults. J Allergy Clin Immunol 1997;100:760–766.
4. Golden DBK, Kagey-Sabotka A, Liechtenstein LM: Survey of patients after discontinuing venom therapy. J Allergy Clin Immunol 2000;105:385–390.
5. Kemp SF, deShazo RD, Moffitt JE, et al: Expanding habitat of the imported fire ant (*Solenopsis invicta*): A public health concern. J Allergy Clin Immunol 2000;105:683–691.
6. Golden DB, Kagey-Sobotha A, Norman PA: Insect sting allergy with negative skin test responses. J. Allergy Clin Immunol 2001;107:897–901.

Other Suggested Reading

Golden DBK, Kwiterovich KA, Addison BA, et al: Discontinuing venom immotherapy: Extended observations. J Allergy Clin Immunol 1998;101:298–305.

Golden DBK, Schwartz HJ: Guidelines for venom immunotherapy. J Allergy Clin Immunol 1986;77:727–778.

Reisman RE: Natural history of insect sting allergy: Relationship of severity of symptoms of initial sting anaphylaxis to resting reactions. J Allergy Clin Immunol 1992;90:335–339.

Reisman RE: Duration of venom immunotherapy: Relationship to the severity of symptoms of initial insect sting anaphylaxis. J Allergy Clin Immunol 1993;92:831–836.

Tankersley MS, Walker RL, Butler WK, et al: Safety and efficacy of an imported fire ant rash immunotherapy protocol with and without prophylactic treatment. J Allergy Clin Immunol 2002;109:556–562.

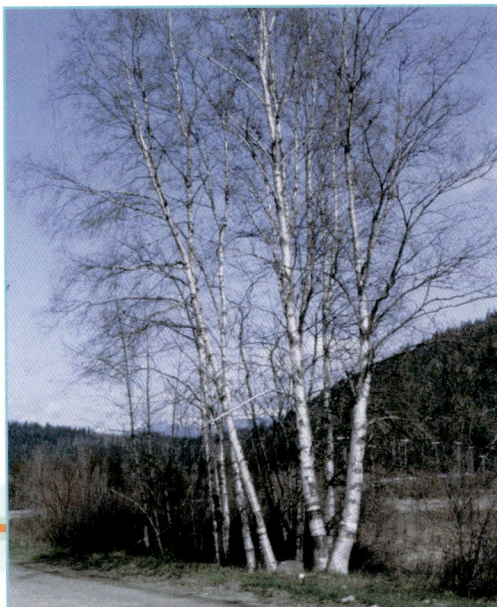

CHAPTER 10
Drug Allergy

Adrian M. Casillas and Marc A. Riedl

I. Introduction

While drug reactions are commonplace in the practice of medicine, identifying a drug allergy may be quite challenging for the practicing physician. Complicating factors of drug reactions include the myriad clinical symptoms and the multiple mechanisms of drug-host interaction, many of which are poorly understood. In addition, the relative paucity of laboratory tests for drug allergy makes the diagnosis heavily dependent on the knowledge and experience of the consulting physician.

The terms drug allergy, drug hypersensitivity, and drug reaction are often used interchangeably. It is important to know the differences between these terms. *Drug reactions* encompass all adverse events related to drug administration, regardless of etiology. Adverse effects to drugs have been documented over many years. Some of the most familiar household medications, such as aspirin (originally prepared by hydrolysis of oils from sweet birch bark) have been used for centuries. *Drug hypersensitivity* is defined as an immunologically mediated response to a drug agent in a sensitized patient. A *drug allergy* is restricted specifically to immunologic IgE-mediated drug reactions.

II. Epidemiology

Adverse drug reactions are a major cause of morbidity and mortality worldwide. They are the most common iatrogenic illness, complicating 5%–15% of therapeutic drug courses.[1,2] In the United States alone, more than 100,000 deaths annually are attributed to serious drug reactions.[3] Some 3%–6% of all hospital admissions are due to adverse drug reactions, and approximately 6%–15% of hospitalized patients (2.2 million individuals in 1994) experience a serious adverse drug reaction.[1,3–7] The majority of these events are due to common, predictable, nonimmunologic mechanisms.

A. Patient-Related Risk Factors

Epidemiologic data support the existence of specific risk factors for both general adverse drug reactions and drug hypersensitivity reactions (Table 10-1).

General adverse drug reactions occur more frequently in seriously ill patients, particularly those with hepatic or renal insufficiency. Other risk factors include polypharmacy, HIV infection, systemic lupus erythematosis (SLE), and alcoholism.

Patient Risk Factors for Adverse Drug Reactions

General drug reactions (nonimmune)

Serious illness
Renal insufficiency
Liver disease
Polypharmacy
HIV infection
Alcoholism
Systemic lupus erythematosus

Hypersensitivity drug reactions (immune)

Adults > children
Female > male
HIV infection
Concomitant viral infection
Previous hypersensitivity to chemically related drug
β-blocker use
Specific genetic polymorphisms
Systemic lupus erythematosus

Particular individuals are at greater risk for *drug hypersensitivity reactions*. These include adult patients, patients with HIV[8–11] or SLE,[12] and patients with previous hypersensitivity reactions to chemically related drugs. Women appear more frequently affected by drug hypersensitivity than men.[13,14]

Although atopic patients do not appear to have a higher rate of sensitization to drugs, they are at increased risk for serious allergic reactions once an IgE response to any drug has developed.[15,16] Certain HLA phenotypes are linked to increased drug reactivity.[17–20] Finally, patients with concomitant viral infections may have a greater risk of drug hypersensitivity.[21,22]

β-blocker use aggravates all allergic and pseudo-allergic reactions, and is a risk factor for pseudo-allergic reactions to radiocontrast media (relative risk = 2.5).[23]

B. Drug-Related Risk Factors

The most important risk factors for drug hypersensitivity are related to the chemical properties and molecular weight of the drug.

1. Drugs with greater structural complexity (e.g., non-human proteins) are more likely to be immunogenic.
2. Drugs must have a sufficient molecular weight (>1000 Da) to be immunogenic in their native state. Most drugs have a smaller molecular weight but become reactive by coupling with carrier proteins, such as albumin, to form haptens.
3. An additional factor affecting the frequency of drug hypersensitivity reactions is the route of drug administration.

a. Topical and intravenous (IV) administration are more likely to cause hypersensitivity reactions.
b. Oral medications are less likely to result in drug hypersensitivity.[16]
c. Intermittent, repeated administrations are more likely to result in sensitization than uninterrupted treatment.

III. Etiology/Pathophysiology

Adverse drug reactions can be classified into immunologic and nonimmunologic etiologies (Table 10-2).

The majority (75%–80%) of adverse drug reactions are due to predictable, nonimmunologic effects.[24] These

Immunologic versus Nonimmunologic Drug Reactions

Type	Example
Immunologic	
Type I hypersensitivity (IgE-mediated)	Anaphylaxis from β-lactam antibiotic
Type II hypersensitivity (cytotoxic)	Hemolytic anemia from penicillin
Type III hypersensitivity (immune-complex)	Serum sickness from anti-thymocyte globulin
Type IV hypersensitivity (Delayed, cell-mediated)	Contact dermatitis from topical antihistamine
Specific T-cell activation	Morbilliform rash from sulfonamides
Fas/Fas-ligand induced apoptosis	Stevens-Johnson syndrome/toxic epidermal necrolysis
Other	Drug-induced lupus-like syndrome, Churg-Strauss syndrome
Nonimmunologic	
Idiosyncratic	Hemolytic anemia in a patient with G-6-PD deficiency after primaquine therapy
Pseudoallergic	Shock after radiocontrast media
Intolerance	Tinnitus after small doses of aspirin
Side-effect due to pharmacologic action	Dry mouth from antihistamines
Secondary effect of drug action	Thrush while taking antibiotics
Drug toxicity	Hepatotoxicity from methotrexate
Drug-drug interactions	Seizure from theophylline while taking erythromycin
Drug overdose	Seizure from excessive lidocaine

include direct effects of the pharmacologic action (predictable side effects), drug toxicity, secondary effects of the drug action, or drug-drug interactions.

Some 20%–25% of adverse drug events are unpredictable effects that may or may not be immune-mediated.[24] The nonimmune-mediated reactions include idiosyncratic reactions, drug intolerance, and pseudo-allergic reactions. Immune-mediated reactions account for 5%–10% of all drug reactions and constitute true drug hypersensitivity.[25,26]

Immune-mediated drug hypersensitivity has traditionally been discussed in the setting of the Gell and Coombs classification system.[27] However, some drug hypersensitivity syndromes do not fit well in a single classification and will be discussed outside of this classification framework.

A. Type I Hypersensitivity Reactions

Immediate hypersensitivity reactions are IgE-mediated and constitute true drug allergy. These reactions are the result of drug binding to specific Fc-epsilon (Fcε) receptors on mast cells, causing mast cell degranulation and release of inflammatory mediators. The development of specific IgE sufficient to produce an immediate hypersensitivity reaction generally requires previous drug exposure. Thus, patients typically develop symptoms with subsequent courses of the medication. Immediate hypersensitivity reactions with a true first dose are distinctly unusual.

The clinical symptoms of type I hypersensitivity include urticaria, angioedema, bronchospasm, pruritus, flushing, rhinoconjunctivitis, vomiting, diarrhea, and the hypotension and tachycardia associated with anaphylaxis. These symptoms frequently appear seconds to minutes after exposure, although they may appear after several hours with oral drugs.

B. Type II Hypersensitivity Reactions

Cytotoxic hypersensitivity reactions are due to the formation of antibodies directed at antigens found on or near cell surfaces. Typically, these specific antibodies are IgG or IgM directed at antigens found in drug molecules or drug-protein haptens. Drugs such as penicillin, the sulfonamides, the phenothiazines, and heparin may form haptens that coat erythrocytes, granulocytes, or platelets. In the presence of preformed drug-specific antibodies, these hapten-coated cells become targets for cytotoxic reactions. The clinical manifestations become apparent with significant depletion of a specific cell type (e.g., anemia, neutropenia, thrombocytopenia).

C. Type III Hypersensitivity Reactions

Immune complex reactions are caused by tissue inflammation and damage mediated by the deposition of circulating drug antigen-antibody complexes.

With ongoing exposure to a drug substance, specific IgG or IgM antibodies are produced that bind the drug antigen in the circulation. These antigen-antibody complexes activate the complement system, resulting in inflammation of surrounding tissues, which commonly include blood vessels, skin, and synovium. Typically, such reactions show up 1–3 weeks after drug administration with symptoms of serum sickness, including fever, rash (Fig. 10-1), arthralgias, and lymphadenopathy.

Type III hypersensitivity may also be involved in drug-induced lupus-like syndromes, with the production of antihistone antinuclear antibodies, resulting in immune complex reactions.

D. Type IV Hypersensitivity Reactions

Delayed-type, cell-mediated reactions are due to major histocompatibility complex (MHC) presentation of drug molecules to CD4+ and CD8+ T-cells. Drug haptens are processed intracellularly or extracellularly and subsequently are recognized by drug-specific T-cells through MHC/T-cell receptor interaction. Activated T-cells release cytokines and other mediators responsible for the inflammatory changes associated with delayed-type reactions, such as contact dermatitis. The skin inflammation typically appears 2–7 days after cutaneous drug exposure.

E. Other Mechanisms

For particular drug reactions, evidence exists for immune mechanisms that do not readily fit into the Gell–Coombs classification system.

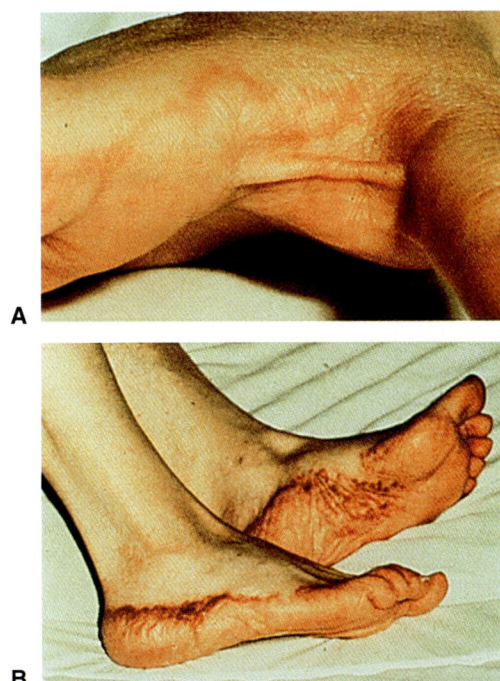

Figure 10-1 A and **B**, Typical rash seen in serum sickness.

1. ***Specific T-Cell Activation***
   Although the immunopathogenesis is not fully delineated, a number of drug reactions appear to be mediated by specific T-cell activation.
   a. These include maculopapular rashes, erythroderma, exfoliative dermatitis, and fixed drug reactions.
   b. A proposed mechanism involves intracellular drug processing by nucleated cells, with MHC I presentation to drug-specific CD8+ T-cells.[28] T-cell directed inflammation is subsequently directed at the skin via cutaneous lymphocyte-associated antigen on circulating T-cells.[29]

2. ***Innate Immune System***
   This system, which contains receptors to recognize characteristic patterns of foreign substances, may play a role in drug reactions. Such reactions may not require a previous exposure to the drug and may be augmented or activated by an intercurrent infectious process such as a viral infection.[30–33]

3. ***Specific Drugs***
   There are specific drugs that may cause characteristic syndromes that do not conform to the Gell-Coombs classification.
   a. Drugs such as hydralazine or procainamide may induce autoantibody activity, resulting in a drug-induced lupus-like syndrome with symptoms of autoimmune disease.
   b. The Churg-Strauss syndrome is a systemic vasculitis associated with glucocorticoids, leukotriene receptor antagonists, and macrolide antibiotics.
   c. Aromatic anticonvulsants such as phenytoin and carbamazepine may cause a life-threatening hypersensitivity reaction characterized by lymphadenopathy and liver and kidney inflammation.
   d. Cutaneous syndromes such as Stevens-Johnson syndrome and toxic epidermal necrolysis induced by sulfonamides and anticonvulsants have been shown to be mediated by Fas and Fas ligand-induced keratinocyte cell death (apoptosis), as well as by activated cutaneous lymphocyte-associated T-cell activity.[34,35]

4. ***Multiple Drug Allergy Syndrome***
   This syndrome has been described in individuals with a hypothetical propensity to develop immune reactions to drug haptens and subsequently express a broad range of immunopathologic responses. Although some data support this hypothesis, further studies have failed to confirm these findings.[36–39] It remains unclear whether such a syndrome exists.

F. Unpredictable, nonimmune-mediated drug reactions can be classified as pseudo-allergic, idiosyncratic, or intolerance.

1. ***Pseudo-Allergic***
   Reactions that are the result of direct mast cell activation and degranulation by a drug are termed *pseudo-allergic*. These reactions may be clinically indistinguishable from type I hypersensitivity; however, they do not involve drug-specific IgE. Rather, medications such as opiates, vancomycin, and radiocontrast media cause direct histamine release, resulting in urticaria, angioedema, bronchospasm, or anaphylactic-like (anaphylactoid) symptoms.

2. ***Idiosyncratic***
   Qualitatively aberrant reactions that cannot be explained by the known pharmacologic action of the drug are termed idiosyncratic. These reactions occur in a small proportion of the population and may be related to individual genetic factors that only become apparent following drug exposure.

3. ***Intolerance***
   Drug intolerance is defined as a lower threshold to the normal pharmacologic action of a drug.

IV. Clinical Manifestations

Adverse drug reactions are great imitators of disease, as they may involve any organ system. Various clinical manifestations may occur due to localized or systemic immune processes. A brief overview of symptoms outlined by organ system follows.

A. Skin

Because of the metabolic and immunologic activity of the skin, drug reactions commonly manifest with cutaneous symptoms. Cutaneous reactions include morbilliform rashes, urticaria, cutaneous vasculitis, eczematous rashes, and fixed drug eruptions. Stevens-Johnson syndrome and toxic epidermal necrolysis represent a more severe form of cutaneous drug reaction that may be life-threatening.

1. ***Urticaria***
   Urticaria (Fig. 10-2) is typically a manifestation of a type I hypersensitivity reaction, although it may appear with type III or pseudo-allergic reactions as well. Urticarial lesions are typically pruritic wheals that last less than 24 hours. Concomitant angioedema may be present. The appearance of urticaria should prompt a thorough evaluation for signs of anaphylaxis resulting from further mast cell mediator release.

2. ***Morbilliform Rashes***
   These rashes (Fig. 10-3) are perhaps the most common drug reaction. Typically, an erythematous, maculopapular rash appears within 1–3 weeks of drug initiation and originates on the trunk, with eventual spread to the limbs. As with most drug rashes, the distribution is generally symmetric, with sparing of

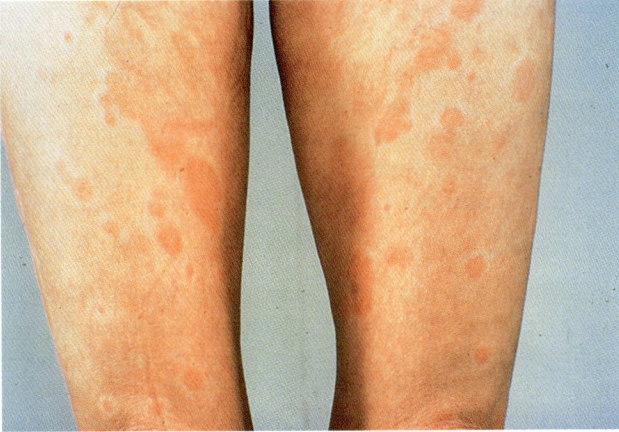

Figure 10-2 Typical pruritic wheal seen in urticaria.

the palms and soles. The rash may be accompanied by fever and pruritus.

3. **Erythema Multiforme, Stevens-Johnson Syndrome (SJS), and Toxic Epidermal Necrolysis (TEN)**

   These conditions represent blistering mucocutaneous skin diseases secondary to drug hypersensitivity reactions.

   a. Erythema multiforme typically presents with target and bullous skin lesions involving the extremities and mucous membranes.

   b. Features of SJS include confluent purpuric macules on the face and trunk, severe mucosal erosions, high fever, and severe constitutional symptoms.

   c. TEN is a more severe form of SJS with epidermal detachment of greater than 30% of skin surface area.[40] TEN patients have widespread areas of confluent skin erythema, followed by epidermal necrosis and detachment. Mucosal surfaces may be severely affected.

4. **Fixed Drug Eruptions**

   These eruptions are well-circumscribed papules or plaques that recur in the same location with each readministration of a drug. Frequently involved areas include the perioral or perianal region. The eruptions may be painful or pruritic.

5. **Eczematous Rashes**

   These rashes are most commonly associated with topical medications and usually represent contact dermatitis (type IV hypersensitivity) to a drug exposure.

6. **Cutaneous Vasculitis**

   This condition may take a variety of appearances.

   a. Typical lesions include purpuric papules or urticarial vasculitis (lesions that are urticarial in appearance but persist longer than 24–48 hours).

   b. The appearance of cutaneous vasculitic lesions should prompt an evaluation for signs of systemic vasculitis, although isolated skin involvement is common. A skin biopsy is warranted if cutaneous vasculitis is suspected.

B. Lung

Pulmonary conditions associated with drug hypersensitivity include eosinophilic pneumonia, and alveolar or interstitial pneumonitis.[41] These reactions typically manifest after 1–2 weeks of drug therapy with a nonproductive cough, dyspnea, fever, and malaise. Findings supporting the diagnosis include eosinophilia and a migratory infiltrate on chest x-ray.

C. Kidney

Interstitial nephritis is the most common renal condition associated with drug hypersensitivity. Patients present with symptoms of tubular dysfunction (azotemia, edema) and may have concomitant fever, rash, and serum or urinary eosinophilia. Membranous glomerulonephritis is a less frequently seen condition that produces a nephrotic clinical picture with edema, proteinuria, and hypoalbuminemia.

D. Liver

Immunologic hepatitis associated with drug hypersensitivity may result in liver function abnormalities and, less commonly, cholestatic jaundice.

E. Systemic Syndromes

1. **Anticonvulsant Hypersensitivity Syndrome**

   This syndrome is a life-threatening syndrome that develops after days to weeks of therapy with aromatic anticonvulsant medications (phenytoin, carbamazepine, phenobarbital). It is characterized by fever, maculopapular rash, and generalized lymphadenopathy.[42] Additional symptoms include facial

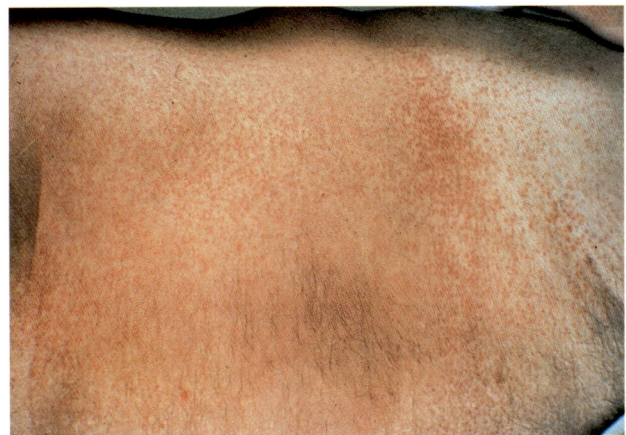

Figure 10-3 Most common morbilliform maculopapular rash seen in drug reactions.

edema, hepatitis, nephritis, and leukocytosis with the presence of atypical lymphocytes and eosinophils. Symptoms may persist for weeks after drug discontinuation. Cross-reactivity between aromatic anticonvulsants may occur.

2. ***Drug-Induced Lupus-like Syndrome***

This syndrome has been associated with numerous drugs but is most commonly observed with procainamide or hydralazine therapy.[43,44] The syndrome generally appears weeks to months into the drug course and manifests with various autoimmune symptoms. These commonly include arthralgias or arthritis, myalgias, serositis, fever, and rash. Symptoms are usually milder than those observed in SLE and resolve within weeks of drug discontinuation.

3. ***Churg-Strauss Syndrome***

This syndrome is a primary vasculitis with eosinophilic infiltration. Multiple organs are affected, including the lungs, heart, intestinal tract, and peripheral nervous system.[45] Patients typically exhibit a symptom pattern of atopic disease (rhinitis, sinusitis) followed by increasingly severe asthma. Ultimately, they develop vasculitis. Vasculitic symptoms may include skin lesions, neuropathy, gastroenteritis, and cardiopulmonary decompensation, all due to extensive organ infiltration by eosinophils. Churg-Strauss syndrome has most recently been associated with leukotriene receptor antagonists, although a causative mechanism has yet to be established.

F. Drug Fever

Drug hypersensitivity may manifest with isolated fever in the absence of other symptoms. Typically, onset occurs 7–10 days into drug treatment. Patients frequently have discordance between fever and constitutional appearance—that is, they look and feel well despite fevers. Discontinuation of the drug results in prompt defervescence within 48 hours.

V. Differential Diagnosis

Since adverse drug reactions may cause innumerable clinical symptoms, an organ system-based approach is useful in considering the differential diagnoses (Box 10-1).

BOX 10-1

Conditions to Be Distinguished from Adverse Drug Reaction, by Organ System

Dermatologic
Viral exanthem
Atopic dermatitis
Contact dermatitis, irritant or allergic other than drug
Angioedema/urticaria due to cause other than drug
Bullous skin disease
Cutaneous infection
Photosensitivity reaction
Psoriasis
Primary autoimmune disease
Lichen planus

Systemic
Anaphylaxis due to food, exercise, insect sting
Autoimmune disease
Infection
Lymphoproliferative disorders

Hematologic
Cytopenias
    Infection
    Autoimmune disease
    Malignancy
    Aplastic anemia
    Nutritional deficiency
Eosinophilia
    Helminthic infection
    Hypereosinophilic syndrome

Pulmonary
Asthma
Hypersensitivity pneumonitis
Interstitial lung disease due to cause other than drug
Infection
Allergic bronchopulmonary aspergillosis
Sarcoidosis
Autoimmune disease
Lymphoproliferative disorders
Wegener's granulomatosis
Hypereosinophilic syndrome
Churg-Strauss syndrome
Pulmonary edema

Renal
Primary glomerular disease
Diabetes
Amyloidosis
Malignancy
Autoimmune disease
Infection
Wegener's granulomatosis

Hepatic
Viral or other infectious hepatitis
Alcoholic hepatitis
Primary biliary cirrhosis
Primary sclerosing cholangitis
Sarcoidosis
Granulomatous hepatitis
Autoimmune hepatitis

VI. History and Physical Examination

Prior to the physical examination, a thorough history should include recording of all possible culprit drugs, dates of administration, and dosage. The relationship between drug intake and the onset of clinical symptoms is critical. Patients should be queried regarding previous drug exposure history. Any underlying hepatic or renal disease affecting drug metabolism or excretion should be identified.

The initial question facing the clinician is whether the symptoms and physical findings are compatible with an immune drug reaction. Because drug reactions may involve any organ system, a complete physical examination is recommended for any patient with suspected drug hypersensitivity.

A. Identify Anaphylaxis

In approaching the patient with a drug reaction, an initial prudent step is to evaluate for signs and symptoms of anaphylaxis, as this is the most immediate life-threatening form of an adverse drug reaction. Dyspnea, wheezing, urticaria, angioedema, tachycardia, or hypotension should be immediately noted and promptly treated with appropriate interventions.

B. Perform a Complete Physical Examination

Drug hypersensitivity reactions may affect virtually any organ system, including the renal, hepatic, pulmonary, musculoskeletal, lymphatic, hematologic, and GI systems. Drug reactions may also present with fever, infrequently in excess of 104°F. A complete physical examination should evaluate for evidence and extent of additional organ involvement. Particular attention should be given to the presence of mucous membrane lesions, lymphadenopathy, hepatosplenomegaly, cardiopulmonary irregularities, and joint tenderness or swelling.

C. Perform a Focused Skin Examination

The skin is the organ most frequently and most prominently affected by adverse drug reactions. Thus, a thorough, detailed examination of the skin is essential.

1. The most common drug-induced skin lesion is a maculopapular rash; however, the spectrum of drug-induced skin lesions includes urticaria, papulovesicular eruptions, bullous lesions, purpura, and exfoliative dermatitis.
2. Cutaneous manifestations should be described accurately with respect to both morphology and distribution. Distinctions should be made between the various types of skin lesions, as this may provide substantial clues to the mechanism of the drug reaction.
3. Specific skin lesions and common underlying immune-mediated diseases are listed in Table 10-3.

TABLE 10-3

Cutaneous Manifestations of Immune Drug Reactions

Type of Skin Lesion	Associated Immune Drug Reaction
Urticaria	IgE-antibody mediated (type I) or anaphylactoid (see Fig. 10-1)
Purpura	Vasculitis
Maculopapular lesions with distribution on the fingers, toes, or soles	Serum sickness (see Fig. 10-2)
Blistering lesions with mucous membrane involvement	Stevens-Johnson syndrome or toxic epidermal necrolysis
Papulovesicular, scaly lesion	Contact dermatitis

4. It is important to remember that skin rashes have multiple alternative drug-independent causes, including common associations with viral or bacterial infections.
   a. Of particular importance is early recognition of Stevens-Johnson syndrome and toxic epidermal necrolysis. These severe skin drug eruptions, which likely represent an overlapping continuum of the same pathologic process, carry a significant mortality rate (SJS 5%, TEN 30%),[40,46] making early detection essential.
   b. Symptoms include purpuric macules, blistering skin lesions, and mucous membrane involvement.
   c. Early drug withdrawal is mandatory in patients who develop such symptoms.

D. Recognize Patterns

Certain patterns of systemic disease may be evident on physical examination and may suggest particular drug-associated syndromes.

1. These include Churg-Strauss syndrome, drug-induced lupus-like syndrome, drug-induced immunologic hepatitis, and interstitial or membranous glomerulonephritis.
2. A severe hypersensitivity syndrome is associated with aromatic anticonvulsants and may lead to complications that include hepatitis, nephritis, toxic epidermal necrolysis, or erythema multiforme. The reported mortality rate in such reactions is 10%,[42] but may be much higher with the development of exfoliative dermatitis.
3. Early recognition of these disease syndromes by the astute clinician will minimize the associated morbidity and mortality.

VII. Laboratory Evaluation

Few laboratory tests are available for suspected drug reactions. The goal of diagnostic testing is to evaluate biochemical or immunologic markers that confirm activation of a particular immunopathologic pathway to explain the suspected adverse drug effect. Laboratory evaluation is guided by the suspected pathologic mechanism (Table 10-4).

A. Type I hypersensitivity reactions require the presence of antigen-specific IgE. Skin testing is a particularly useful diagnostic procedure to test for antigen-specific IgE in select instances (see Chapter 12). Skin testing is standardized for penicillin, and well-described for local anesthetics[47,48] and muscle relaxants.[49–52] It may also be informative when testing high-molecular-weight protein substances such as insulin, vaccines, streptokinase, polyclonal or monoclonal antibodies, and latex.[48,53] Positive skin testing to such reagents confirms the presence of antigen-specific IgE and is supportive of a type I hypersensitivity reaction in the appropriate clinical setting. Negative skin testing is helpful only in penicillin skin testing, because the test specificity has been adequately established.[54] With other drug agents, a negative skin test does not effectively rule out the presence of specific IgE.

1. Penicillin skin testing should include testing for both the major and minor determinants to achieve maximal sensitivity in identifying patients at-risk for IgE-mediated reactions to penicillins. The major determinant, benzylpenicilloyl, comprises 95% of tissue-bound penicillin metabolites.

   a. However, skin testing with native penicillin and the major determinant alone will identify only 80%–85% of patients at risk for type I hypersensitivity reactions. The remaining 15%–20% react only to the minor determinants[55–57] and may actually suffer the most severe clinical reactions.[58]

   b. Patients with positive skin tests have a significant risk (>50%) of experiencing a hypersensitivity reaction if given penicillin.[59] Skin testing for both major and minor determinants is highly specific (97%–99%),[54] and life-threatening reactions in patients with negative skin tests are extremely rare.

2. It is important to recognize the minimal but real risk of systemic reactions with skin testing procedures.

   a. For this reason, skin-prick testing followed by intradermal testing is advisable. Medical treatment for anaphylaxis should be readily available in the procedure setting.

   b. Skin testing should optimally be performed more than 4 weeks after the adverse event to minimize false negative results due to depletion of mast cell mediators or specific IgE.

   c. Drug-specific skin testing is contraindicated in patients with a history of drug-induced SJS or TEN, because of the risk of inducing recurrence.

3. In vitro testing for IgE is available for a limited number of drugs in the form of radioallergosorbent testing (RAST).[60] Although such serologic testing is commonly referred to as RAST testing, enzyme-linked immunosorbent assay (ELISA) techniques are frequently used (see Chapter 13).

TABLE 10-4

Diagnostic Testing for Drug Hypersensitivity

Immunologic Reaction	*Clinical Manifestation*	*Laboratory Tests*
Type I	Anaphylaxis Angioedema Urticaria	Skin testing RAST testing Serum tryptase
Type II	Hemolytic anemia Thrombocytopenia Neutropenia	Direct/indirect Coombs test
Type III	Serum sickness Vasculitis Glomerulonephritis	Immune complexes ESR Complement studies ANA/ANCA C-reactive protein Tissue biopsy for immunoflourescence studies
Type IV	Allergic contact dermatitis Maculopapular drug rash*	Patch testing Lymphocyte proliferation assay†

*Suspected type IV reaction; mechanism not fully elucidated.
†Investigational test.

a. Caution should be used in interpreting drug RAST results. RAST tests are historically less sensitive than skin testing for determining specific IgE levels.[48] In addition, because the immunogenic determinant is undefined for the majority of drug agents, a negative RAST result may not include testing for the relevant antigen, and therefore may be falsely reassuring (i.e., it has a poor negative predictive value).[61]

b. Further, it is important to realize that drug-specific IgE antibody tests (in vitro or in vivo) are not diagnostic of cytotoxic, immune complex, or cell-mediated drug-induced immune reactions.

4. Because type I hypersensitivity reactions involve the IgE-mediated degranulation of mast cells, laboratory tests measuring mast cell activation may be helpful if done at the time of the adverse event.

a. Although serum histamine levels peak 15 minutes after anaphylaxis and return to baseline within 30 minutes, serum β-tryptase levels peak 1 hour after anaphylaxis and remain elevated for 2–4 hours after the event.[62]

b. Elevation of 24-hour urine histamine/*N*-methylhistamine levels may also indicate massive mast cell activation, although this is a less sensitive test than serum β-tryptase.[63]

B. Type II immune reactions to a drug result in destruction of cells due to cytotoxic reactions mediated by drug haptens that adhere to the cell membrane. Hemolytic anemia is the most frequently observed manifestation; however, thrombocytopenia or neutropenia may also occur and may be documented with a complete blood cell count. Hemolytic anemia may be confirmed with a positive direct or indirect Coombs test, reflecting the presence of complement or drug hapten on the red cell membrane. Additional specific testing for immunocytotoxic thrombocytopenia and granulocytopenia is available at some medical centers.

C. Type III immune reactions involve immune complex deposition in tissues with resultant complement activation, inflammation, and tissue damage.

1. The classic presentation is a serum sickness picture that develops 10–21 days after drug administration. Associated symptoms include fever, arthralgias, rash, and lymphadenopathy. Vasculitis and glomerulonephritis are also evident at times.

2. Laboratory tests to detect circulating immune complexes are helpful to support the clinical diagnosis. These include general screening tests such as cryoglobulins and more specific immune complex assays utilizing C1q binding, polyethelene glycol, or Raji cell binding. Positive tests are helpful. Negative tests

do not exclude the diagnosis of immune complex disease.

3. Other useful laboratory studies include nonspecific inflammatory markers such as erythrocyte sedimentation rate, C-reactive protein, and complement levels, including CH_{50}, C3, and C4. Systemic vasculitides induced by medication may be detected by autoantibody tests such as antinuclear antibody, antihistone antibody (associated with drug-induced lupus syndrome),[64,65] and antinuclear cytoplasmic antibody (associated with Churg-Strauss syndrome).[66]

D. Type IV immune reactions involve delayed hypersensitivity, cell-mediated reactions.

1. The classic presentation of a type IV reaction is allergic contact dermatitis caused by topical medications.

2. Patch testing for specific drug agents is an appropriate diagnostic step for such reactions.[67] Erythema, induration, and a pruritic vesiculopapular rash that develops 48 hours after patch application support a type IV immune reaction (see Chapter 20). Recent research has suggested that cell-mediated hypersensitivity may be responsible for the typical cutaneous morbilliform rash seen in reactions to drugs such as sulfonamides or penicillins.[28,29] While some evidence supports a positive correlation between patch testing and morbilliform drug reactions,[68] the diagnostic utility is controversial.[69] Chapter 20 covers this topic in greater detail.

3. Lymphocyte proliferation testing may hold promise as a diagnostic test to confirm type IV immune reaction to drugs.[70]

4. These in vitro testing results have been inconsistent to date and cannot be recommended for routine clinical use.[69]

E. Other Diagnostics

When necessary, tissue biopsies may be valuable diagnostically. Biopsies of affected organs such as skin, kidney, or liver may show patterns associated with a specific immunopathologic process. Such information may or may not be helpful in implicating a particular drug.

1. The definitive diagnostic test for drug hypersensitivity is a provocative challenge procedure with observed readministration of the suspected offending agent. Such testing is useful in situations when an allergic reaction to a drug is improbable and diagnostic testing is not available.[48]

2. The initial test dose is usually a fraction (0.1%–1% of therapeutic dose) of what would be expected to cause a serious reaction. If tolerated, threefold escalated doses are given until a reaction occurs or a therapeutic dose is achieved. IgE-mediated reactions usually occur within 30 minutes of dosing, so the

dose interval can be relatively short. However, late reactions such as maculopapular rash may occur 24–48 hours after administration, therefore requiring dose escalation over a period of days in testing for such reactions.

3. A drug challenge is contraindicated in patients with a history of Stevens-Johnson syndrome, toxic epidermal necrolysis, or serious anaphylactic reactions to a drug.

VIII. Approach to Final Diagnosis

Due to the lack of definitive, confirmatory drug-specific testing, the diagnosis of drug hypersensitivity is largely based on the physician's clinical judgment. In general, conditions that should be met for the diagnosis include the following:

- The patient's symptoms are consistent with an immunologic drug reaction.
- The patient was administered a drug known to cause the symptoms.
- The temporal sequence of drug administration and appearance of symptoms is consistent with a drug reaction.
- Other causes of the symptoms are effectively excluded.
- Laboratory data support an immunologic mechanism to explain the drug reaction. This is not present or available in all cases.

A. Familiarity with the suspected drugs and their propensity to cause the observed reactions is essential. Consultation with reference materials, such as the *Physician's Desk Reference* or MEDLINE search literature, is often necessary. Every effort should be made to differentiate between immunologic drug hypersensitivity and other adverse drug reactions.

1. *Predictable nonimmune-mediated drug-related reactions* to be considered include overdosage or toxicity, side effects due to pharmacologic action, drug-drug interactions, and secondary effects (e.g., yeast overgrowth during antibiotic therapy).
2. *Unpredictable nonimmune-mediated reactions* include drug intolerance, idiosyncratic reactions, and anaphylactoid reactions. While certainly problematic, these effects do not constitute true drug hypersensitivity and the appropriate distinction should be made by the consulting physician.

B. Upon making the diagnosis, an effort should be made to include appropriate documentation in the medical record specifying which drug or drug class is problematic for the patient, and specifying the nature of the adverse effect. Recommendations for discontinuation or continuation of the agent should be given, along with suggestions for substitute medications. The risk of cross-reactivity with other drugs or environmental agents should also be addressed.

IX. Therapy and Management

Once a diagnosis of drug hypersensitivity has been made, the most important and effective therapeutic measure is discontinuation of the offending medication, if possible. Alternative medications with unrelated chemical structures should be substituted when available. It is important to observe the consequences of stopping or substituting candidate medications. With rare exceptions, symptom resolution should be prompt if the diagnosis of drug hypersensitivity is correct.

A. Besides avoidance of the offending drug, specific therapy for drug reactions is largely supportive and symptomatic.

1. Type I hypersensitivity reactions include anaphylaxis, urticaria, angioedema, and bronchospasm. Appropriate treatment of anaphylaxis should include subcutaneous epinephrine, antihistamines, intravenous fluids, supplemental oxygen, and systemic corticosteroids. Airway patency should be closely monitored, particularly in patients with angioedema. Patients with less severe type I hypersensitivity reactions should be observed for a minimum of 6 hours to monitor for severe, life-threatening late-phase reactions (see Chapter 6).
2. Type II (cytotoxic) reactions usually require no further therapy beyond discontinuation of the offending drug. Systemic corticosteroids may speed recovery, and supportive transfusion therapy may be required in severe cases.
3. Treatment of type III reactions consists of discontinuation of the offending drug and symptomatic treatment with nonsteroidal anti-inflammatory agents and antihistamines. More severe cases of immune complex–mediated disease may respond to a short course of systemic corticosteroids or plasmapheresis.
4. Type IV reactions typically present as allergic contact dermatitis. Avoiding further contact with the culprit agent is the primary therapy. Topical corticosteroids and oral antihistamines may provide symptomatic relief and speed resolution of symptoms. Systemic corticosteroids may be considered in severe cases of dermatitis (see Chapter 4).
5. The management of SJS or TEN includes withdrawal of the causative medication as soon as possible. In moderate to severe cases, patients should be hospitalized and provided with supportive therapy. Patient

management should be comparable to care for major burns, with fluid replacement, antibiotic therapy, nutritional support, and appropriate skin care.[71] The use of systemic corticosteroids remains controversial, although their use should be avoided in advanced cases because of an increased risk of infection.[72] Treatment with cyclophosphamide[73] or intravenous immune globulin[34] may halt disease progression, though large trials are lacking.

B. With avoidance measures, the prognosis is excellent for most patients with drug hypersensitivity. Patients who experience a drug reaction should be informed about the specific risks of taking future doses of the offending medication.

1. Those with a history of anaphylactic reaction should be instructed in emergency treatment measures, such as the prompt use of self-administered epinephrine and antihistamines.
2. The use of medical alert bracelets is a reasonable recommendation.

C. In addition to avoiding the specific drug, patients should be educated regarding chemically related medications that may potentially cross-react.

1. Examples include imipenem avoidance in the penicillin-allergic patients, or carbemazepine avoidance in the patient with a hypersensitivity syndrome to phenytoin.
2. Providing a written list of cross-reacting drugs to the patient is particularly helpful.
3. IgE-mediated hypersensitivity may not be lifelong, as specific IgE levels wane over time in certain individuals. Approximately 80% of adults with documented skin-test-positive penicillin allergy have no detectable specific IgE when skin-tested 10 years later.[56] However, patients with a previous history of type I hypersensitivity reaction should be retested for specific IgE if readministration of the offending drug is being considered.

D. Patients should be instructed to inform their personal clinicians of all drug allergies. In addition, they should pay close attention to the contents of all prescription medications or over-the-counter formulations that they take. Patients who suffer adverse effects due to drug toxicity, intolerance, or drug side effect should be specifically educated that this does not constitute a "drug allergy." Such effects may not be reproducible on readministration and in general do not constitute a serious health risk. Classifying all adverse drug reactions as "allergies" and subsequently excluding these medications from use does a disservice to both the patient and the clinician in terms of providing effective medical therapy.

X. Special Considerations in Patient Subsets

A. Drug Discontinuation

Drug discontinuation may be problematic in certain scenarios, when no suitable alternative agent exists. For instance, patients with HIV frequently develop maculopapular rashes with sulfonamide therapy.[74,75] However, sulfa drugs remain the best alternative for the prevention and treatment of *Pneumocystis carinii* pneumonia.

1. In such instances, graded challenge protocols may be appropriate and successful.[76] Initiation of treatment begins with a fractional dose (typically 1% of desired dose) of the medication. The dose is then slowly increased over a period of days to weeks until a therapeutic level is achieved. Using published protocols, approximately 80% of patients with prior skin reactions tolerate TMP-SMX therapy.[77–80]
2. Graded challenges should not be attempted in patients with a history of Stevens-Johnson syndrome or toxic epidermal necrolysis because of the high mortality risk in such patients.

B. Patients with Reactions to β-Lactam Antibiotics

Occasionally, patients with IgE-mediated reactions to β-lactam antibiotics require penicillin therapy (e.g., neurosyphilis). If no satisfactory alternative treatment is available, and if the disease is serious enough to risk possible anaphylaxis from the treatment, a desensitization procedure should be considered.

1. This involves the administration of an initial dose, typically 10^{-4} to 10^{-5}, of the therapeutic dose. Dose escalation is then performed, with doubling of the dose every 15–30 minutes until a therapeutic dose is achieved.[63,81]
2. Premedication with antihistamines or corticosteroids is not advised, as it may mask early anaphylactic symptoms and allow continued hazardous dose escalation.
3. Both oral and parenteral routes appear equally effective for desensitization procedures. Although the oral approach is arguably safer,[82] it is not always possible. Desensitization should be performed in the hospital setting with close monitoring and prompt medical treatment in the event of a serious reaction. It is highly advisable to proceed under the consultative supervision of clinicians experienced in this area. With appropriately managed desensitization, the patient will often tolerate therapy for a course of continuous treatment. However, once the penicillin is discontinued, the patient is at-risk for a type I hypersensitivity reaction on readministration of the

drug. Desensitization procedures are drug specific- and do not confer tolerance to an entire drug class or to cross-reactive medications.

C. Penicillin-Allergic Patients

A frequent question that arises in the management of penicillin-allergic patients is the degree of cross-reactivity between penicillins and structurally related compounds.

1. Carbapenems (e.g., imipenim) are cross-reactive with penicillin.[83]
2. Aztreonam cross-reactivity is extremely rare in penicillin-allergic patients.[84,85]
3. Varying degrees of cross-reactivity between cephalosporins and penicillins have been documented.
   a. Prior to 1980, reaction rates to cephalosporins in patients with positive penicillin skin tests were reported as 5%–16%.[86,87] It is unclear whether this high degree of reported cross-reactivity is attributable to side-chain similarities of penicillin and first-generation cephalosporins or to questionable surveillance methods used in retrospective observational studies.
   b. Since 1980, the rate of cross-reaction between penicillin and second- or third-generation cephalosporins has been found to be 2% or less.[55,88,89] The degree of cross-reactivity appears to be greater for first-generation cephalosporins than for second- or third-generation cephalosporins.[57]
4. While the incidence of true cross-reactivity between penicillins and cephalosporins is low, the possible reactions include anaphylaxis, which may be fatal.[90]
5. Therefore, patients with a history of penicillin allergy who need cephalosporin therapy should preferably undergo skin testing to penicillin (major and minor determinants).[24] If skin tests are negative, the patient can receive a cephalosporin at no greater risk than the general population. Positive skin tests for penicillin IgE confer a small but increased risk for a cross-reactive hypersensitivity reaction.
6. In these instances, if no acceptable alternative to the cephalosporin exists, a cautious graded challenge with appropriate monitoring is recommended.

D. Pretreatment Protocol for Radiocontrast Media (RCM) Reactions

For the patient who has a history of a prior anaphylactoid reaction with RCM and who requires RCM, medical pretreatment may minimize the risk of a recurrent adverse event.

1. Ensure proper hydration.
2. Use a nonionic, low-osmolar RCM.

3. Pretreat with prednisone, 50 mg, 13 hours, 7 hours, and 1 hour before the procedure, plus diphenhydramine, 50 mg, 1 hour before the procedure, plus ephedrine, 25 mg, 1 hour before the procedure; *or* pretreat with an H_2-receptor antagonist 1 hour before the procedure.[48]

There is no evidence that sensitivity to seafood or "iodine" is predictive of RCM reactions.

XI. When to Obtain Consultation

Referral to a specialist in allergy/immunology should be considered for any patient who has a serious adverse drug reaction requiring hospitalization or manifesting as anaphylaxis. In addition, referral is appropriate for the recommendation, performance, and interpretation of particular diagnostic tests, including skin testing or other immunologic studies. Medication desensitization protocols should be performed only under the supervision of a specialist experienced in the procedure. Specialist consultation may also be helpful in patients who have complex drug histories or reactions, and those who fail to respond appropriately to initial treatment.

XII. Practice Guidelines

Guidelines for the management of drug reactions have been published recently by the Joint Task Force for Practice Parameters in Allergy, Asthma, and Immunology:

Disease Management of Drug Hypersensitivity: A Practice Parameter. Ann Allergy Asthma Immunol 1999;83:665–700.

www.jcaai.org/Param/Drug.htm

XIII. Internet Resources

www.theallergyreport.org/reportindex.html
A general reference for health care providers, intended to improve an understanding of drug allergy and other allergic conditions.

www.jcaai.org/Param/
Practice parameters for drug allergy as established by the Joint Council for Allergy, Asthma, and Immunology.

www.aaaai.org/patients/search_allergic_conditions.stm
On-line library of patient educational materials for drug allergy and other allergic conditions.

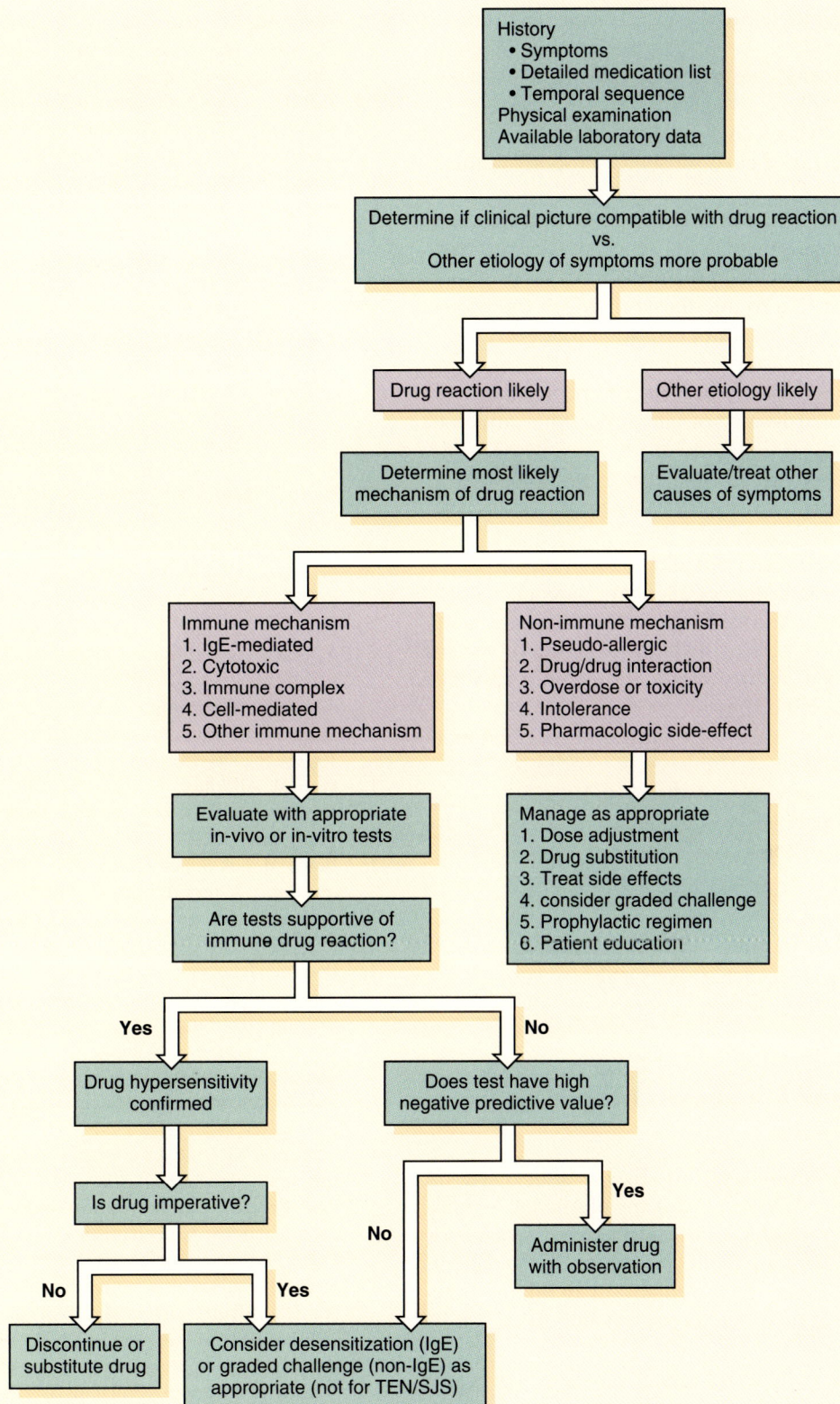

Figure 10-4 Algorithm for the management of drug allergy.

XIV. ICD-9 Codes

692.3	Dermatitis due to drugs and medicines in contact with skin
693.0	Dermatitis due to drugs and medicines taken internally
995.0	Anaphylaxis NOS or due to adverse effect of correct medicinal substance properly administered
995.2	Unspecified adverse effect, allergic reaction, hypersensitivity, or idiosyncracy to correct medicinal substance properly administered
995.3	Shock due to anesthesia in which the correct substance was properly administered
V14	Personal history of allergy to medicinal agent
V14.0	Personal history of allergy to penicillin
V14.1	Personal history of allergy to other antibiotic agent
V14.2	Personal history of allergy to sulfonamides
V14.3	Personal history of allergy to other anti-infective agent
V14.4	Personal history of allergy to anesthetic agent
V14.5	Personal history of allergy to narcotic agent
V14.6	Personal history of allergy to analgesic agent
V14.7	Personal history of allergy to serum or vaccine
V14.8	Personal history of allergy to other specified medicinal agent
V14.9	Personal history of allergy to unspecified medicinal agent
V15.07	Personal history of allergy to latex
V15.08	Personal history of allergy to radiographic dye

XV. Diagnosis and Management Algorithm *(Fig. 10-4, p. 149)*

XVI. Patient Education Materials and Handouts

Patient education handouts on adverse drug reactions, published by the American Academy of Allergy, Asthma, and Immunology (AAAAI), are available at www.aaaai.org. This educational information can be found in the Patients & Consumers Center and is available in an on-line printable format or in more traditional brochures that can be ordered from AAAAI.

Refer to the patient education CD, which is provided with this text, for additional patient education information. It has been formatted to provide readily accessible, easy-to-understand handouts for adult patients and the parents of pediatric patients. These handouts can be easily modified to fit specific practice requirements.

REFERENCES

1. DeSwarte RD: Drug allergy. In Patterson R (ed): Allergic Diseases: Diagnosis and Management, 3rd ed, p 505. Philadelphia: JB Lippincott; 1989.
2. Jick H: Adverse drug-reactions: The magnitude of the problem. J Allergy Clin. Immunol 1984;74:555–557.
3. Lazarou J, Pomeranz BH, Corey PN: Incidence of adverse drug reactions in hospitalized patients: A meta-analysis of prospective studies. JAMA 1998;279:1200–1205.
4. Jick H: Adverse drug reactions: The magnitude of the problem. J Allergy Clin Immunol 1984;74:555–557.
5. Einarson TR: Drug-related hospital admissions. Ann Pharmacother 1993;27:832–840.
6. Bates DW, Cullen DJ, Laird N, et al: Incidence of adverse drug events and potential adverse drug events: Implications for prevention. ADE Prevention Study Group. JAMA 1995;274:29–34.
7. Demoly P, Bousquet J: Epidemiology of drug allergy. Curr Opin Allergy Clin Immunol 2001;1:305–310.
8. Carr A, Cooper DA, Penny R: Allergic manifestations of human immunodeficiency virus (HIV) infection. J Clin Immunol 1991;11:55–64.
9. Roujeau JC, Stern RS: Severe adverse cutaneous reactions to drugs. N Engl J Med 1994;331:1272–1285.
10. Bayard PJ, Berger TG, Jacobson MA: Drug hypersensitivity reactions and human immunodeficiency virus disease. J AIDS 1992;5:1237–1257.
11. Coopman SA, Johnson RA, Platt R, Stern RS: Cutaneous disease and drug reactions in HIV infection. N Engl J Med 1993;328:1670–1674.
12. Petri M, Allbritton J: Antibiotic allergy in systemic lupus erythematosus: A case-control study. J Rheumatol 1992; 19:265–269.
13. Bigby M, Jick S, Jick H, Arndt K: Drug-induced cutaneous reactions: A report from the Boston Collaborative Drug Surveillance Program on 15,438 consecutive inpatients, 1975 to 1982. JAMA 1986;256:3358–3363.
14. Barranco P, Lopez-Serrano MC: General and epidemiological aspects of allergic drug reactions. Clin Exp Allergy 1998; 28(Suppl 4):61–62.
15. Idsoe O, Guthe T, Willcox RR, de Weck AL: Nature and extent of penicillin side-reactions, with particular reference to fatalities from anaphylactic shock. Bull WHO 1968;38: 159–188.
16. Adkinson NF Jr: Risk factors for drug allergy. J Allergy Clin Immunol 1984;74:567–572.
17. Park BK, Pirmohamed M, Kitteringham NR: Idiosyncratic drug reactions: A mechanistic evaluation of risk factors. Br J Clin Pharmacol 1992;34:377–395.
18. Stein HB, Patterson AC, Offer RC, Atkins CJ, Teufel A, Robinson HS: Adverse effects of D-penicillamine in rheumatoid arthritis. Ann Intern Med 1980;92:24–29.
19. Romano A, De Santis A, Romito A, et al: Delayed hypersensitivity to aminopenicillins is related to major histocompatibility complex genes. Ann Allergy Asthma Immunol 1998;80:433–437.
20. Kowalski ML, Woszczek G, Bienkiewicz B, Mis M: Association of pyrazolone drug hypersensitivity with HLA-DQ and DR antigens. Clin Exp Allergy 1998;28:1153–1158.

21. Descamps V, Valance A, Edlinger C, et al: Association of human herpesvirus 6 infection with drug reaction with eosinophilia and systemic symptoms. Arch Dermatol 2001;137:301–304.

22. Sullivan JR, Shear NH: The drug hypersensitivity syndrome: What is the pathogenesis? Arch Dermatol 2001;137:357–364.

23. Lang DM, Alpern MB, Visintainer PF, Smith ST: Increased risk for anaphylactoid reaction from contrast media in patients on beta-adrenergic blockers or with asthma. Ann Intern Med 1991;115:270–276.

24. Bernstein IL, Gruchalla RS, Lee RE, et al: Disease management of drug hypersensitivity: A practice parameter. Ann Allergy Asthma Immunol 1999;83:VIII–700.

25. deShazo RD, Kemp SF: Allergic reactions to drugs and biologic agents. JAMA 1997;278:1895–1906.

26. Anderson JA, Adkinson NF Jr: Allergic reactions to drugs and biologic agents. JAMA 1987;258:2891–2899.

27. Gell PGH, Coombs RRA, Lachman R: Clinical Aspects of Immunology, 3rd ed. Oxford: Blackwell Scientific Publications, 1975.

28. Hertl M, Merk HF: Lymphocyte activation in cutaneous drug reactions. J Invest Dermatol 1995;105:95S–98S.

29. Yawalkar N, Egli F, Hari Y, Nievergelt H, Braathen LR, Pichler WJ: Infiltration of cytotoxic T cells in drug-induced cutaneous eruptions. Clin Exp Allergy 2000;30:847–855.

30. Park BK, Kitteringham NR, Powell H, Pirmohamed M: Advances in molecular toxicology: Towards understanding idiosyncratic drug toxicity. Toxicology 2000;153:39–60.

31. Park BK, Naisbitt DJ, Gordon SF, Kitteringham NR, Pirmohamed M: Metabolic activation in drug allergies. Toxicology 2001;158:11–23.

32. Uetrecht JP: New concepts in immunology relevant to idiosyncratic drug reactions: The "danger hypothesis" and innate immune system. Chem Res Toxicol 1999;12:387–395.

33. Gruchalla RS: Drug metabolism, danger signals, and drug-induced hypersensitivity. J Allergy Clin Immunol 2001;108: 475–488.

34. Viard I, Wehrli P, Bullani R, et al: Inhibition of toxic epidermal necrolysis by blockade of CD95 with human intravenous immunoglobulin. Science 1998;282:490–493.

35. Le Cleach L, Delaire S, Boumsell L, et al: Blister fluid T lymphocytes during toxic epidermal necrolysis are functional cytotoxic cells which express human natural killer (NK) inhibitory receptors. Clin Exp Immunol 2000;119:225–230.

36. Asero R: Detection of patients with multiple drug allergy syndrome by elective tolerance tests. Ann Allergy Asthma Immunol 1998;80:185–188.

37. Smith JW, Johnson JE, Cluff LE: Studies on the epidemiology of adverse drug reactions. II. An evaluation of penicillin allergy. N Engl J Med 1966;274:998–1002.

38. Sullivan TJ, Ong RC, Gilliam LK: Studies of the multiple-drug allergy syndrome. J Allergy Clin Immunol 1989;83:270.

39. Khoury L, Warrington R: The multiple drug allergy syndrome: A matched-control retrospective study in patients allergic to penicillin. J Allergy Clin Immunol 1996;98: 462–464.

40. Bachot N, Roujeau JC: Physiopathology and treatment of severe drug eruptions. Curr Opin Allergy Clin Immunol 2002;1:293–298.

41. Rosenow EC III: Drug-induced pulmonary disease. Dis Month 1994;40:253–310.

42. Bocquet H, Bagot M, Roujeau JC: Drug-induced pseudolymphoma and drug hypersensitivity syndrome (drug rash with eosinophilia and systemic symptoms: DRESS). Semin Cutan Med Surg 1996;15:250–257.

43. Pramatarov KD: Drug-induced lupus erythematosus. Clin Dermatol 1998;16:367–377.

44. Price EJ, Venables PJ: Drug-induced lupus. Drug Safety 1995;12:283–290.

45. Gross WL: Churg-Strauss syndrome: Update on recent developments. Curr Opin Rheumatol 2002;14:11–14.

46. Wolkenstein P, Revuz J: Drug-induced severe skin reactions: Incidence, management and prevention. Drug Safety 1995;13:56–68.

47. deShazo RD, Nelson HS: An approach to the patient with a history of local anesthetic hypersensitivity: Experience with 90 patients. J Allergy Clin Immunol 1979;63:387–394.

48. Patterson R, DeSwarte RD, Greenberger PA, et al: Drug Allergy and Protocols for Management of Drug Allergies, 2nd ed. Providence, RI: OceanSide Publications; 1995.

49. Fisher M: Intradermal testing after anaphylactoid reaction to anaesthetic drugs: Practical aspects of performance and interpretation. Anaesth Intensive Care 1984;12:115–120.

50. Moscicki RA, Sockin SM, Corsello BF, Ostro MG, Bloch KJ: Anaphylaxis during induction of general anesthesia: Subsequent evaluation and management. J Allergy Clin Immunol 1990;86:325–332.

51. Nicklas RA, et al: Anaphylaxis during general anesthesia, the intraoperative period, and the postoperative period. J Allergy Clin Immunol 1998;101:S512–S516.

52. Haddi E, Charpin D, Tafforeau M, et al: Atopy and systemic reactions to drugs. Allergy 1990;45:236–239.

53. Hamilton RG, Adkinson NF Jr: Natural rubber latex skin testing reagents: Safety and diagnostic accuracy of non-ammoniated latex, ammoniated latex, and latex rubber glove extracts. J Allergy Clin Immunol 1996;98:872–883.

54. Sogn DD, Evans R III, Shepherd GM, et al: Results of the National Institute of Allergy and Infectious Diseases collaborative clinical trial to test the predictive value of skin testing with major and minor penicillin derivatives in hospitalized adults. Arch Intern Med 1992;152:1025–1032.

55. Shepherd G: Allergy to beta-lactam antibiotics.: Immunol Allergy Clin North Am 1991;11:611.

56. Sullivan TJ, Wedner HJ, Shatz GS, Yecies LD, Parker CW: Skin testing to detect penicillin allergy. J Allergy Clin Immunol 1981;68:171–180.

57. Lin RY: A perspective on penicillin allergy. Arch Intern Med 1992;152:930–937.

58. Torres MJ, Mayorga C, Pamies R, et al: Immunologic response to different determinants of benzylpenicillin, amoxicillin, and ampicillin: Comparison between urticaria and anaphylactic shock. Allergy 1999;54:936–943.

59. Weiss ME, Adkinson NF Jr: Beta-lactam allergy. In Mandell LD, Douglas RG Jr, Bennett JE (eds): Principles and Practice of Infectious Disease, 3rd ed, p 264. New York: Churchill-Livingstone; 1989.

60. Weiss ME, Adkinson NF: Diagnostic testing for drug hypersensitivity. Immunol Allergy Clin North Am 1998; 18:731.

61. Gruchalla RS, Sullivan TS: In vivo and in vitro diagnosis of drug allergy. Immunol Allergy Clin North Am 1991;11:595.

62. Schwartz LB, Metcalfe DD, Miller JS, Earl H, Sullivan T: Tryptase levels as an indicator of mast-cell activation in systemic-anaphylaxis and mastocytosis. N Engl J Med 1987;316:1622–1626.

63. Adkinson NF Jr: Drug allergy. In Middleton E Jr, Reed CE, Ellis EF, et al (eds): Allergy: Principles and Practice, 5th ed, p 1212. St. Louis: Mosby-Year Book; 1998.

64. Adams LE, Hess EV: Drug-related lupus: Incidence, mechanisms and clinical implications. Drug Safety 1991;6:431–449.

65. Monestier M, Kotzin BL: Antibodies to histones in systemic lupus erythematosus and drug-induced lupus syndromes. Rheum Dis Clin North Am 1992;18:415–436.

66. Jennette JC, Falk RJ: Small-vessel vasculitis. N Engl J Med 1997;337:1512–1523.

67. Bernstein IL, Storms WW: Practice parameters for allergy diagnostic testing. Joint Task Force on Practice Parameters for the Diagnosis and Treatment of Asthma. The American Academy of Allergy, Asthma and Immunology and the American College of Allergy, Asthma and Immunology. Ann Allergy Asthma Immunol 1995;75:543–625.

68. Barbaud A, Reichert-Penetrat S, Trechot P, et al: The use of skin testing in the investigation of cutaneous adverse drug reactions. Br J Dermatol 1998;139:49–58.

69. Primeau M, Adkinson NF: Recent advances in the diagnosis of drug allergy. Curr Opin Allergy Clin Immunol 2001;1:337–341.

70. Nyfeler B, Pichler WJ: The lymphocyte transformation test for the diagnosis of drug allergy: Sensitivity and specificity. Clin Exp Allergy 1997;27:175–181.

71. Craven NM: Management of toxic epidermal necrolysis. Hosp Med 2000;61:778–781.

72. Halebian PH, Corder VJ, Madden MR, Finklestein JL, Shires GT: Improved burn center survival of patients with toxic epidermal necrolysis managed without corticosteroids. Ann Surg 1986;204:503–512.

73. Arevalo JM, Lorente JA, Gonzalez-Herrada C, Jimenez-Reyes J: Treatment of toxic epidermal necrolysis with cyclosporin A. J Trauma 2000;48:473–478.

74. Lee BL, Safrin S: Interactions and toxicities of drugs used in patients with AIDS. Clin Infect Dis 1992;14:773–779.

75. Carr A, Cooper DA: Pathogenesis and management of HIV-associated drug hypersensitivity. In Volberding P, Jacobson MA (eds): AIDS Clinical Review 1995/1996, p 773. New York: Marcel Dekker;1996.

76. Para MF, Finkelstein D, Becker S, Dohn M, Walawander A, Black JR: Reduced toxicity with gradual initiation of trimethoprim-sulfamethoxazole as primary prophylaxis for *Pneu-mocystis carinii* pneumonia: AIDS Clinical Trials Group 268. J AIDS 2000;24:337–443.

77. Absar N, Daneshvar H, Beall G: Desensitization to trimethoprim-sulfamethoxazole in HIV- infected patients. J Allergy Clin Immunol 1994;93:1001–1005.

78. Rich JD, Sullivan T, Greineder D, Kazanjian PH: Trimethoprim/sulfamethoxazole incremental dose regimen in human immunodeficiency virus-infected persons. Ann Allergy Asthma Immunol 1997;79:409–414.

79. Moreno JN, Poblete RB, Maggio C, Gagnon S, Fischl MA: Rapid oral desensitization for sulfonamides in patients with the acquired immunodeficiency syndrome. Ann Allergy Asthma Immunol 1995;74:140–146.

80. White MV, Haddad ZH, Brunner E, Sainz C: Desensitization to trimethoprim sulfamethoxazole in patients with acquired immune deficiency syndrome and *Pneumocystis carinii* pneumonia. Ann Allergy 1989;62:177–179.

81. Gruchalla RS: Acute drug desensitization. Clin Exp Allergy 1998;28(Suppl 4):63–64.

82. Stark BJ, Earl HS, Gross GN, Lumry WR, Goodman EL, Sullivan TJ: Acute and chronic desensitization of penicillin-allergic patients using oral penicillin. J Allergy Clin Immunol 1987;79:523–532.

83. Saxon A, Adelman DC, Patel A, Hajdu R, Calandra GB: Imipenem cross-reactivity with penicillin in humans. J Allergy Clin Immunol 1988;82:213–217.

84. Saxon A, Hassner A, Swabb EA, Wheeler B, Adkinson NF Jr: Lack of cross-reactivity between aztreonam, a monobactam antibiotic, and penicillin in penicillin-allergic subjects. J Infect Dis 1984;149:16–22.

85. Adkinson NF Jr: Immunogenicity and cross-allergenicity of aztreonam. Am J Med 1990;88:12S–15S.

86. Petz LD: Immunologic reactions of humans to cephalosporins. Postgrad Med J 1971;47(Suppl):9.

87. Petz LD: Immunologic cross-reactivity between penicillins and cephalosporins: A review. J Infect Dis 1978; 137(Suppl):S74–S79.

88. Shepherd GM, Burton DA: Administration of cephalosporin antibiotic to patients with a history to penicillin. J Allergy Clin Immunol 1993;91:262.

89. Anne S, Reisman RE: Risk of administering cephalosporin antibiotics to patients with histories of penicillin allergy. Ann Allergy Asthma Immunol 1995;74:167–170.

90. Pumphrey RS, Davis S: Under-reporting of antibiotic anaphylaxis may put patients at risk. Lancet 1999;353:1157–1158.

OTHER SUGGESTED READING

Pichler WJ: Drug allergy. Curr Opin Allergy Immunol 2001;1: 285–341.

SECTION II
Procedures in the Practice of Allergy

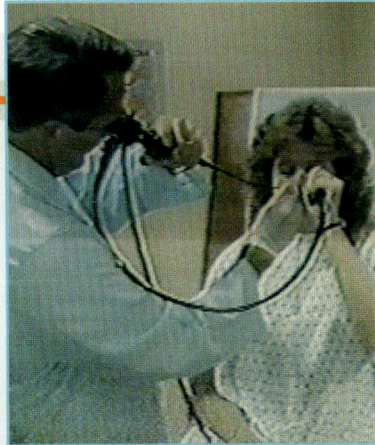

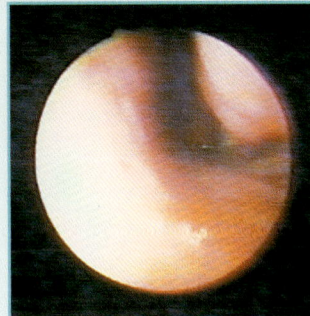

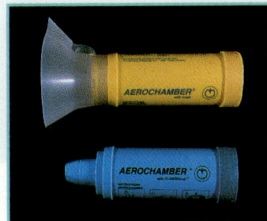

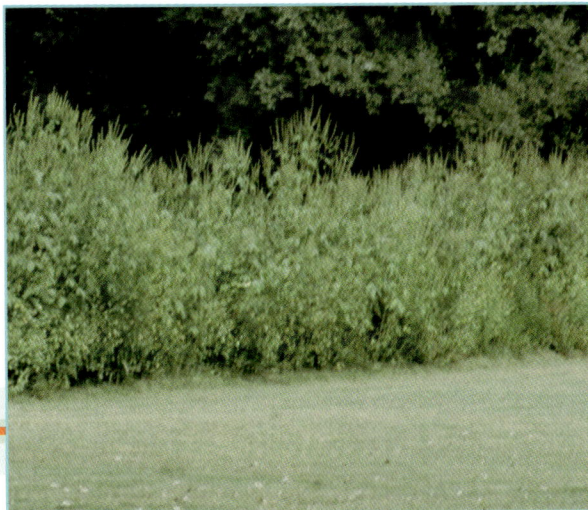

CHAPTER 11
Allergen Immunotherapy for the Primary Care Physician

Joann Blessing-Moore

I. Introduction

Allergic diseases are common throughout the world and affect all age groups. In the United States, approximately 20%–30% of the general population and 10%–15% of the pediatric population are atopic.[1,2] Allergic rhinitis can appear at any age but is usually evident before age 30 years. Allergies can significantly affect quality of life and impair both physical and cognitive functioning. It is not surprising that allergic rhinitis accounts for $1.9 billion in annual direct health care spending, plus a significant amount in undetermined indirect costs.[3] Furthermore, the incidence and frequency of allergic rhinitis and asthma have increased dramatically over the last few years, and the morbidity and mortality from these diseases are significant.

Allergen immunotherapy is the only available treatment that can reduce symptoms, improve quality of life, alter the course of disease, and induce long-term clinical remission safely and effectively in patients with allergic rhinitis, asthma, and insect venom sensitivity.[3,4] Immunotherapy has been shown to decrease the development of sensitization in children to other antigens, the risk of development of asthma[5] (by threefold), bronchial hyperreactivity, and the need for medications. With our present knowledge of potential remodeling (chronic changes) in asthmatic patients' lungs, it becomes important, if not essential, to consider immunotherapy early in the course of treatment. Specific allergen immunotherapy (SIT) can modify the immune response of this disease process.

This chapter recapitulates the most recent guidelines for safe, effective administration of therapy and outlines some of the basics of SIT administered by subcutaneous (SC) injection. This is a rapidly advancing field, which makes the teamwork of the generalist and specialist even more essential.

II. Immunopathology: "Mechanism of Action" of Immunotherapy

Allergic rhinitis, or hay fever, was first described in 1819 by Joan Bostock (and later by Charles Blackely in 1873[6]). Forty years later, Noon and Freeman[7] introduced grass pollen immunotherapy for patients with allergic rhinitis. Initially immunotherapy had been applied for the treatment of infectious diseases. Later, allergen immunotherapy was considered for protection against the "pollen toxin." Cooke and his colleagues proposed that immunotherapy worked by the development of blocking antibodies, and they later demonstrated serum antibodies (IgE, IgG).[8] By the mid-1970s it was recognized that IgG-blocking antibodies did not necessarily correlate with clinical improvement.[9] In 1976, Rocklin and colleagues proposed that immunotherapy increased the suppressor T-cells that controlled IgE antibody production.[10]

The allergic response is characterized by (1) the production of antigen-specific IgE antibodies that bind to mast cells and basophils, resulting in the release of mediators and the recruitment of eosinophils by cytokines, and (2) specific cytokines which are released from CD4+ Th2 cells (Il-4, Il-5, and Il-13, but not the Il-2 or IFN-γ of the Th1 cells). Immunotherapy induces several modifications of the immune system, including a specific rise in IgG, a variable change in IgE, and a modification of the Th1/Th2 response.[11,12] The mechanism of allergen-specific immunotherapy is complex but has been shown to modify the immune response by an increase in Th0/Th1 or a decrease in Th2/Th1 (or both), with a reduction in mediator release and tissue inflammation.[13] This form of therapy provides long-term benefits with continued control of symptoms several years after the individual stops therapy.[14,15]

III. Efficacy of Antigen/Vaccine Immunotherapy

Allergen immunotherapy studies have shown the clinical efficacy of treatment with specific antigens, including (1) inhalants; tree, grass, and weed pollen; fungi; house dust mite; cockroach; and animal (dog and cat) danders; and (2) bee venom. Immunotherapy is not indicated at this time for food allergy. Immunotherapy not only controls symptoms of rhinitis, it also decreases the risk of developing asthma in these allergic patients.

The efficacy of SIT in asthma and allergic rhinitis is evidenced-based, with data available from randomized placebo-controlled trials and meta-analysis of these clinical trials. SIT acts on several sites, and allergy often affects multiple organs. Asthma and rhinitis often coexist. Grembiale et al. noted a significant decrease in methacholine sensitivity after 1 year of SIT in monosensitized patients with allergic rhinitis due to *Dermatophagoides pteronyssinus*. At the end of the study the methacholine sensitivity was within normal range. Their conclusion was that SIT, when administered to carefully selected monosensitized patients with perennial allergic rhinitis, reduces airway responsiveness in subjects with rhinitis and may be appropriate prophylactic treatment for allergic rhinitis in patients with hyperreactive airways.[16] Similar studies have been done in children (see discussion of immunotherapy for young children under Special Treatment for Specific Populations).

Specific studies have shown SIT to be effective in the treatment of patients with allergic rhinitis and asthma, and to be effective in some patients with allergic conjunctivitis or atopic dermatitis.[17] There are no data to support its use for hives or non-IgE-mediated symptoms of asthma or allergic rhinitis.

A. Allergic Rhinitis

The most recent meta-analysis of 16 double-blind, placebo-controlled prospective studies found that in 759 patients with allergic rhinitis, immunotherapy treatment was effective in 94% of the studies, with improvement in symptoms and a reduction in the use of medication.[18] Settipane et al. noted a threefold decrease in the risk for development of asthma in college students who were treated with SIT for allergic rhinitis symptoms.[19] Immunotherapy can decrease the risk for the development of asthma in both adults and children.[19]

B. Asthma

The following meta-analyses are of note:

1. A 1995 meta-analysis of the clinical efficacy of immunotherapy in asthma clearly demonstrated its effectiveness.[20] In 20 studies of immunotherapy in asthmatic patients, the combined odds of symptomatic improvement from immunotherapy with any allergen were 3.2. The combined odds of a reduction in bronchial hyperreactivity were 6.8. The mean corresponded to a mean 7.1% improvement in forced expiratory volume in 1 second (FEV$_1$) from immunotherapy. This figure could be overestimated because of unpublished negative results, but an additional 33 studies would be necessary to overturn these results. Allergen immunotherapy is an option in the treatment of selected patients with asthma.

2. In the 2000 meta-analysis of 24 double-blind, prospective, controlled studies of allergen immunotherapy in 962 patients with asthma and documented allergy, immuotherapy was effective in 71% of the studies as indicated by improvement in the symptoms of asthma, a reduction in medication, improved pulmonary function, and protection against bronchial challenge.[21]

3. A systematic review of the Cochrane collaboration examined 54 trials of SIT in asthma involving more than 1000 patients. This report emphasized the decrease in symptom scores and medication requirements, as well as decreased allergen and nonspecific bronchial hyperresponsiveness.[22]

C. Multiple System Involvement

1. A more recent double-blind, prospective, controlled study of SIT for dust mite allergy conducted over 3 years in patients with allergic rhinitis and/or asthma revealed significant reductions in allergen-specific

skin and conjunctival reactivity, improvement in methacholine-induced bronchial hyperreactivity, and reduced use of medications for asthma and rhinitis. Patients responded within the first 12 months of treatment and continued to improve over the next 2 years.[23] A similar case-control study in young children less than 5 years old who were treated with house dust mite immunotherapy resulted in a decrease in asthma attacks during the first year of therapy.[24]

2. Furthermore, in the 3-year Preventive Allergy Treatment (PAT) study of grass and/or birch pollen immunotherapy in 205 children ages 6–14 years with rhinoconjunctivitis, there was a reduction in the development of asthma. All children in this study had moderate to severe hay fever symptoms, but at the conclusion of the study, none reported asthma symptoms requiring daily treatment. At the end of the study period, the actively treated children had significantly fewer asthma symptoms when evaluated clinically. Methacholine bronchial provocation test results improved significantly in the active group.[25]

D. Negative Studies

Despite the large number of positive studies, two highly publicized "negative" studies have been reported.

1. Creticos et al. treated 53 patients with monoallergy to ragweed with monotherapy for 2 years. Within the first year (but not the second year) there was a small but significant reduction in medication use and an increase in peak flow.[26] This study suggests that monotherapy may not be adequate and may not add to good medical management. This is not surprising, because mold, dust, cockroach, animal dander, and other pollen sensitivities are also significant in atopic patients.

2. Adkinson studied 121 children ages 5–12 years with moderate to severe asthma. The children were treated with ideal medical management (maximum environmental controls, with medication adjusted every 2–3 weeks) plus immunotherapy to include up to seven extracts versus placebo. After 2 years, bronchial sensitivity to methacholine decreased in both groups; however, the difference in the peak expiratory flow rates between the two groups did approach significance in favor of immunotherapy. Also, the younger age group (<8.5 years) and those with mild asthma (medication score <5) showed the most significant effect of treatment in favor of immunotherapy.[27] It has been questioned whether the antigen dose was optimal and whether the treated patients needed the same level of medication for adequate control.

In summary, the studies presently available reveal overwhelming evidence of the efficacy of immuno-

therapy for allergic rhinitis and asthma (and bee venom therapy).

E. Bee Venom Immunotherapy

Bee venom immunotherapy has been shown to be highly effective. Bee, vespid, mosquito, and fire ant immunotherapy is recommended for patients who have had systemic anaphylaxis involving the cardiovascular or respiratory system to a sting and have positive skin test or RAST results in response to a clinically relevant venom. Immunotherapy is not required for children who have only had cutaneous symptoms, such as urticaria.[1] Bee venom immunotherapy treatment is recommended for a total course of approximately 3–5 years and provides significant protection in 97% of treated patients. Rush therapy or a modification of rush therapy, cluster therapy, is often recommended because of the risk of anaphylaxis. This chapter discusses primarily immunotherapy for allergic rhinitis and asthma, but brief notes on venom immuno-therapy are included.

IV. Guidelines for SIT

Allergen immunotherapy is defined as the repeated administration of specific allergens to patients with IgE-mediated conditions, for the purpose of providing protection against the allergic symptoms and inflammatory reactions associated with natural exposure to the allergen.[28,29] In 1998, an international panel of allergists and immunologists published the WHO position paper, "Allergen Immunotherapy: Therapy Vaccines for Allergic Disease."[30] In 1996, the Task Force of the American Academy, American College, and Joint Council of Asthma, Allergy and Immunology published practice parameters for allergen immunotherapy.[28] This document has been revised (2003) and provides the most complete and up-to-date reference-based guideline for the standardization of the immunotherapy treatment program for patients with allergic rhinitis and asthma.[31]

V. Treatment and Management Basics (Box 11-1)

A. Patient Selection

1. Allergen immunotherapy is a very effective form of therapy for individuals with a history of allergic rhinitis, asthma, and stinging insect hypersensitivity.[32]

BOX 11-1

Determinants of Efficacy

Patient selection (history, testing)
Selection of specific vaccines
Maintenance antigen dose/frequency

Allergic rhinitis and asthma frequently coexist in the same individual, and many people with allergic rhinitis have increased bronchial sensitivity to methacholine or histamine. It is considered by many that the upper and lower airways may be considered as a unique single entity susceptible to a common inflammatory process. SIT offers unique advantages for treatment. Also, the clinician considering SIT should remember that conjunctivitis may be associated with asthma and allergic rhinitis.

2. Indications for immunotherapy from the European and American guidelines include the following:
   a. A history of allergen sensitization playing a predominant role in eliciting symptoms and in the overall severity of the disease.
   b. A history of inadequate control of symptoms, excessive need for medications, or side effects from medications.
   c. The demonstration of specific IgE antibodies to clinically relevant antigens.
   d. The availability of a high-quality allergen extract and the administration of a proper dose.
   e. The willingness of the patient to comply with long-term treatment.
3. Factors favoring the use of immunotherapy include the following:
   a. Better symptom control for allergic rhinitis and asthma, and a decreased progression of the allergic symptoms.
   b. Decreased development of new sensitivities.
   c. A possibly decreased incidence of progression from rhinitis to other allergic problems, including asthma.
4. In general, referral to a specialist for immunotherapy should be considered if:
   a. A patient does not respond to adequate environmental control measures and medications.
   b. Adequate environmental control is not possible.
   c. The patient experiences substantial side effects from medications.
   d. The patient has an inadequate response to medications or requires corticosteroids.
   e. Comorbid medical conditions such as allergic rhinitis and asthma exist.
   f. The patient has symptoms for a significant part of the year.
   g. The patient experiences severe symptoms.
   h. The patient prefers immunologic control of symptoms.
   i. The patient has recognized complications of allergic rhinitis such as sinusitis, sinus headaches, recurrent otitis media, and sleep apnea.[33,34]
      1) The preceding criteria have been well established; however, as it becomes more evident that the immunologic changes induced by immunotherapy occur over time in the atopic patient, including remodeling of the lungs in the asthmatic patient, early immunotherapy intervention will become even more important.
      2) Patients who meet the preceding criteria for immunotherapy must be made aware of the risks and benefits of appropriate management options (medications with or without immunotherapy). Both forms of treatment can result in symptom control, and in asthmatics there may be a decrease in bronchial hyperreactivity.[35,36] Environmental controls are essential, regardless of other medical management techniques.[37]
5. Patient preference and compliance are essential issues with this type of treatment program. Regular visits are required over several years to provide optimal treatment. The antigen dosage is advanced on a rush, cluster, or traditional weekly or biweekly basis (build-up phase) and then maintained with an optimal dose at regular intervals (maintenance program). Medications are usually required through the initial phases of this program but over time can often be decreased as symptom control improves.
6. Patients must be aware of the severity of their symptoms to help in the evaluation of when shots are appropriate and whether symptoms are triggered by the shots.
7. Patients who are unable or unwilling to communicate clearly with the allergist and who have a history of noncompliance are frequently not good candidates for immunotherapy. (However, the rush build-up program is often preferred for patients who have difficulty with compliance with weekly shots and regular medications but who can adhere to a monthly shot program) (Boxes 11-2 and 11-3).
8. The goal of early aggressive treatment of asthma is to reduce the remodeling of the lungs. SIT may modify the disease course in the atopic patient by preventing the development of new sensitization or by altering the progression of disease before damage has occurred.[38,39]

BOX 11-2

Patient Considerations for Immunotherapy

Aware of medical treatment options
   Environmental controls
   Medications
   Immunotherapy
Preferences; compliance with therapy
Response to prior treatment and side effects
Severity of disease

B. Individual Antigen/Vaccine Mix (SIT) (Box 11-4)

1. *Antigen Classification*
   a. The effectiveness of treatment depends on proper patient selection as well as on proper selection of antigens. Commercially available allergens include pollen, molds, house dust mite, animal dander protein, and insect venoms.
   b. Allergen formulation is classified by weight per volume (wt/vol), protein nitrogen units (PNU), or, most recently, standardized allergy units or bioequivalent allergy units (AU or BAU).
      1) Allergens are classified by the World Health Organization (WHO) and the International Union of Immunological Societies (IUIS) so that investigators throughout the world can standardize research in this area. Now, clinicians are able to standardize treatment.
      2) The Center for Biologics Evaluation and Research (CBER) of the Food and Drug Administration (FDA) has established reference vaccines and reference serum pools[40] of cat, short ragweed, and house dust mite, which has resulted in more consistent and hopefully more potent dosing.[41] Certain antigens are standardized by measuring content of the major antigen in the vaccine (e.g., Cat Fel d 1 protein, Der p 1). Other antigens are standardized by actual testing of the individual antigen dilutions on the back of patients sensitive to the specific antigen to determine the biologically active unit (BAU). In addition, individual vaccines can be compared to the CBER reference vaccine using RAST or ELISA.

2. *Antigen Selection*
   a. Allergen cross-reactivity is well recognized and adds to the complexity of specific antigen selection. There is rarely significant cross-allergenicity between families, but variable cross-reactivity among tribes and genera of a family is well recognized, and there is a high degree of cross-reactivity between species of the same genus.
      1) Cross-reactivity can be noted for some grasses, trees, and weeds. Treatment with a mix of timothy and bermuda grasses can suppress reactivity to 10 different grasses.[42] Similar cross-reactivity has been demonstrated for tree and weed antigens.
      2) There are two families (Northern pasture grass and bermuda) that do not cross-react with their cross-reacting native prairie grasses.[43]
   b. It is essential to take a careful history with knowledge of all the environmental exposures and correlate this information with the skin test or RAST data to determine the appropriate mix of antigens. The omission of a clinically relevant allergen from an extract vaccine may contribute to decreased effectiveness of allergen immunotherapy vaccine. On the other hand, the inclusion of irrelevant allergens can dilute the individual antigen content of extracts.
   c. Certain antigens contain proteases and enzymes that may disrupt the proteins of other allergens. It is best to avoid mixing fungal or insect (cockroach) antigens with pollens and danders. However, house dust mite antigens have had no effect on other antigens, possibly because of being mixed with 25% glycerin.[44]
      1) Vaccines of fungi (molds) and insects (cockroach) contain high protease activity.
      2) Pollens are considered low protease activity antigens but may also contain enzymes that affect the potency of an antigen. Grass pollen proteins are susceptible to the proteolytic enzymes.[41]
      3) In general, it is recommended to separate the high and low protease activity vaccines (Box 11-5).

3. *Antigen Preparation and Storage* (Box 11-6)
   a. Lower dilution antigens are more susceptible to more rapid loss of potency, which may partially relate to the fact that with the lower protein content there is a greater risk of adsorption to the vial walls. But this is not totally blocked by the use of human serum albumin as a diluent, and not all antigens are equally affected.
   b. Diluents for allergen vaccines are designed to preserve potency as well as to provide antibacterial activity.

1) Glycerin may inhibit some of the proteolytic enzymes.[45]
2) Human serum albumin theoretically decreases the adsorption of antigen to the vial surface[46] and may protect against the effects of phenol.
3) Phenol is used as an antibacterial agent but may break down the antigen protein.
4) Other diluents have been tried, but the most common are the three listed. The choice of diluents would be easy if it were not for the irritation associated with 50% glycerin. Standardized vaccines are available in a lyophilized state in 50% glycerin-saline. Nonstandardized solutions are available in either glycerin or aqueous solution with phenol.[47]

c. Temperature control is essential. At room temperature, proteolytic enzymes may be more active, and at higher temperatures the vaccine proteins may be more labile.[48–50] Repeated freezing and thawing can also decrease the potency of some antigens. It is best to store antigens in the refrigerator and use a refrigerated tray when exposed to room temperature.

4. *Optimal Dose, Optimal Interval*
   a. The formulation of antigen is based on a dose that will provide adequate symptom control, with consideration of cross-reactivity of the antigens to which the patient is sensitive and compatibility of the components, as well as the diluents to be used.
   b. Symptom control has been demonstrated in patients with increased dosages of antigen.[51,52] From these studies it appears that an approximately 0.5-mL dose of the 1:5 or 1:10 dilution of the concentration provided by the company or a therapeutic dose of purified major allergen, which would range from 5 to 10 µg,[53] should provide an adequate maintenance dose for the patient.
   c. The optimal interval for allergen immunotherapy is not standardized. Studies by DiBerardino[54] and Feeling et al.[55] of aqueous preparations and alum-precipitated preparations in experimental animals showed that 80% is left at the injection site during the first 4 days, 90% within 14 days, and the remaining 10% disappears within 28 days. Their recommendation is to administer SIT before the end of the 4-week interval during which the antigen disappears. A general recommendation for maintenance is 2–6 weeks (Box 11-7).

5. *Vaccine Dilutions*
   a. Antigens are routinely diluted for treatment in four or more serial dilutions. The manufacturer's stock mix may be 1:10 wt/vol of standardized antigens in AU or BAU. The first dilution, which is usually a 10-fold dilution of the stock mix, is often considered as the maintenance dose. The maintenance dose is also based on recommended concentrations of standardized antigen. Often multiple antigens are used, so it is not an exact dilution for each of the antigens but a relative term for the dilution.
   b. To standardize the treatment protocols, the Task Force of the AAAAI and ACAAI has established the guidelines shown in Table 11-1.[31] Note that the maintenance concentrate is listed first, the volume/volume (vol/vol) dilution is 1:1, and the recommended lid color is red. Tenfold dilutions can be easily prepared with 4.5 mL diluent plus 0.5 mL antigen or antigen mix.
   c. Vial labels should include the following basic data (there is some redundancy, but it is

TABLE 11-1
Antigen Dilution

Dilution	Vol/Vol	Number	Lid Color
Maintenance concentrat.	1:1	1	Red
10-fold	1:10	2	Yellow
100-fold	1:100	3	Blue
1,000-fold	1:1,000	4	Green
10,000-fold	1:10,000	5	Silver

important that the appropriate dose be easily recognized):

1) Antigen "name" (i.e., tree, dust, or appropriate abbreviations)
2) Dilution number (1 to 4 or 1 to 5)
3) Vol/vol dilution (i.e., 1:1, 1:10, 1:100, 1:1000 . . .)
4) Appropriate lid color
5) Physician's name
6) Date of expiration of the antigen[31,41]

The expiration date for a maintenance concentration of mixed antigens would be the earliest expiration date of the antigens included. The expiration date for the diluted antigens depends on the dilution. The greater the dilution, the shorter the shelf-life (Table 11-2).

6. ***Dosing Schedule***

The immunotherapy schedule is divided into two phases, a build-up phase and a maintenance phase. During the build-up phase it is essential that the patient maintain a regular schedule (weekly or more often). Once maintenance is reached, the schedule may be more flexible.

a. The advancing schedule—build-up phase—can be one of three basic types:

1) A rush schedule, with antigens given repeatedly and in increasing doses over 1 or 2 days, with appropriate intervals between shots (at least 20–30 minutes) until the maximum dose is reached.

a) Premedication is often recommended to reduce the rate of systemic reactions.[56] Premedication may be with H_1-receptor antagonists, H_2-receptor antagonists, and corticosteroids. Premedication is not considered routinely necessary for venom rush immunotherapy because the risk of a systemic reaction is relatively low.[57]

b) This program has the advantage that the patient can be on maintenance therapy within 1–2 days. This program can be time- and cost-effective for the patient.

2) Traditional/conservative schedules involve advancing the dose 1–2 times a week. This schedule is important for the severe asthmatic or other patients extremely sensitive to the antigen mix.

3) A cluster schedule involves giving more than one shot during each visit, so that the patient advances to a maintenance level more quickly.[58] The wait between shots remains 20–30 minutes or longer.

4) Basically, the immunotherapy schedule is a stepwise advance in antigen concentration that proceeds from the most dilute concentration to a maintenance concentration. The first dose is from bottle No. 4 (green cap) of a 1000-fold dilution of maintenance concentration of antigen/vaccine (or a weaker dilution) and proceeds as the dose is advanced from 0.1 mL to 0.2 mL to 0.3 mL, and then to the next vial, with similar dosage increases. The next vial would be vial No. 3, a 100-fold dilution (blue cap), then vial No. 2, a 10-fold dilution (yellow cap), and finally the maintenance vial No. 1 of antigen/vaccine (red cap) (Table 11-3).

TABLE 11-2
Antigen Expiration

Antigen Concentration	Expiration
Maintenance concentrat.	6–12 mo
1:10 (vol/vol)	6 mo
1:100	6 mo
1:1,000	6 wk
1:10,000	Unknown

TABLE 11-3
Antigen Dosing Schedule

Dose	Dilution	Vial No.	Cap Color	mL
1	1,000-fold	4	Green	0.1
2		4		0.2
3		4		0.3
4		4		0.5
5	100-fold	3	Blue	0.1
6		3		0.2
8		3		0.3
9		3		0.4
10		3		0.5
11	10-fold	2	Yellow	0.1
12		2		0.2

b. When patients reach their maintenance concentrate dose they can receive their allergy shots every 4–6 weeks, depending on sensitivities and symptom control.

   1) The effectiveness of immunotherapy is dose-dependent. An optimal maintenance dose is established for the patient based on current studies. However, for many extremely allergic patients, the maintenance dose may be lower and yet the patient may note significant symptom control.

      a) The documented, optimal clinically effective dose for house dust mite (Der P 1 antigen) is 7.0–11.9 µg. Standardized *Dermatophagoides pteronyssinus* house dust mite extract (Der P 1) is available in a 10,000 BAU concentration. This solution contains 132–114 µg of Der P 1/mL. Thus, an optimal dose could be 0.05–0.1 mL of the 10,000 BAU standardized antigen solution. Three or four 10-fold dilutions of this concentration could be used as the starting dose.[59]

      b) Controlled studies have demonstrated effective doses for 0.5 mL of the following antigens: dust mite (1200 BAU/mL),[60] cat allergen (4000–6000 BAU/mL),[61] grass (8000 BAU/mL),[62] and short ragweed. (Early symptom improvement has been demonstrated with these doses but long-term benefits are assumed to be related to the cumulative dose.)

      c) Patients usually note clinical improvement on therapy within 1 year after reaching the maintenance dose.

      d) Appendix 1 contains all the necessary materials for a state-of-the-art immunotherapy program.

7. ***Replacement Antigen Vials***

The traditional expressions of vaccine potency (wt/vol, PNU) do not provide specific information about antigen potency from lot to lot; however, the standardization of antigen is designed to minimize such differences. Second, antigen stability is based on many factors, including diluent and temperature control. For these reasons, the first dose from a new replacement antigen vial is generally dropped back for patient safety (i.e., one-third to one-half of the original dose of same dilution: original vial No.1—0.3 mL—to new vial No.1—0.15 mL).

C. Safety of Specific Allergen Immunotherapy

1. The rate of severe reactions in the United States from antigens/vaccine when appropriately administered is very low.[63–65] In a review of systemic reactions from

TABLE 11-4
Safety for Immunotherapy

Parameter Measured	Oklahoma	Atlanta
Visits for injections	104,101	162,436
Number of reactions	22 (in 18 pts.)	98 (in 96 pts.)
Rate of reactions	1/4700	1/1600
Reactions during build up	17	36
Reactions during maintenance	5	62
Respiratory reaction rate	19/22	72/98
Hypotension rate	0/22	7/98

Data from Wells J: Systemic reactions to immunotherapy: Comparisons between two large allergy practices. J Allergy Clin Immunol 1996;97:1031–1032.

immunotherapy in two large clinics, the reaction rate was also low (Table 11-4).[63,66]

2. The major risk of allergen immunotherapy is anaphylaxis, which is extremely rare[67,68] but can be fatal despite optimal medical management. Therefore, allergen immunotherapy should be administered under the supervision of an appropriately trained physician.[69,70]

   a. The health care provider and staff should be able to recognize early signs and symptoms of anaphylaxis and administer emergency medications as necessary.

   b. One study reported that fatal reactions to immunotherapy occurred once in every 2.8 million injections (1980–1984) to once in every 2 million injections (1985–1989). Four of the seventeen reported events occurred while the patient was on maintenance therapy. It is essential that patients wait in a controlled environment where medical help is available. In this report, 76% of the reactions occurred in asthmatics.[71] However, not all studies have found an increased risk of reactions in asthmatic patients.

3. Tinkleman[66] reported a systemic reaction rate of 1.3 per 100 injections during the build-up phase and 1.6 per 100 injections during weekly immunotherapy maintenance. Patients at increased risk for reactions should carry an EpiPen and be able to recognize the early warning signs of a reaction, so that they can get medical assistance in time.

4. Patients taking β-blockers may be at increased risk for inadequate control of anaphylaxis, because epinephrine is first-line therapy for anaphylaxis.[72]

5. Patients taking ACE inhibitors may theoretically be at increased risk of inadequate control because of interactions with emergency medication, but data on this problem are not readily available.

6. Large local reactions do not predict a systemic reaction.

7. Antihistamines are recommended as premedication for the rush and cluster immunotherapy protocols. There is no evidence that antihistamines mask the early warning signs or delay the onset of systemic reactions.

8. Patients considered at high risk for a reaction include patients with unstable asthma, patients taking β-blockers, and "those with a seasonal exacerbation and exquisite sensitivity."[65]

9. Prompt recognition of a systemic reaction and the use of epinephrine are the mainstays of therapy.[73]

D. Monitoring Treatment

1. The only way to assess the clinical efficacy of aeroallergen immunotherapy is by clinical evaluation, which includes subjective and objective parameters.

2. Follow-up on a regular basis is essential to ensure that symptoms are controlled or reduced, the need for medication is reduced or the medication has greater efficacy, the complications of allergy (e.g., sinusitis) decrease, and quality of life improves. Patient follow-up visits allow further time for patient education and evaluation, as well as time to evaluate whether the patient's goals are being met and whether the immunotherapy program is clinically effective.

3. In vivo data (i.e., specific IgG[74]) are not a reliable indicator of program success. Skin tests may or may not show decreased antigen sensitivity and are not essential in patient monitoring. However, repeat skin tests may be necessary if symptoms are not well controlled on immunotherapy or if there is a question of new environmental sensitivities.

4. For patient follow-up, evaluation of quality of life is important. Health-related quality-of-life (HRQL) measures can be used to better understand and clinically assess treatment programs. HRQL can be measured in both children and adults.[75] The Short Form 36(SF-36), developed by the New England Medical Center, has questions divided among the following categories:
   a. Physical functions
   b. Problems with work or other daily activities due to physical health
   c. Pain
   d. Nervousness and depression
   e. Problems with work/daily activities due to emotional problems
   f. Social functioning
   g. Energy
   h. General health[76]

5. Allergen immunotherapy is also cost-effective.[77] It is important to review patient medication needs and occurrences of acute allergic problems.

6. For patients on venom immunotherapy, 3–5 years may be adequate duration of therapy for some patients. Skin testing and serum IgG testing for the specific vespid venoms have been well studied, and the results often correlate with control of the patient's symptoms control.[78]

7. The follow-up visit allows further opportunity to review with the patient the basics of this treatment program, including:
   a. The importance of compliance with regular shot visits and follow-up.
   b. Safety monitoring to reduce the risk of systemic reactions from immunotherapy. Monitoring involves the patient as well as the medical team. Patients should have verbal and written information available and reviewed at regular intervals.

E. Duration of SIT

1. Pollen immunotherapy is usually effective within the first year and provides long-term clinical efficacy after 3–4 years of treatment. Immunotherapy induces remission as well as a persistent alteration in immunologic reactivity.[79–82]
   a. Durham demonstrated a sustained remission for at least 3 years after stopping a 3- to 4-year course of immunotherapy.
   b. Hedlin's studies revealed that patients remained well for at least 5 years after 3 years of immunotherapy (28/30 patients).
   c. Ebner et al. found that 70% of patients remained well for at least 3 years after 3–4 years of immunotherapy.[83]

2. Given these results, it becomes pertinent to consider immunotherapy early in the course of the allergic disease in order to prevent progression and the possible development of multiple allergies.[84]

3. The decision to discontinue venom immunotherapy in a patient who has had a previous life-threatening reaction from a sting requires special consideration. Factors to consider include the potential frequency of stings, the severity of the original reaction, and whether reactions to immunotherapy occurred during the treatment course, as well as the patient's age and the existence of any underlying medical conditions that could complicate a reaction or the treatment of a reaction.

   The risk of a systemic sting reaction when venom immunotherapy is stopped after 5 years or longer is in the range of 5%–15% in the 5–10 years after stopping treatment. The clinical protection does not appear to decline with time despite the progressive decline in skin test positivity and the decline in venom-specific IgE responses.[85] There is also no evidence of a rebound effect after therapy is stopped. Long-term studies have revealed an incidence of 10% reactivity with each sting even 10–15 years after stopping immunotherapy. Patients may not react to one sting but may react to a subsequent sting, resulting in a cumulative 17% incidence of reactions after stopping therapy for 10 years.

Negative skin tests do not occur in 25% of patients even after 5 years of treatment and do not provide a guarantee of negative reactivity. There is almost a 10% frequency of reactions in patients who appear to lose sensitivity.

Children who are mild reactors may be considered lower risk, and discontinuation of treatment may be considered after just 3 years of treatment.[86]

VI. Special Treatment for Specific Populations

A. Older Patients

The proportion of older adults among the U.S. population is increasing. In a recent survey of allergists (ACAAI members), virtually all responders indicated that they provided inhalant allergen immunotherapy to patients ages 40–54 years, and frequently to older adults (>55 years).[87]

1. The prevalence of atopic disease in the older population is significant, and allergen immunotherapy can offer the advantage of better control of symptoms, plus avoidance of possible secondary effects of allergy medications.[88]
2. In general, atopy can be more difficult to treat in the elderly. Nasal structural changes occur naturally with aging, resulting in increased nasal airflow resistance and airway drying and atrophy of the mucous membranes, in addition to pulmonary symptoms. Environments may be more difficult to control, especially with respect to house dust mite, cockroach, mold, and animal dander antigens.
   a. In one study, mold sensitization increased in parallel with age and was the greatest in the 60- to 69-year-old age group.[89]
   b. Patients may also be on medications that contribute to nasal congestion and membrane dryness. In addition, other medications may contribute to metabolic breakdown.
3. It is of note that systemic reactions from immunotherapy have not been age related.[90]
   a. For all patients on immunotherapy, anaphylaxis is a rare event. However, older patients are often taking medications that can make treatment of anaphylaxis more difficult (e.g., β-blockers).
   b. In addition, comorbid conditions such as severe hypertension or cardiac instability, cerebrovascular disease, and arrhythmias are relative contraindications to the use of epinephrine.[91]
   c. Anaphylaxis is a rare complication of treatment but must always be considered.

4. In summary, age is not a limiting factor in initiating immunotherapy. Immunotherapy can help control atopic symptoms, thereby reducing the need for medications, and can improve the individual's quality of life.

B. Pregnant Women

Immunotherapy during pregnancy is not contraindicated and may be considered first-line therapy for allergic rhinitis[92] and allergic asthma. Allergy symptoms during pregnancy may worsen as a result of physical, hormonal, and environmental changes.

1. For many of the commonly used allergy medications, there are no safety data from controlled trials during pregnancy. Appropriate use of maintenance immunotherapy can afford significant symptom control during pregnancy, thereby optimizing the health of both mother and baby.[93,94]
2. There is no direct evidence that immunotherapy has an adverse effect on the unborn child. In one retrospective study of 109 pregnancies in 81 Indian women taking SIT, there was no difference in the rate of abortions, perinatal mortality, prematurity, toxemia, or congenital malformations. A control group of 60 patients who had refused SIT had higher rates of abortion, prematurity, and toxemia.[95]
3. Furthermore, in a 10-year follow-up study, pollen immunotherapy during pregnancy was shown to have no effect on pollen skin tests or on the development of asthma or allergic rhinitis in the offspring.[96]
4. In general, immunotherapy should be continued at a maintenance dose and should not be advanced during pregnancy.[97] Allergen immunotherapy ordinarily should not be initiated during pregnancy.[98] The major risk associated with allergen immunotherapy during this time period is the usual risk of anaphylaxis.
5. The continuation of venom immunotherapy during pregnancy is an important consideration. There is a 3%–5% risk of a serious reaction from a natural sting in any vespid-allergic patient who has not been treated with immunotherapy. In one study of 43 pregnancies in 26 women on venom immunotherapy, there was no increased risk for reactions or birth problems. One patient had anaphylaxis from a natural insect sting, but the pregnancy was normal. Two patients had shot reactions, neither of which required treatment. One child among the 43 live births was born with multiple congenital anomalies of unknown cause (same frequency of birth anomalies as in the general population).[99]

C. Children

Specific immunotherapy may be more effective in children and young adults than later in life.[100] Immunotherapy is safe in young children,[89,101] and inhalant sensitivity is often an issue at 4–5 years of age.[102]

1. In a 3-year study of 1053 children on SIT, 3.7% had mild allergic reactions and one serious reaction (0.08% of a total 47,247 injections). All the reactions occurred within 30 minutes.[103]
2. In previous studies children with allergic rhinitis who were placed on immunotherapy had a decreased risk of developing asthma.[104]
   a. The Preventive Allergy Treatment (PAT-ESACI [European Society of Allergy and Clinical Immunology]) study includes 208 children, ages 6–14 years, with allergic rhinoconjunctivitis who have been randomized to receive 3 years of SIT or medication only. Among those children on SIT without any clinical signs of asthma prior to the initiation of SIT, the treated children have less asthma and decreased bronchial hyperreactivity after 2, 3, and 5 years of study.[105]
   b. Bauer reported that SIT prevented the development of nonspecific bronchial hyperreactivity in a group of children with only allergic rhinitis from pollen or house dust mite allergens.[106] Hedlin et al. noted reduced bronchial hyperreactivity as well as a reduced allergen sensitivity in 29 children (7–16 years old) with asthma after 3 years of SIT and inhaled corticosteroids, which persisted 5 years after stopping SIT.[107,108]
   c. A 5-year study by Pajino et al. of 123 children and controls found that after 3 years of treatment with standardized mite extract, 75% of treated children had no new sensitivities at 2-year follow-up, versus 33% of controls.[109] Des Roches et al. also noted a reduced number of new sensitizations in children who had been on SIT for a year.[110]
   d. In the study by Adkinson et al. of 121 children with allergic rhinitis and moderate to severe asthma on SIT or maximum medical control, all improved. Children younger than 8.5 years and those with mild asthma exhibited a more significant treatment effect with SIT.[111]
   e. In a 9-year study by Cools et al. of children with asthma who had received SIT for 4–5 years, there was a threefold decrease in asthmatic symptoms compared with controls.[112] Calvo et al., in a 10-year follow-up study of children who had been treated with SIT, noted a decrease in the number of asthma drugs needed.[113] Johnstone reported that two-thirds of children with asthma on SIT had complete resolution of their asthma symptoms (versus 7% of controls) and a decrease in allergic rhinitis symptoms.[110,114]
3. In summary, SIT is safe and effective in children. It helps control symptoms of allergic rhinitis and asthma,

---

BOX 11-8

Benefits of Immunotherapy in Children

Improved symptom control for asthma and allergic rhinitis (Johnstone)

Increased PC20 to allergens; increased tolerance of cat dander (Hedlin)

Decreased risk of developing asthma (Cools, Valovirta)

Decrease in development of new sensitivities (Des Roches)

---

it prevents new sensitivities, and it decreases the risk of asthma in children with allergic rhinitis (Box 11-8).

D. Autoimmune Deficiency Patients

Data on the effectiveness of or risks associated with immunotherapy in patients with immunodeficiency or autoimmune diseases are limited. There is no evidence that such treatment is harmful. The decision to treat must be made on an individual basis.

VII. Guidelines for Administration of Antigen Vaccine Outside of the Allergist's Office

A. Away from Home

Allergen immunotherapy is best administered in the prescribing allergist's office. However, in many cases it is preferable to have the patient receive the vaccine in another physician's office nearer the patient's home or place of work.

1. In 1994, 86% of 1415 allergists reported that they were willing to send, or had on occasion sent, extracts to another physician's office for administration.[115]
2. The allergy vaccine should be administered under the supervision of an appropriately trained physician and staff, regardless of location. The antigen must be stored properly, administered according to the recommended schedule with adjustments as appropriate, and reactions should be recognized early and treated appropriately.[31]
3. The prescribing physician will provide:
   a. Vaccines well labeled with the name of the patient, the name of the antigen/vaccine, the dilution, the expiration date, and the name of the prescribing physician.
   b. The treatment protocol and schedule.
   c. Dosage adjustment guidelines for:
      1) Build-up phase (1–2 injections per week, usually at least 2 days apart)
      2) Maintenance phase (injections every 4–8 weeks)

3) Start of each new vial (dose reduction)
4) Seasonal peaks (maintain without advancing or reducing the dose)
5) Missed injections (dose depends on time since the last shot)
6) Adjustment of doses if any reaction occurs

d. General procedures and equipment recommendations for treatment of an anaphylactic reaction.

4. In addition, the patient's responsibilities are the same in any office and include the following:

a. Maintain a regular shot schedule.

b. Inform the staff of conditions that may make the patient high risk:

1) Acute illness or allergy/asthma exacerbations
2) New medications (especially β-blockers)
3) Any reaction related to the last shot

c. Carry an Epi-Pen to all visits if recommended by the specialist.

d. Wait 20–30 minutes or longer in the office after each shot.

e. Return to the prescribing physician's office for regular follow-up visits.

5. If there are questions about the schedule or if the patient has a systemic reaction to the vaccine, the prescribing physician must be contacted and the patient seen as appropriate by the prescribing physician.

6. Patients at high risk should be treated in an allergist's office, because the allergist and the staff have more experience and training and are more likely to recognize the signs and symptoms of a reaction earlier and initiate early treatment, which may decrease the possibility of a serious outcome.[116]

B. Home Therapy

Immunotherapy is best provided in the prescribing allergist's office. In exceptional cases in which allergen immunotherapy cannot be administered at a medical facility, very careful consideration of the potential benefits and risk of at-home administration of an allergenic extract therapy must be made on an individual patient basis. It should be noted, however, that the FDA package insert that accompanies all allergenic extracts implies that allergy injections should be given in a clinical setting, under the supervision of a physician, with the patient waiting at least 20 minutes after each injection. Patients who are at greater risk of reactions from immunotherapy may need to wait longer.[28]

VIII. Future Therapies

A. The preceding discussion referred to the use of aqueous extracts for SC administration only. A variety of new formulations delivered by various routes are under study and will be available in the very near future. Some examples include:

- Anti IgE[117,118]
- Peptide formulations[119–121]
- Anticytokine treatments[122]
- DNA-based immunotherapy[123]

B. Over the past 10 years the most important allergens from house dust mites, pollens, animal dander, insects, and food have been cloned, sequenced, and expressed. Recombinant allergens will enable new strategies for allergen immunotherapy. These strategies include short linear allergen-derived peptides, corresponding to T-cell epitopes, that will offer the possibility of a safer approach; engineered hypoallergens with reduced reactivity for IgE antibodies; nucleotide-conjugated vaccines that promote Th1 responses; and the possibility of developing prophylactic allergen vaccines.[124]

C. Alternative routes of therapy that are under investigation include intranasal,[125] sublingual, swallow, or oral immunotherapy. In the future, these routes may afford a "viable alternative to parenteral injection therapy."[29] Intranasal immunotherapy has been shown to improve nasal symptoms of rhinitis.[126] This form of therapy is not currently available in the United States but has gained some acceptance elsewhere in the world.

D. The key issue is that with treatment, patients can lead more comfortable and productive lives, and with control of sensitization and inflammation, chronic changes may be avoided. Early treatment with the presently available vaccines can result in symptom control, decreased sensitization, a decreased risk of disease progression, and a decreased risk of complications. Allergen-specific immunotherapy—SIT (as well as avoidance)—can modify the immune response, modify the disease process, and potentially alleviate symptoms for the long term, even after injections are discontinued.

Immunologic control is possible with early intervention with environmental controls and antigen-specific vaccine.

IX. Internet Resources

www.aaaai.org

www.acaa.org

www.jcaai.org

X. ICD-9 Codes

95115   Single injection
95117   Two or more injections
95165   Single dose of antigen (excluding venom antigen)

95130   Single venom antigen dose (not injection fee)
95131   Two venoms
95132   Three venoms
95133   Four venoms
95134   Five venoms
94160   Peak flow testing

If shots are being given outside the office and the allergist has supplied the antigen, the fee for shot injection is usually used (codes 95115, 95117). For asthmatic patients, a peak flow may be needed before the shot is given.

For patients on immunotherapy, regular follow-up visits are also required. The allergist providing the extract sets this visit schedule.

XI. Patient Education Material

A. See Appendix 1.

B. Refer to patient education CD, which is provided with this text, for additional patient education information. It has been formatted to provide readily accessible, easy-to-understand handouts for adult patients and the parents of pediatric patients. The handouts can be easily modified to fit specific practice requirements.

REFERENCES

1. Nimmagadda SR, Evans R III: Allergy: Etiology and epidemiology. Pediatr Rev 1999;20:111–116.
2. Sly RM: Changing prevalence of allergic rhinitis and asthma. Ann Allergy Asthma Immunol 1999;82:233–248.
3. Ray NF, Baraniuk JN, Thamer M, et al: Direct expenditures for the treatment of allergic rhinoconjunctivitis in 1996, including the contributions of related airway illnesses. J Allergy Clin Immunol 1999;103:401–407.
4. TePas ED, Umetsu DT: Immunotherapy of asthma and allergic diseases. Curr Opin Pediatr 2000;12:574–578.
5. Adkinson NF: Immunotherapy for allergic rhinitis (editorial). N Engl J Med 341;341:522–525.
6. Blackley DE: Experimental Research on the Causes and Nature of Catarrhus Aestivas (Hay-Fever or Hay-Asthma). London: Balliere, Tindall, and Cox, 1873.
7. Freeman J: Vaccination against hayfever: report of results during the last 3 years. Lancet 1914;1:1178.
8. Cooke RA, Barnard J, Hebald S, Stull A: Serological evidence on immunity with coexisting sensitization in a type of human allergy, hay fever. J Exp Med 1935;62:733–750.
9. Finegold E: Immunotherapy: Historical perspective. Ann Allergy Asthma Immunol 2001;87:3–4.
10. Rocklin RE, Sheffer AL, Greineder DK, Melmon KL: Generation of antigen-specific suppressor cells during allergy sensitization. N Engl J Med 1980;302:1213–1219.
11. Creticos PS: The consideration of immunotherapy in the treatment of allergic asthma. Ann Asthma Allergy Immunol 2001;87:13–27.
12. Yang X: Does allergen immunotherapy alter the natural course of allergic disorders? Drugs 2001;61:365–375.
13. Bosquet J: Am J Respir Crit Care Med 2002;164:2139–2142.
14. Corren J: Allergic rhinitis: Treating the adult. J Allergy Clin Immunol 2000;105:10–15.
15. Durham SR, Walker SM, Varga EM, et al: Long-term efficacy of grass pollen immunotherapy. N Engl J Med 1999;341:468–475.
16. Grembiale RA, Camporota L, Saveno N, et al: Specific immunotherapy may reduce asthma risk in allergic rhinitis patients. Am J Respir Crit Care Med 2000;162:2048–2052.
17. Bodtger U, Poulsen LR, Jacoti HH, Malling HJ: The safety and efficacy of subcutaneous birch pollen immunotherapy: A one-year randomized, double-blind, placebo-controlled study. Allergy 2002;57:297–305.
18. Ross R, Nelson H, Finegold I: Effectiveness of specific immunotherapy in the treatment of allergic rhinitis: An analysis of randomized, prospective, single- or double-blind placebo-controlled studies. Clin Ther 2000;22:342–350.
19. Settipane RJ, Hagy GW, Settipane GA: Long-term risk factors for developing asthma and allergic rhinitis: A 23-year follow-up study of college students. Allergy Proc 1994;15:21–25.
20. Abramson MJ, Puy RM, Weiner JM: Is allergen immunotherapy effective in asthma? A meta-analysis of randomized controlled trials. Am J Respir Crit Care Med 1995;151:969–974.
21. Ross R, Nelson H, Finegold I: Effectiveness of specific immunotherapy in the treatment of asthma: A meta-analysis of prospective, randomized, double-blind, placebo-controlled studies. Clin Ther 2000;22:329–341.
22. Abramson M, Puy R, Weiner J: Immunotherapy in asthma: An updated systematic review. Allergy 1999;54:1022–1041.
23. Pichler CE, Helbling A, Pichler WJ: Three years of specific immunotherapy with house dust-mite extracts in patients with rhinitis and asthma: Significant improvement of allergen-specific parameters and nonspecific bronchial hyperreactivity. Allergy 2001;56:301–306.
24. DiBernardino C, DiBernardino F, Colombo R, Angrisano A: A case-control study of *Dermatophagoides* immunotherapy in children below 5 years of age. Allergy Immunol 2002;34:56–59.
25. Moller C, Dreborg S, Ferdousi HA, et al: Pollen immunotherapy reduces the development of asthma in children with seasonal rhinoconjunctivitis (the PAT study). J Allergy Clin Immunol 2002;109:251–256.
26. Creticos P, Reed CE, Normal P, et al: Ragweed allergy in adult asthma. N Engl J Med 1996;334:301–306.
27. Adkinson NF Jr, Eggleston PA, Eney D, et al: A controlled trial of immunotherapy for asthma in allergic children. N Engl J Med 1997;336:324–331.
28. Nicklas RA, Bernstein IL, et al: Practice parameters for allergen immunotherapy. J Allergy Clin Immunol 1996;98:1001–1011.
29. Theodoropoulos DS, Lockey RF: Allergen immunotherapy: Guidelines, update, and recommendations of the World Health Organization. Allergy Asthma Proc 2000;21:159–166.

30. Bosquet J, Lockey R, Malling HJ: Allergen immunotherapy: Therapeutic vaccines for allergic diseases (World Health Organization paper, Executive Summary). Ann Allergy Asthma Immunother 1998;00:401–404.

31. Li J, Bernstein IL, Nicklas R, et al: Practice parameter for allergen immunotherapy. Ann Allergy Asthma Immunol 2003;90:S1–S40.

32. Malling HJ: Allergen-specific immunotherapy in allergic rhinitis. Curr Opin Allergy Clin Immunol 2001;1:43–46.

33. Spector S, Nicklas R: Practice parameters for the diagnosis and treatment of asthma. J Allergy Clin Immunol 1995; 96:707–870.

34. Dykewicz M, Fineman S, Skoner DP, et al: Diagnosis and management of rhinitis. Ann Allergy Asthma Immunol 1998;81:478–518.

35. Lichtenstein ALM, Ishizaka K, Norman P, et al: IgE antibody measurement in ragweed hay fever: Relationship to clinical severity and the results of immunotherapy. J Clin Invest 1973;52:472–482.

36. Burrows BM, Martinez FD, Halonen M, et al: Association of asthma with serum IgE levels and skin test reactivity to allergens. N Engl J Med 1989;320:271–277.

37. Platts-Mills TAE, Vaughan JW, Carter MC, Woodfolk JA: The role of intervention in established allergy: Avoidance of indoor allergens in the treatment of chronic allergic disease. J Allergy Clin Immunol 2000;106:787–804.

38. Walker D, Virchow CJ, Bruinjnzeel P, Blaser K: T cell subsets and their soluble products regulate eosinophilia in allergy and nonallergic asthma. J Immunol 1991;146:1829–1835.

39. Malling J-J, Weeke B: EAACI immunotherapy position paper. Allergy 1993;48:9–35.

40. http://www.fda.gov/cber/vaccine/vacpubs.htm

41. Nelson H: Preparing and mixing allergen vaccines. In Lockey R, Bukantz S (eds): Allergens and Allergen Immunotherapy, pp 401–422. New York: Marcel Dekker, 1999.

42. Leavengood DC, Renard RL, Maertin B, Nelson JS: Cross-allergenicity among grasses determined by tissue threshold changes. J Allergy Clin Immunol 1985;76:789–794.

43. Esch RE: Grass pollen allergens. In Lockey R, Bukantz S (eds): Allergens and Allergen Immunotherapy, p 115. New York: Marcel Dekker, 1999.

44. Kordash A, Williamson JP: Effect of mixing allergenic extracts containing *Helminthosporium, D. farinae,* and cockroach with perennial ryegrass. Ann Allergy 1993;71: 240–246.

45. Nelson HS, Ikle D, Buchmeier A: Studies of allergen extract stability: The effects of dilution and mixing. J Allergy Clin Immunol 1996;98:382–388.

46. Norman PS, Marsh DG: Human serum albumin and Tween 80 as stabilizers of allergen solutions. J Allergy Clin Immunol 1978;62:314–319.

47. VanMetre TEJR, Rosenberg GL, Vaswanki SK, Zeigler SR, Adkinson NF Jr: Pain and dermal reaction caused by injected glycerin in immunotherapy solutions. J Allergy Clin Immunol 1996;97:1033–1039.

48. Nelson HS: Effect of preservatives and conditions of storage on the potency of allergy extracts. J Allergy Clin Immunol 1981;67:64–69.

49. Nelson J, Ikle D, Buchmeier A: Studies of allergen extract stability: The effects of dilution and mixing. J Allergy Clin Immunol 1996;98:382–388.

50. Baer H, Anderson MC, Hale R, Gleich GH: The heat stability of short ragweed pollen extract and the importance of individual allergens in skin reactivity. J Allergy Clin Immunol 1980;66:2281–2285.

51. Johnstone DE, Crump L: Value of hyposensitization therapy for perennial bronchial asthma in children. Pediatrics 1961;27:39–44.

52. Franklin W, Lowell FC: Comparison of two dosages of ragweed extract in the treatment of pollenosis. JAMA 1967; 201:915–917.

53. DuBuske LM: Appropriate and inappropriate use of immunotherapy. Ann Allergy Asthma Immunol 2001; 87:56–67.

54. DiBerardino L: The optimal interval for allergen immunotherapy: An open question. ACI Int 2002;14(2):78–79.

55. Feeling LI, Muni IA, Helms RJ: Rates of release of subcutaneously injected antigens in the rat. Allergy 1979;34: 339–344.

56. Portnoy J, King K, Kanaerk J: Premedication reduces the incidence of systemic reactions during rush immunotherapy. Ann Allergy 1994;73:409–418.

57. Bernstein J, Kagen S, Bernstein D, Bernstein I: Rapid venom immunotherapy is safe for routine use in the treatment of patients with Hymenoptera anaphylaxis. Ann Allergy 1994;73:423–428.

58. Tabar AI, Muro MD, Garcia BE, et al: D. pter cluster immunotherapy: A controlled trial of safety and clinical efficacy. J Invest Allergol Clin Immunol 1999;3:155–164.

59. Grammer L, Shaughnessy M, Patterson R: Administration of inhalant allergen vaccines. In Lockey R (ed): Allergens and Allergen Immunotherapy, p 423. New York: Marcel Dekker, 1999.

60. Ewan P, Alexander M, Snape C, et al: Effective hyposensitization in allergic rhinitis using a potent partially purified extract of house dust mite. Clin Allergy 1988;18:501–508.

61. Alvarez-Cuesta E, Cuesta-Herranz J, Puyuna-Ruiz J, et al: Monoclonal antibody-standardized cat extract immunotherapy: Risk benefit effects from a double-blind placebo study. J Allergy Clin Immunol 1994;93:456–466.

62. Dole I, Martin-Cocera D, Bartolome J, Cinarra M: A double-blind, placebo-controlled study of immunotherapy with grass-pollen extract, Alutard SQ during a 3-year period with initial rush immunotherapy. Allergy 1996;51:489–500.

63. Wells J: Systemic reactions to immunotherapy: Comparisons between two large allergy practices. J Allergy Clin Immunol 1996;97:1030–1032.

64. Lin M, Tanner E, Lin J, Friday G: Nonfatal allergic reactions induced by skin testing and immunotherapy. Ann Allergy 1993;71:557–562.

65. Lockey RF, Nicoara-Kasti GL, Theodoropoulos DS, Bukantz SC: Systemic reactions and fatalities associated with allergen immunotherapy. Ann Allergy Asthma Immunol 2001;87:47–55.

66. Tinkelman DG: Immunotherapy: A one-year prospective study to evaluate risk factors for systemic reactions. J Allergy Clin Immunol 1995;95:8–14.

67. Turkeltaub P: Deaths associated with allergenic extracts. FDA Med Bull 1994/7.

68. Reid M, Lockey RF, Turkeltaub PD, Platts-Mills TAE: Fatalities from immunotherapy and skin testing. J Allergy Clin Immunol 1990;92:6–15.

69. Stewart GE, Lockey R: Systemic reactions from allergen immunotherapy (editorial). J Allergy Clin Immunol 1992;90:567–579.

70. AAAAI Board of Directors: Guidelines to minimize the risk from systemic reactions caused by immunotherapy with allergenic extracts: Physician reference materials. Position Statement 25. J Allergy Clin Immunol 1994;93:811–812.

71. Reid M: Survey of fatalities from skin testing and immunotherapy 1985–89. J Allergy Clin Immunol 1993;92(1 Pt 1):6–15.

72. Frazier C: Epinephrine for anaphylaxis (guest editorial). Ann Allergy 1994;72:393–394.

73. Executive Committee, American Academy of Allergy and Immunology: Personnel and equipment to treat systemic reactions caused by immunotherapy with allergenic extracts. J Allergy Clin Immunol 1986;77:271–273.

74. Gehlhar K, Schlaak M, Becker W, Bufe A: Monitoring allergen immunotherapy of pollen-allergic patients: Ratio of allergen-specific IgG4 to IgG1 with clinical outcomes. Clin Exp Allergy 1999;29:497–506.

75. Bender BG: Measurement of quality of life in pediatric asthma trials. Ann Allergy Asthma Immunol 1996;77:438–444.

76. Juniper EF: Measuring health-related quality of life for persons with asthma: An overview. In Weiss DB, Buist AS, Sullivan SD (eds): Asthma's Impact on Society, pp 99–126. New York: Marcel Dekker, 2000.

77. Bernstein J: Pharmacoeconomic immunotherapy. In Lockey R (ed): Allergens and Allergen Immunotherapy, 2nd ed, p 445. New York: Marcel Dekker, 1999.

78. Portnoy JM, Moffit JE, Golden DB, et al: Stinging insect hypersensitivity: A practice parameter. J Allergy Clin Immunol 1998;102:S107–S149.

79. Greenberger J: Allergy Clin Immunol 1986;77:865–870.

80. Durham SR, Walker S, Varga E-M, et al: Long-term efficacy of grass pollen immunotherapy. N Engl J Med 1999;341:468–475.

81. Robinson DS: Allergen immunotherapy: Does it work, and if so, how and for how long? Thorax 2000;55(Suppl 1):S11–S14.

82. Hedlin G, Heilborn H, Lilja G, et al: Long-term follow-up of a patient treated with a three-year course of cat and dog immunotherapy. J Allergy Clin Immunol 1995;96(6 Pt 1):879–885.

83. Ebner C, Seimann U, Bohle B, et al: Immunological changes during specific immunotherapy of grass pollen allergy. Clin Exp Allergy 1997;27:1007–1115.

84. Des Roches A, Paradis L, Menardo JL, et al: Immunotherapy with a standardized *Dermatophagonides pteronyssinus* extract: VI. Specific immunotherapy prevents the onset of new sensitization in children. J Allergy Clin Immunol 1997;99:450–453.

85. Golden D, Kagey-Sobotk A, Lichtenstein LM: Survey of patients after discontinuing venom immunotherapy. J Allergy Clin Immunol 2000;105:385–390.

86. Golden DB: Discontinuation of venom immunotherapy. Curr Opin Allergy Clin Immunol 2001;1:353–355.

87. Lange DW, Visintainer PF, Howland WD, Stein M, Villareal M: Survey of the extent and nature of care for adults and older adults by allergy/immunology practitioners. Ann Allergy Asthma Immunol 2000;85:85–86.

88. Armentia A, Fernandez A, Tapias JA, et al: Immunotherapy with allergenic extracts in geriatric patients: Evaluation of effectiveness and safety. J Allergol Immunopathol 1993;21:193–196.

89. Erel F, Karaayvaz M, Calisdaner Z, et al: The allergen spectrum in Turkey and the relationships between allergens and age, sex, birth month, birthplace, blood group and family history of atopy. J Invest Allergol Clin Immunol 1998;8:226–233.

90. Karaayvas M, Erel F, Calisdaner Z, et al: Systemic reactions due to allergen immunotherapy. J Invest Allergol Clin Immunol 1999;9:39–44.

91. Coren J: Allergic rhinitis: Treating the adult. J Allergy Clin Immunol 2000;105:S610–S615.

92. Mazzotta P, Loebstein R, Koren G: Treating allergic rhinitis in pregnancy: Safety considerations. Drug Safety 1999;20:361–375.

93. Schatz M, Aeiger RS: Asthma and allergy in pregnancy. Clin Perinatol 1997;24:407–432.

94. Metzger WJ: Indications for allergen immunotherapy during pregnancy. Compr Ther 1990;16:17–26.

95. Shaikh WA: A retrospective study on the safety of immunotherapy during pregnancy. Clin Exp Allergy 1993;23:857–860.

96. Settipane RA, Chafee FH, Settipane GA: Pollen immunotherapy during pregnancy: Long-term follow-up of offspring. Allergy Proc 1988;9:555–561.

97. Metzger WJ, Turner E, Patterson R: The safety of immunotherapy during pregnancy. J Allergy Clin Immunol 1978;61:268.

98. Portnoy JM: Immunotherapy for inhalant allergies: Guidelines for why, when and how to use. Postgrad Med 2001;109(5):89.

99. Schwartz HJ, Golden DB, Lockey RF: Venom immunotherapy in the Hymenoptera-allergic pregnant patient. J Allergy Clin Immunol 1990;85:709–712.

100. Demoly P, Dhivert-Donnadieu H, Bousquet J: Vaccination with allergens in children. Allergy Immunol (Paris) 2000;32:397–401.

101. Akcakaya N, Hassanzadeh A, Camcioglu Y, Cokugras H: Local and systemic reactions during immunotherapy with absorbed extracts of house dust mites in children. Ann Allergy Asthma Immunol 2000;85:317–321.

102. Bosquet J, Demoly P, Michel FB: Specific immunotherapy in rhinitis and asthma. Ann Allergy Asthma Immunol 2001;87:38–42.

103. Buscino L, Zannino L, Cantani A, et al: Systemic reactions to specific immunotherapy in children with respiratory allergy: A prospective study. Pediatr Allergy Immunol 1995;6:44–47.

104. Valovirta E: Capacity of specific immunotherapy in preventing allergic asthma in children: The Preventive Allergy Treatment study (PAT). J Invest Allergol Clin Immunol 1997;7:369–370.

105. Jacobson L: Preventive aspects of immunotherapy: Prevention for children at risk of developing asthma. Ann Allergy Asthma Immunol 2001;87(Suppl):43–46.

106. Bauer CP: Untersuchung zur Asthmaprevention durch die spezifische Immuntherapie bei Kindern. Allergologic 1993;x:468.

107. Hedlin G, Wille S, Browaldh L, et al: Immunotherapy in children with allergic asthma. J Asthma Allergy Clin Immunol 1999;103:609–614.

108. Hedlin G, Heilborn H, Lilja G, et al: Long-term follow-up of patients treated with a three-year course of cat or dog immunotherapy. J Allergy Clin Immunol 1995;96:879–885.

109. Pajino GB, Morabito L, Barbaerio O: Specific immunotherapy with standardized dist mite extract prevents the onset of new sensitizations in monosensitized children: An updated review and personal experience of five years' follow-up. Paper presented at the annual meeting of the AAAAI, March 3, 1999.

110. Des Roches A, Paradis L, Menardo JL, et al: Immunotherapy with a standardized *Dermatophygoides pteromyssinum* extract. J Allergy Clin Immunol 1997;99:450–453.

111. Adkinson HF Jr, Effleston PA, Eney D, et al: Comment. N Engl J Med 1997;336:324–331.

112. Cools M, Van Bever HP, Weyler JJ, et al: Long-term effects of specific immunotherapy, administered during childhood, in asthmatic patients allergic to either house dust mite or to both house dust mite and grass pollen. Allergy 2000; 55:69–73.

113. Calvo M, Marin F, Grob K, et al: Ten-year follow-up in pediatric patients with allergic bronchial asthma: Evaluation of specific immunotherapy. J Invest Allergol Clin Immunol 1994;4:126–131.

114. Johnstone SE: Study of the role of antigen dose in the treatment of pollinosis and pollen asthma. Am J Dis Child 1957; 94:1–5.

115. aaaaj/evals/zeitz.rpt.

116. American College of Asthma, Allergy and Immunology: Position statement on the administration of immunotherapy outside of the prescribing allergist facility. Ann Allergy Asthma Immunol 1998;81(2).

117. Milgrom H, Fick RB, Su JQ, et al: Treatment of allergic asthma with monoclonal anti-IgE antibody. N Engl J Med 1999;341:1966–1973.

118. Kreuhr J, Brauberger J, Zielen S, et al: Efficacy of combination treatment with anti-IgE plus specific immunotherapy in polysensitized children and adolescents with seasonal allergic rhinitis. J Allergy Clin Immunol 2002; 109:274–280.

119. Lichtenstein LM, Creticos PS, Norman PS, et al: Initial clinical experience with T-cell epitope-defined peptides from ragweed allergen Amb a 1. J Allergy Clin Immunol 1995; 95:390.

120. Chapman MD, Smith AM, Vailes LD, Pomes A: Recombinant allergens for immunotherapy. Allergy Asthma Proc 2002;23:5–8.

121. Ali FR, Kay AB, Larche M: The potential of peptide immunotherapy in allergy and asthma. Curr Allergy Asthma Rep 2002;2(2):151–158.

122. Borish LC, Nelson HS, Lanz M, et al: Phase I/II study of interleukin-4 receptor in moderate asthma (abstr). J Allergy Clin Immunol 1998;101:A35.

123. Broide D: Immunostimulatory DNA sequences inhibit IL-5 eosinophilic inflammation and a hyperresponsiveness in mice. J Immunol 1998;161:7054–7062.

124. Kline JM: Modulation of airway inflammation by CpG oligodeoxynucleotides in a murine model. J Immunol 1998;160:2555.

125. Georgitis JW, Clayton WF, Wypych JI, et al: Further evaluation of local intranasal immunotherapy with aqueous and allerginoid grass extracts. J Allergy Clin Immunol 1984; 74:694–670.

126. Pomes A, Chapman MD: Can knowledge of the molecular structure of allergens improve immunotherapy? Curr Opin Allergy Clin Immunol 2001;6:549–554.

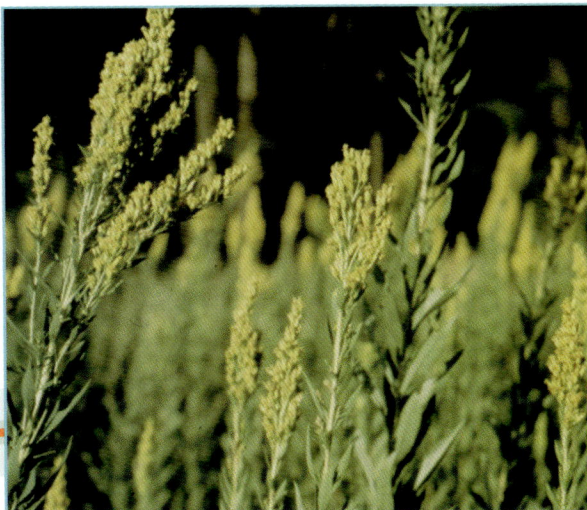

Goldenrod 2 *Courtesy of Hollister-Stier Laboratory*

CHAPTER 12
Skin Testing

Etan C. Milgrom and William W. Storms

I. Introduction

Allergy testing should be considered for patients with seasonal allergic rhinitis, perennial allergic rhinitis, asthma, sinusitis, recurrent upper respiratory tract infections, atopic dermatitis (eczema), chronic urticaria, bee/wasp/hornet allergy, food allergy, latex allergy, occupational asthma, and various other allergic conditions (Table 12-1).[1,2] The indications for allergy testing vary from patient to patient and depend on the severity of the disease, individual patient considerations, and the availability of testing. The two forms of IgE-mediated allergy testing are skin tests (the term skin or prick tests refers the same procedure and can be used interchangably) and serum in vitro IgE-specific antibody tests (see Chapter 13, Radioallergosorbent Testing, for more information). Skin testing for IgE-mediated sensitivity is the most widely used technique to identify allergic triggers. Skin testing is more sensitive and specific than serum in vitro testing (Table 12-2). However, when skin testing is either unavailable or contraindicated, serum in vitro allergen-specific testing, or RAST, should be considered. It is a relatively reliable second choice.

In the evaluation of perennial and environmental allergies, the number of skin tests performed will vary in different areas of the country. Children should be tested with a fewer number of skin tests to minimize the discomfort (relatively small) from the procedure.[3] Specific individual tests are required for allergen-specific conditions (e.g., drug allergy, latex allergy, Hymenoptera sensitivity, anesthetic allergy). Food allergy evaluation may require a larger number of skin tests, depending on the patient's history.

II. Allergy Skin Testing

A. General Principles

1. Antihistamines must be stopped 5–7 days prior to skin testing because they will block any IgE-mediated immune reaction occurring on the skin.
2. Long-term oral steroid use can partially suppress skin test reactions; short-burst oral steroid therapy will not.
3. There is no age limit for performing skin tests, but they will generally show diminished reactivity in infants and the elderly.
4. Skin testing is usually not performed in children younger than 5 years of age unless special circumstances prevail, such as children with severe atopic dermatitis, anaphylactic food allergies, and severe asthma.

171

TABLE 12-1

Disease Indications for Allergy Testing

Inhaled Allergens	Drugs	Food Allergy	Other
Allergic rhinitis	Penicillin allergy	Severe atopic dermatitis	Stinging insect anaphylaxis
Asthma	Local anesthetic reactions	Food-induced skin, respiratory, or GI symptoms	Latex allergy
Occupational asthma		Urticaria (usually chronic)	
Sinusitis		Anaphylaxis	

5. Testing should be performed and interpreted by individuals who have had both training and experience with this procedure.[1,2]

6. The choice of inhalant allergens for testing should be made according to the pollen-producing plants of the region in which the individual resides.

7. Although skin testing is considered to be a safe procedure, large local reactions may occur, as well as occasional systemic symptoms. Therapy for anaphylaxis should be available in case of a severe reaction. Epinephrine injections almost always will reverse any severe reaction. Chapter 6 covers this topic in greater detail.

8. Pregnant patients should only be skin tested if it is believed that the results will have substantial and immediate therapeutic implications; otherwise the testing should be postponed until after childbirth.

9. Positive skin test results do not necessarily confirm a diagnosis of allergy. Skin test results must be correlated with the patient's history in order to determine whether there is a significant allergic etiology.

III. The Skin Test Procedure

A. Materials

1. **Screening Skin Test Tray**
   This tray should include vials of individual allergen extracts consisting of common pollens in the local area, dust mites, animal dander, mold spores, and common foods. This skin test screening panel is comprehensive enough to determine the need for implementation of environmental control measures. The

TABLE 12-2

Comparison of Skin Tests with RAST

Factor Evaluated	Skin Tests	RAST
Accuracy	Excellent	Good
Cost	$3–5 per test	$10–15 per test
Skills	Required	NA
Risk	Minimal	None
Patient education tool	Excellent	Good

TABLE 12-3

Typical Skin Testing Screening Panel (for Southern California)

	Wheal (mm)	Flare (mm)
Positive histamine control	_____	_____
Negative diluent control	_____	_____

Trees (spring)

Elm		
Oak		
Maple		
Ash		

Grasses (summer)

Timothy		
Bermuda		
Rye		

Weeds (fall)

Ragweed		
Kochia		
Pigweed		
Scale		
Russian thistle		

Perennial allergens

Dust mite		
D. farinae		
D. pteronyssinus		
Feather		
Cat		
Dog		
Molds		
Alternaria		
Hormodendrum		
Aspergillus		

Foods

Milk		
Soy		
Egg		
Wheat		
Shrimp		
Peanut		

antigen vials can be ordered from several companies (see Appendix 3). The extracts used are usually 1:10 or 1:20 wt/vol extracts in 50% glycerin and should be standardized whenever possible. Each screening tray should also have a negative (diluent only) and a positive (histamine [1.0 mg/mL] only) control vial. These two vials are critical for proper interpretation of the allergic skin test results (Table 12-3). Figures 12-1 and 12-2 show partial contents of a typical screening skin test tray and device.

2. ***Skin Test Devices***

   Many commercially available devices can be used to break the skin superficially. Some examples are sterile needles, sterile sewing needles, sterile Morrow-Brown needles, Dermapik plastic devices from Greer Laboratory, and Quintest skin test devices from Hollister-Stier Laboratory (Fig. 12-3).

B. Procedure[1]

1. ***Skin (Prick) Testing***

   a. Patients should be instructed on the risks and benefits of the procedure and sign a consent form verifying this interaction (Box 12-1).

   b. Cleanse the skin with 70% isopropyl or ethyl alcohol and allow to dry.

   c. With a pen or stamp, mark the arm or back with lines at least 2–3 cm apart to prevent coalescence of positive skin reactions (Fig. 12-4). The marks should correspond with the order of antigens on the skin test tray that is being used for testing (see Figs. 12-1 and 12-2).

   d. Allergy test antigens are applied either to the arm or the back. Some clinicians prefer to perform the testing on the patient's arm so that the patient can see the results. Direct visualization of allergic reactions can promote patient education and compliance. Other clinicians may prefer the back because it is a large, flat surface that affords a greater number of skin test sites.

   e. The correct droplets of antigen should be placed next to the appropriate marked line in an aseptic manner. This step can be omitted with devices that allow direct placement of the antigen on the device just before the skin is punctured. The latter technique is preferable.

   f. The skin test device can puncture the skin by either the scratch or prick technique. The device is placed through the droplet at a 90-degree angle and the device is either twisted on the skin surface (scratch test) or gently lifted with a flick-like motion on the skin surface as the device is withdrawn (prick test). Alternatively, some skin test device systems place the device in a vial containing the desired antigen prior to skin testing. The device is then placed directly on the skin and the skin is punctured by gently pushing the device into the skin (Figs. 12-5 and 12-6).

   g. The device was inserted too deeply if blood is drawn with puncture of the skin.

   h. Each device should be discarded directly into a sharps container and not reused.

   i. The Dermapik (not shown) and Quintest (see Fig. 12-1) systems allow for placement of the antigen on the tip of the device prior to puncturing the skin. These devices are advantageous in that there is no need to first place the antigen

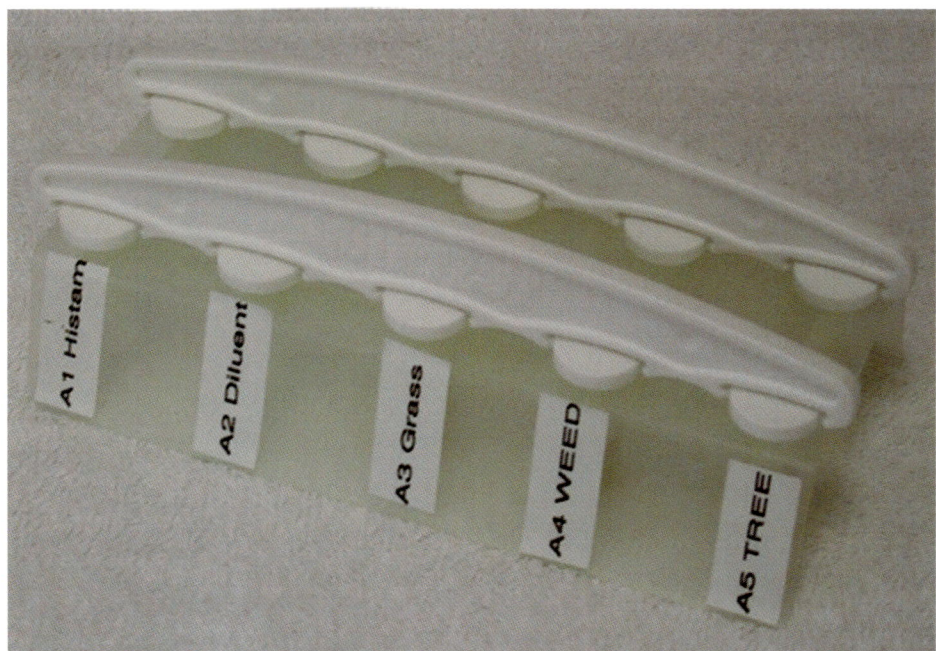

Figure 12-1 Skin test tray and device from Hollister-Stier Laboratories with prelabeled antigen from skin test screening panel. Note that the multiple skin test device is immersed in antigen vials on the tray and is ready for the next skin test patient.

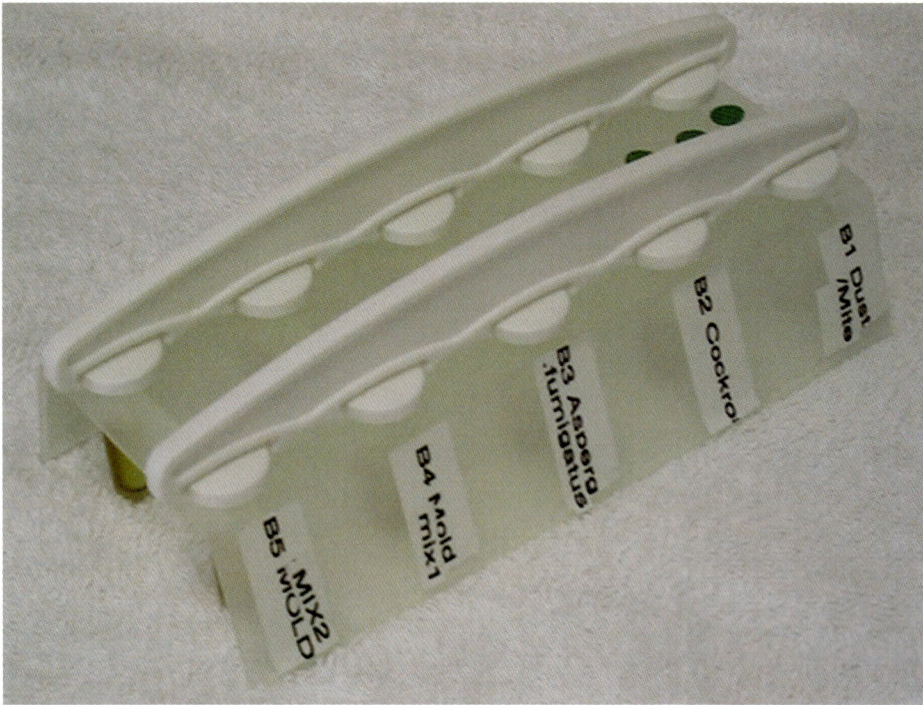

Figure 12-2 Another example of a skin test tray and device from Hollister-Stier Laboratories with prelabeled antigen from a skin test screening panel.

directly on the skin. Furthermore, the depth of the device insertion is also consistent with each skin puncture, minimizing procedural variability from test to test.

j. The size of the wheal (induration) and flare (erythema) at each skin test site is measured in millimeters 15–20 minutes after the skin testing is completed, at the peak of the allergic reaction; the results are then recorded on the skin test sheet (Fig. 12-7). The larger the size of the reaction, the stronger the allergic response. The average diameter (width × length) of each wheal and flare is recorded. If the width is 8mm and the length is 12mm, the recorded measurement is 10mm ($[8 + 12]/2 = 10$). The appearance of pseudopod-like extensions from any wheal generally indicates a stronger allergic response as well (see Table 12-4 for skin test grading.).

2. ***Intradermal (Intracutaneous) Testing***

Intradermal (intracutaneous) testing can be performed when the prick testing results are inconclusive, that is, when suspected allergens are clinically significant but are skin test negative. When the antigen is introduced intracutaneously, the risk of a severe allergic reaction is much greater, and therefore the antigen used must be prepared at 1:1000 wt/vol concentration, and no more than 0.02 mL

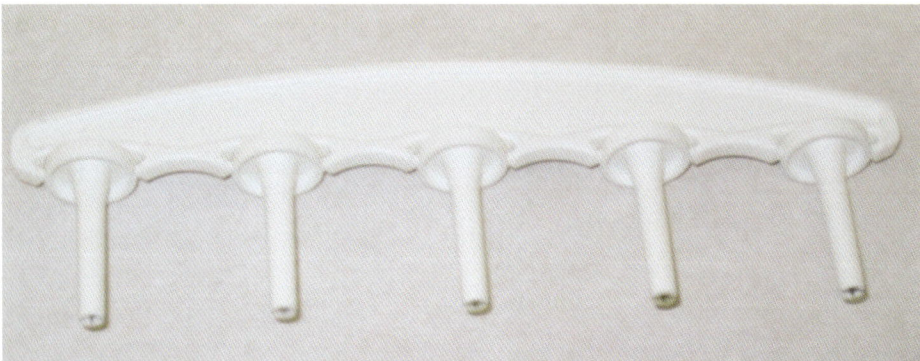

Figure 12-3 Multiple skin test device from Hollister-Stier Laboratories.

BOX 12-1

Sample Consent Form

USC–University Park Health Center

Allergy Testing
Patient Information Sheet

Patient: _____ Social Security #: _____/_____/_____

Address: _____

Date of Birth: _____/_____/_____ Telephone # (Local): _____

Patient Information:

1. Limit your physical activity for the first 4 hours following your allergy testing. After 4 hours, you may resume regular activity.
2. Upon completing your allergy testing, you may resume your regular diet and medication intake.
3. Some local swelling, redness, and itching may persist for 1–2 hours if you have had a positive reaction to your testing. Apply a cold pack intermittently to these areas should this become troublesome.

Remember to:

1. Report any of the following symptoms to the physician or Allergy Clinic Nurse at the University Park Health Center.

   4 to 6 hours after testing you experience an increase in the following at the test site:
   - redness
   - localized heat
   - swelling
   - discomfort

   (note: you may apply a cool compress for relief of these symptoms.)

2. Immediately report any of the following symptoms to emergency medical services:
   - hives
   - difficulty swallowing
   - wheezing
   - feeling faint
   - chest tightness

Call Emergency Medical Services at:

On Campus .... The Department of Public Services

Off Campus .... Los Angeles Emergency Services "911"

I have received and read the Allergy Testing Patient Information Sheet that contains information regarding allergy testing restrictions, possible reactions to the testing, and important telephone numbers to call for questions or immediate assistance.

I have been given the opportunity to ask questions and to have those questions answered to my satisfaction.

Signature: _____ Date: _____/_____/_____

　　　　　　　　　　patient, parent, or legal guardian

Relationship: ☐ Self　　☐ Parent　　☐ Legal Guardian　　☐ Other: _____

Witness: _____ Date: _____/_____/_____

Modified with permission from USC–University Park Health Center.

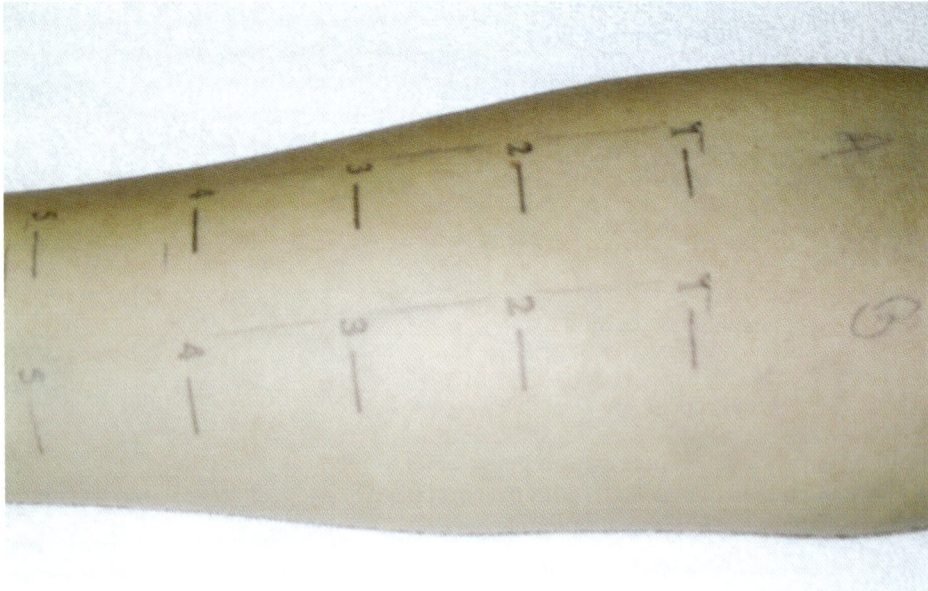

Figure 12-4 Premade ink stamp with numbers corresponding to skin test antigens on the skin test tray.

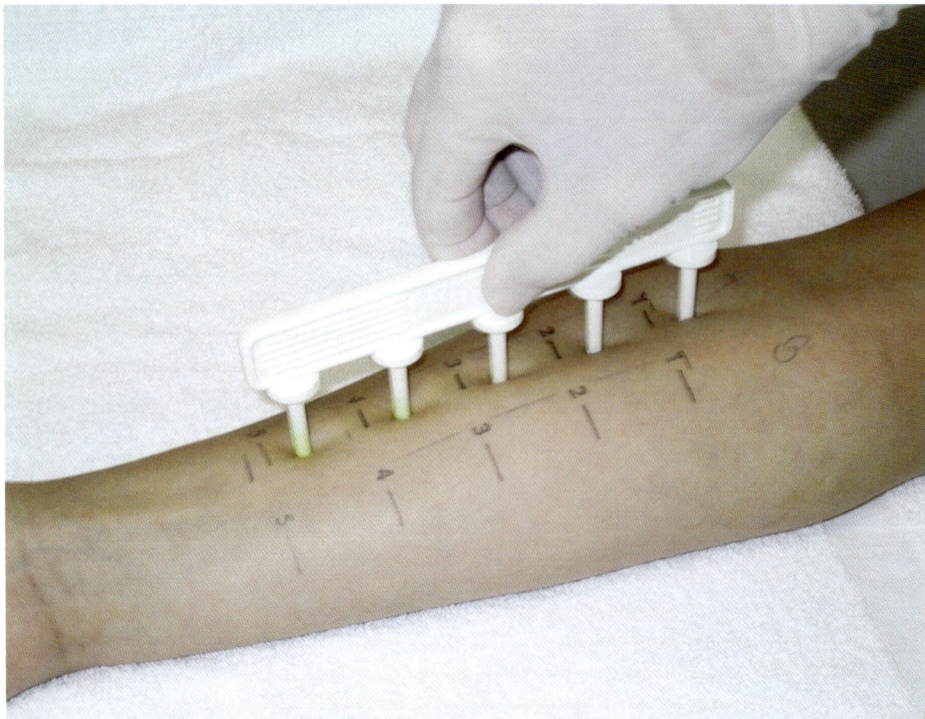

Figure 12-5 Technique for direct placement of antigen on the skin with a multiple skin test device already dipped in antigen vials.

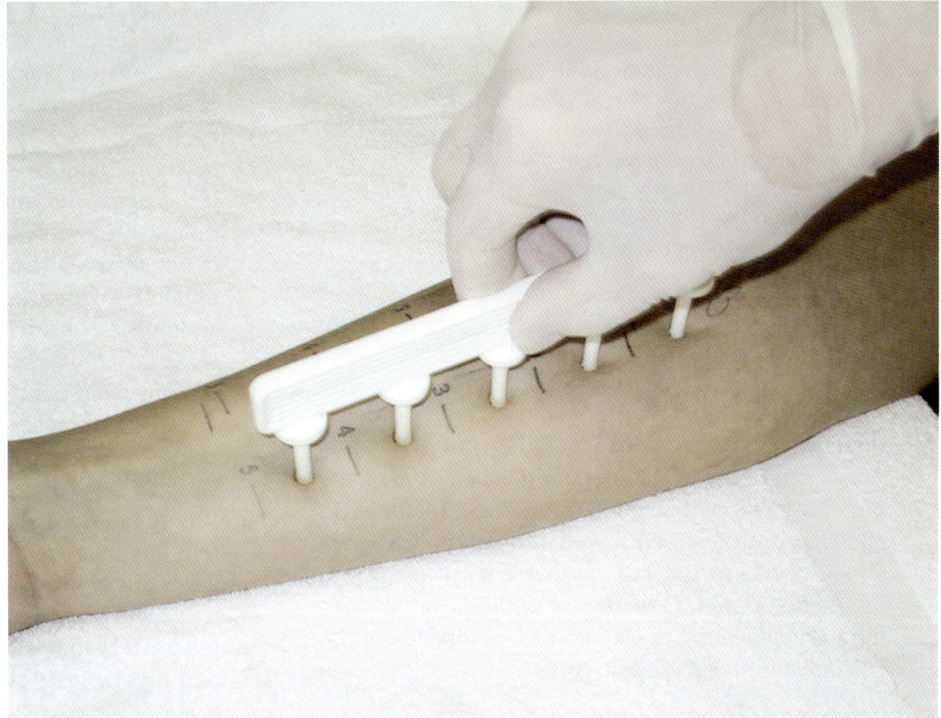

Figure 12-6 Direct placement of antigen on the skin with the second multiple skin test device from the skin test tray.

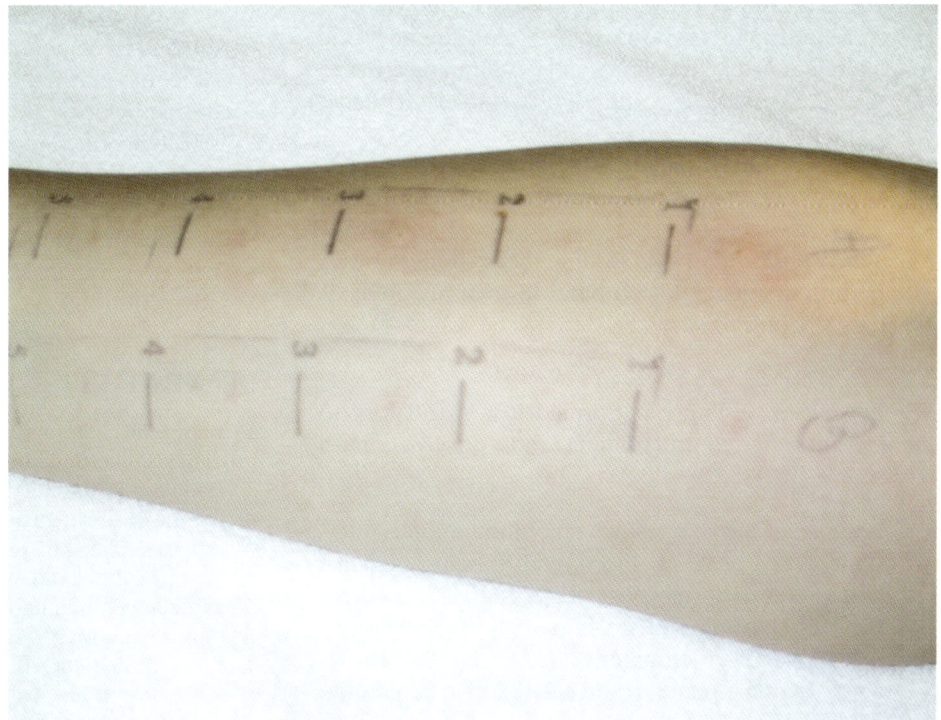

Figure 12-7 Note wheal-and-flare reaction to A1: histamine (4+), A3: grass mix (2+) antigens, and A2: (0) negative control (see Table 12-4 for skin test grading).

TABLE 12-4	
Skin Test Grading	
0	All reactions equal to negative control
+	Erythema (flare) and 2-mm wheal (induration)
++	Erythema and 4-mm wheal without pseudopods (pseudopod-like extension of induration)
+++	Erythema, >5-mm wheal with or without pseudopods
++++	Erythema, >10-mm wheal with or without pseudopods

should be injected. These preparations can be ordered directly from different manufacturers (see Appendix 3, Allergic Extract Manufacturers). Because of the increased risk to patients and increased liability to clinicians, professionals well trained in this area should perform the intradermal tests. It is recommended and preferable to rely on RAST rather than intradermal testing to clarify any discrepancy in the prick testing results.

C. Important Rules of Allergy Skin Testing

1. Do not perform intradermal skin testing unless properly trained.
2. Never perform intradermal skin tests with any allergen unless previous prick tests to same allergen were negative. A positive prick test to any one allergen is a major and absolute contraindication to the performance of an intradermal skin test with that same allergen.
3. Prick tests are usually graded after 15–20 minutes. In cases of dermagraphism (hyperirritable skin) allow 25–30 minutes.
4. When performing skin testing, there should always be an emergency kit on hand to treat anaphylaxis (see Chapter 6).

D. Interpretation of Skin Test Results[1]

Whenever skin tests are performed it is mandatory to include a negative control (diluent) and a positive control (histamine).

1. The size of the skin test wheal or induration is interpreted on a scale of 0 to 4, with 0 being negative and 4+ being strongly positive. A result of 1+ is equivocal, and a result of 2+ to 4+ is significantly positive (see Table 12-4 for grading scale). Figure 12-7 shows a 4+ histamine reaction and a 2+ allergic reaction to grasses.

2. The wheal and flare can also be recorded in millimeters.
3. All results should be compared to the negative and positive control skin test reaction to develop a point of reference and assess the allergic response with each patient. Figure 12-7 shows a 4+ histamine reaction and a 0+ negative response.
4. If the negative control develops a positive reaction, then the allergen results may be invalid due to dermagraphism. When dermagraphism occurs, it is more difficult to interpret the results, and RAST testing should be considered.
5. If the histamine control is negative, the test results are probably being inhibited by the prior ingestion of antihistamines, and testing should be rescheduled once the patient has refrained from all antihistamine-like product for at least 5–7 days.
6. When it is difficult to visually interpret the reaction (e.g., hyperpigmented skin), it is helpful to palpate the induration to assess the degree of allergic reactivity. Additionally, shining a flashlight on the test field can help create shadows on the indurated skin and highlight subtle allergic reactions.

E. Special Considerations in Patient Subsets

Evaluation of the Oral Allergy Syndrome

Occasionally, patients with oral allergy syndrome will not exhibit positive reactivity on either skin testing or RAST testing despite an obvious history of oral allergic hypersensitivity. In these patients, it is possible to confirm the allergic reactivity by performing the prick-prick test.[4] This test involves applying a sterile needle directly to the suspected food product and then immediately pricking the patient's skin directly with the same needle. The results of this test are interpreted much like ordinary skin testing (i.e., need to compare skin test results to positive and negative controls).

REFERENCES

1. Bernstein L, Storms WW: Practice parameters for allergy diagnostic testing. Ann Allergy 1995;75:553–625.
2. Hamilton RG, Adkinson NF Jr: Clinical laboratory methods for the assessment and management of human allergic diseases. Clin Lab Med 1986;6:117–138.
3. Ownby DR, Adinoff AD: The appropriate use of skin testing and allergen immunotherapy in young children. J Allergy Clin Immunol 1994;94:662–665.
4. Frieri M, Kettelhut B: Food Hypersensitivity and Adverse Reactions: A Practical Guide for Diagnosis and Management. New York: Marcel Dekker, 1998.

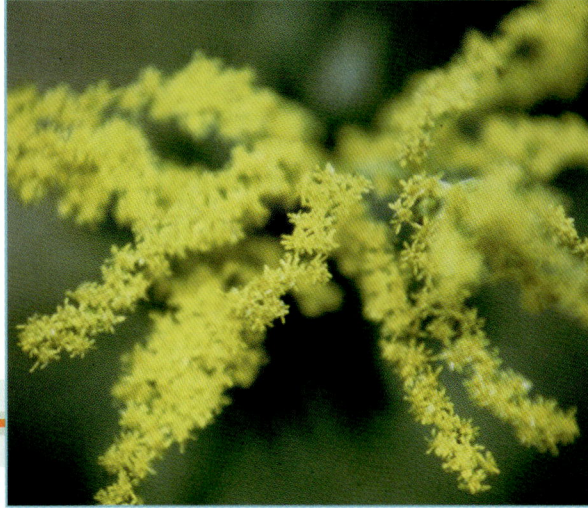

CHAPTER 13
Radioallergosorbent Testing (RAST)

Etan C. Milgrom and William W. Storms

I. Introduction

Many in vitro radioallergosorbent tests, or RAST, have been developed over the past 30 years to help identify IgE-mediated disease. All RAST tests are based on the same principles. The patient's serum, containing allergen-specific IgE immunoglobulin, is allowed to interact with allergen that is bound to a solid phase. The specific IgE that binds to the allergen is detected and quantified by adding labeled anti-IgE antibody to the solid phase (Fig. 13-1).[1] The labeled anti-IgE antibody is measured either by a gamma counter (radioactive anti-IgE, phadebas RAST, or modified RAST), or by colorimetry or fluorometry (enzyme-labeled anti-IgE antibody), or by monoclonal and polyclonal anti-IgE antibodies.

For most diagnostic evaluations, in vitro testing is considered a second choice to skin testing. The average sensitivity of an in vitro test as compared to a prick test is about 75%, and therefore skin tests are preferred to in vitro tests.[1] RAST can be a helpful adjunct in evaluating allergic disorders, especially in patients with severe atopic dermatitis who have no disease-free skin available on which to perform skin tests and in patients who exhibit significant dermagraphism during skin testing (see Table 12-2, which compares skin testing and RAST). In vitro testing may also be preferable to skin testing in patients who cannot refrain from taking antihistamines (required to perform skin testing), in uncooperative patients with mental or physical impairments, and when the clinical history suggests a greater risk of anaphylaxis from skin testing.

It should be noted that measurement of total serum IgE is of modest clinical value (see Appendix 4, Total Serum IgE by Age, for data on IgE levels). The total serum IgE of allergic patients can be elevated but is not pathognomonic. Total serum IgE is not a good predictor of allergic disease unless it is strongly positive. Furthermore a normal total serum IgE does not rule out atopy. Total serum IgE is more significant in the evaluation of patients with suspected allergic bronchopulmonary aspergillosis, congenital immunodeficiencies, hyper-IgE syndrome, parasitosis, and other uncommon diseases.[2]

II. Interpretation of RAST Test Results

A. Meaningful Interpretation

Interpretation of in vitro RAST tests is similar to interpretation of skin tests in that a positive result is not necessarily diagnostic. A positive test should always

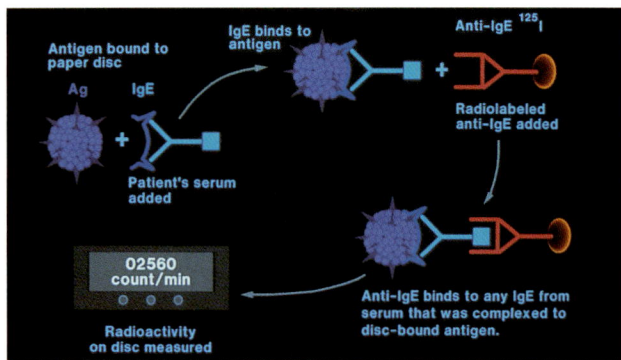

Figure 13-1 RAST for IgE. (Reprinted with permission from the American Academy of Allergy, Asthma and Immunology.)

be correlated with the patient's history. As with any laboratory value, the clinician should use the normal reference ranges provided by the laboratory to determine abnormal results.

B. Specifying the Test

The practitioner should also make sure that the IgE allergen-specific antibody test is performed, not an IgG antibody test. The IgG antibody does not correlate with clinical disease, even though it is available for testing in different laboratories (see Chapter 21).[3]

C. Use of Individual Allergens

It is important that the in vitro IgE antibody tests be performed to individual allergens rather than to mixtures.

REFERENCES

1. Bernstein L, Storms WW: Practice parameters for allergy diagnostic testing. Ann Allergy 1995;75:553–625.
2. VanArsdel PP Jr, Larson EB: Diagnostic tests for patients with suspected allergic disease: Utility and limitations. Ann Intern Med 1989;110:304–312.
3. American Academy of Allergy and Immunology: Measurement of specific and nonspecific IgG4 levels as diagnostic and prognostic tests for clinical allergy. Position statement. J Allergy Clin Immunol 1995;94:652–654.

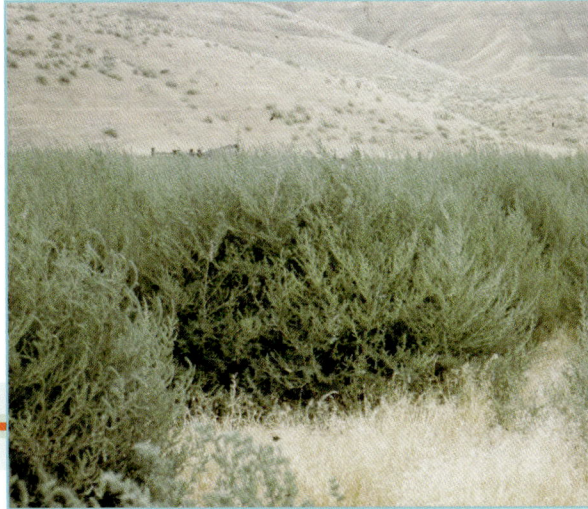

Kochia Courtesy of Hollister-Stier Laboratory

CHAPTER 14
Nasal and Conjunctival Smears
Etan C. Milgrom

I. Introduction

The laboratory workup of the allergic patient is not that helpful (see Chapter 21). The IgE level is elevated in only one-third of allergic patients. Peripheral eosinophilia is more diagnostic in parasitic diseases. Nasal and conjunctival smears,[1] if performed properly, can be of assistance in the diagnosis of allergic disease, although in today's cost-saving health care environment, ordering this procedure may not be fiscally prudent.

Eosinophils are the typical cells found in allergic reactions, especially in the submucosa of the nasal passageway and conjunctivae in allergic rhinitis and conjunctivitis. The purpose of the nasal and conjunctival smear is to identify the degree of eosinophilia infiltration within nasal and ophthalmologic secretions.

II. Method

A. Specimen Collection

Instruct the patient to blow his or her nose into a piece of sterile gauze, or place a cotton-tipped applicator into the anterior nasal cavity for a couple of minutes. The cotton-tipped applicator can be placed, for a second, in the submucosa of the lower lid for the eye smear.

B. Smear and Stain

Smear the mucus onto a microscope slide with the cotton-tipped applicator.

1. ***Staining the Smear with Hansel's Stain***
   a. Cover the slide with methyl alcohol and allow to air dry.
   b. Submerge the slide in Hansel's stain for 30 seconds.
   c. Add five drops of distilled water to the slide and let stand for 30 seconds.
   d. Pour off the stain and rinse with distilled water.
   e. Rinse and decolorize the slide with methyl alcohol until the stained material appears pale green.
   f. Air dry.
2. ***Staining the Smear with Wright's Stain*** (Fig. 14-1)[2]
   a. Cover the slide with methyl alcohol and allow to air dry.
   b. Submerge the slide in Wright's stain for 2–3 minutes.
   c. Rinse and decolorize the slide with methyl alcohol for 1 minute.
   d. Restain with 1% methylene blue for 1 minute.
   e. Rinse with distilled water.
   f. Air dry and examine.

181

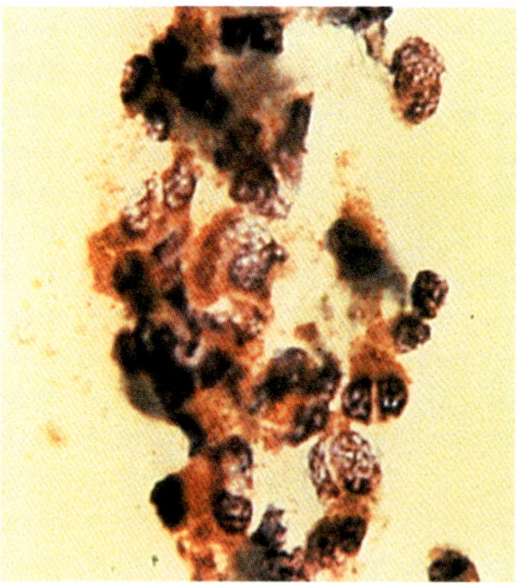

Figure 14-1 Procedure for nasal smear: (1) Patient blows nose into plastic wrap; (2) smear specimen on slide; (3) stain with Wright's stain; (4) decolorize with methanol; (5) restain with 1% methylene blue (1 minute); and (6) rinse, air dry, and examine. ≥25% eosinophils = nasal smear eosinophilia. (Adapted from Mullarkey MF, Hill JS, Webb DR: Allergic and nonallergic rhinitis: their characterization with attention to the meaning of nasal eosinophilia. J Allergy Clin Immunol 1980;45(2):122–126, with permission.)

3. ***Interpreting the Results***
   a. Examine under a high power lens and oil immersion (1000×).

b. Interpretation of the smear can be attained by quantitating an eosinophil to neutrophil ratio (E/N).

c. An E/N ratio greater than 1 is suggestive of allergic disease. Allergic disease is also suspected if there are 25% or more eosinophils. (Rarely, these findings may be consistent with nonallergic rhinits with eosinophilia syndrome, or NARES. See Chapter 1, Allergic Rhinitis, for further explanation.)

d. An E/N ratio of less than 1 may indicate infectious rhinitis or sinusitis.

e. Nasal smears lacking both eosinophils and neutrophils suggest vasomotor rhinitis (see Chapter 1 for more information on this topic).

REFERENCES

1. Meltzer ED, Jalowayski AP: Nasal cytology in clinical practice. Am J Rhinol 1988;2.
2. Mullarkey MF, Hill JS, Webb DR: Allergic and nonallergic rhinitis: their characterization with attention to the meaning of nasal eosinophilia. J Allergy Clin Immunol 1980;45(2): 122–126.

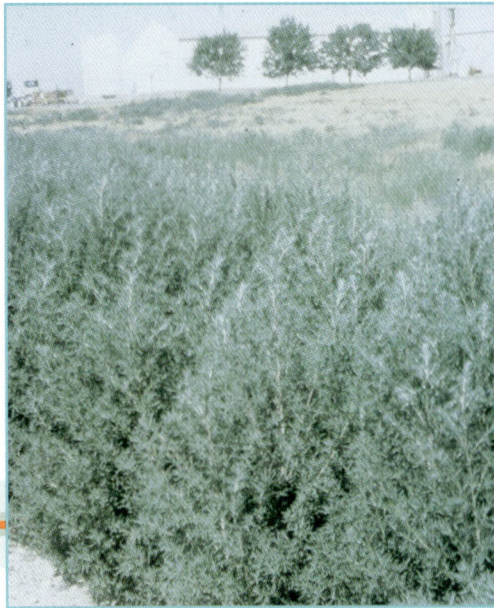

CHAPTER 15
Inhalers and Spacers

Ricardo A. Tan and Etan C. Milgrom

I. Inhalers

A. Metered-Dose Inhalers

With the advent of metered-dose inhalers (MDI) to administer β-agonists, cromolyn, ipatropium, and corticosteroids, a delivery system became available that allowed direct deposition of medication into the lungs, avoiding significant systemic side effects, in particular with oral steroids. Other devices have since been developed (such as dry-powder inhalers and breath-actuated inhalers), all of which require a particular skill that needs to be mastered in order to maximize the effectiveness of the medication that is delivered by the device (Fig. 15-1).

1. The MDI system allows only 10%–15% of the inhaled medication to reach the airway. Therefore, perfecting the MDI technique is vital to maximizing therapy:
   a. Remove the cap and hold the inhaler upright.
   b. Shake the inhaler to mix the medication with the propellant.
   c. Tilt the head back slightly to open and straighten the oral airway.
   d. Exhale a normal breath of air, not a forced one (to avoid airway constriction).
   e. Position the MDI 2–3 inches away from the open mouth. Distancing the inhaler from the mouth will promote aerosolization of the medication and enhance respiratory deposition. The use of spacers (see next section) serves the same function. The MDI may also be positioned inside the mouth to help with coordination, if needed.
   f. Take a deep slow breath and in less than 1 second press down on the canister to release the medication, while continuing to breath in.
   g. Breathe in slowly and deeply for 3–5 seconds.
   h. Hold your breath for 10 seconds to allow the medicine to reach the alveoli.
   i. Wait 1 minute between puffs (as prescribed) and repeat the preceding technique.
2. As with most skills, use of the MDI needs to be taught very carefully by health care professionals and must be mastered by patients before a maximal therapeutic response can be attained. There are several recurring faulty MDI techniques that need to be avoided:
   a. Not continuing to inhale after actuation of the inhaler.
   b. Not holding the breath for 10 seconds after actuation of the MDI.
   c. Poor hand-to-mouth coordination.

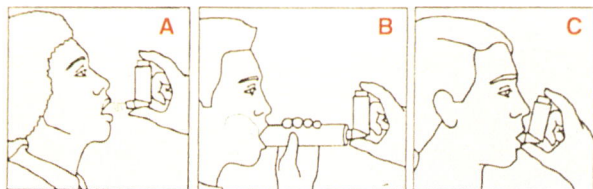

Figure 15-1 Steps for using the metered-dose inhaler: (1) Remove the cap and hold the inhaler upright; (2) shake the inhaler; (3) tilt your head back slightly and breathe out; (4) position the inhaler in one of ways shown in **A**–**C** (**A** and **B** are optimal but **C** is acceptable for those who have difficulty with **A** or **B**.); (5) press down on the inhaler to release medication as you start to breathe in slowly; (6) breathe in slowly (3–5 seconds); (7) *hold* breath for 10 seconds to allow medicine to reach deeply into lungs; (8) repeat puffs as directed (Waiting 1 minute between puffs may permit second puff to penetrate the lungs better.); and (9) spacers are useful for all patients. (They are particularly recommended for young children and older adults and for use with inhaled steroids.) *Note:* Inhaled dry powder capsules require a different inhalation technique. To use a dry powder inhaler, it is important to close the mouth tightly around the mouthpiece of the inhaler and inhale rapidly.

    d. Actuation of the MDI at the end of inhalation.
    e. Inability or failure to remove the cap from the MDI.
    f. Using an empty canister (see later discussion).
3. Gauging the remaining medication in an MDI (Fig. 15-2): Actuating the canister will continue to produce propellant material even when it is void of medication. This can give patients a false impression that the inhaler is still full. To determine how much medication remains in the inhaler, the patient should follow these steps:
    a. Place the medication canister in a small container of tepid water.
    b. An empty canister will float on top of the water. A full canister will sink to the bottom. A partially full canister will float somewhere at mid-depth. The emptier the canister, the higher it will ride in the water.

Note: Nedocromil sodium is chemically distinct from other aerosol asthma medications and should not be measured with the flotation test just described. Nedocromil sodium should be measured by tracking the number of actuations.

B. Rotahaler Inhalation Device

The rotahaler inhalation device is an inhalation system that uses inhaled dry powder capsules. This device is advantageous in that the inhaler can be placed directly in the mouth and does not require aerosolization. The powder has, however, been reported to cause airway irritation in some patients. This system requires completely different administration skills to maximize deposition of the prescribed medication.

1. Insert the capsule into the rotahaler as directed by the manufacturer.
2. Rotate the rotahaler as directed by the manufacturer to open the capsule.
3. Exhale a normal breath of air, not a forced one (to avoid airway constriction).
4. Close the mouth tightly around the mouthpiece of the inhaler and breathe in through the mouth as quickly and deeply as possible.
5. Hold the breath briefly, then remove the rotahaler from mouth and exhale.
6. Repeat the preceding steps after 1 minute as directed by the clinician.
7. Clean the rotahaler as recommended by the manufacturer.

C. Diskus Inhaler

The diskus inhaler is another powder inhalation device manufactured by GlaxoWellcome for the inhalation of fluticasone and salmeterol (Fig. 15-3). Like the rotahaler, this device can be placed directly in the mouth, obviating use of a spacer, and does not require aerosolization. It also has a built-in dose indicator to keep track of remaining doses.

1. Hold the diskus in one hand and place the thumb of the other hand on the marked thumb grip on the diskus.
2. Push the thumb away until the mouthpiece appears and snaps into position.
3. Hold the diskus horizontally and slide the lever away, toward the thumb grip, until it clicks into place.
4. Exhale a normal breath of air, not a forced one (to avoid airway constriction).
5. Place the mouthpiece directly between the lips and breathe in steadily and deeply through the diskus.
6. Remove the diskus from mouth and hold breath for 10 seconds.

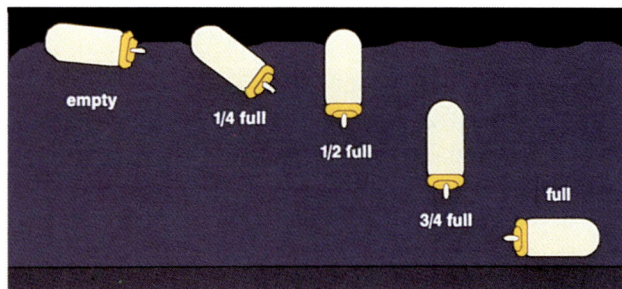

Figure 15-2 How to gauge the remaining medication in an MDI: Drop the canister into a pan of water. The position in the water will indicate how much medication is left.

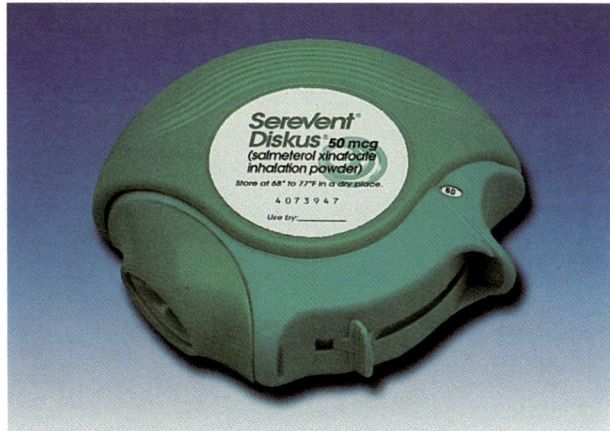

Figure 15-3 Diskus inhaler.

7. Repeat the preceding steps in 1 minute as directed by clinician.
8. To close the diskus, place thumb on the thumb grip and slide it back to its original position until it clicks shut.

II. Spacers

A. Mechanism of Action

Spacers are devices consisting of a hollow tube, with or without a valve, that is attached to the mouthpiece of an MDI. A spacer is used to improve penetration of the inhaled medication into the lungs and to decrease the incidence of side effects (such as oral thrush from inhaled steroids). Extending the distance from the MDI to the mouth decreases particle velocity and allows more evaporation of the propellant. Although spacers are most helpful for patients who have difficulty coordinating their inhalation with pressing down on the MDI, they are also beneficial for the majority of asthmatics. New delivery devices such as dry-powder inhalers and breath-actuated inhalers do not necessitate spacers.

B. Spacer Devices

Spacers with valves block exhaled air from reentering the spacer and increasing the humidity in the chamber. Spacers are available in a wide variety of shapes and sizes. The most commonly used devices include tube spacers such as the Aerochamber (Fig. 15-4), the Optihaler (Figs. 15-5 and 15-6), and the Nebuhaler, as well as collapsible chambers such as the InspirEase device (Fig. 15-7). Even makeshift plastic bottles and cardboard tubes (even toilet paper rolls!) have been used in developing countries, with proven efficacy. In a comparative study of different spacers, the larger the volume of the spacer (>750 mL), the greater the clinical improvement, presumably owing to better delivery of medication.[1] Volume, rather than shape or presence of valves, appears to be the primary factor determining the efficacy of the device.

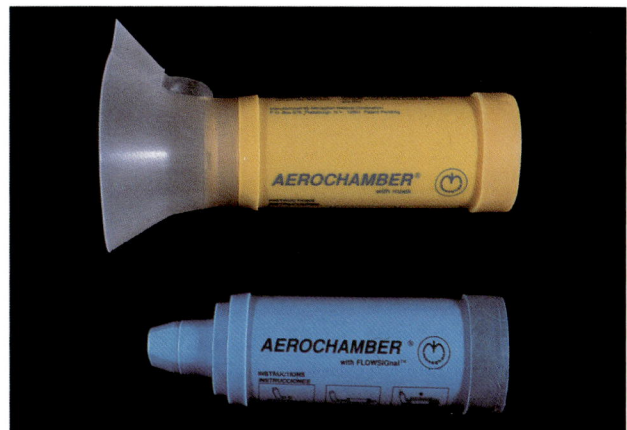

Figure 15-4 The Aerochamber (tube spacer attaches to an MDI).

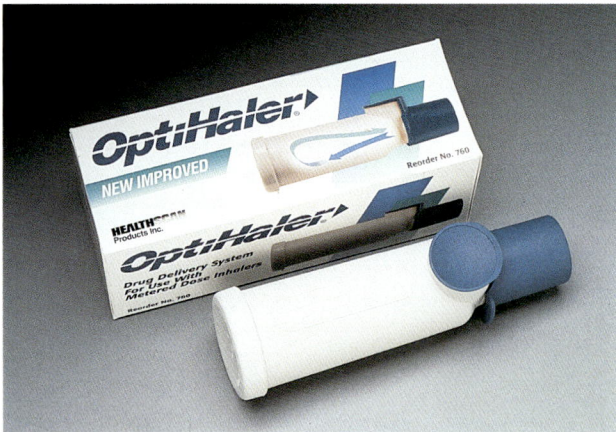

Figure 15-5 The Optihaler (tube spacer attaches to an MDI). (Reprinted with permission from Respironics, Inc. and its affiliates. Respironics, Asthma, and Allergy Products, Cedar Grove, NJ).

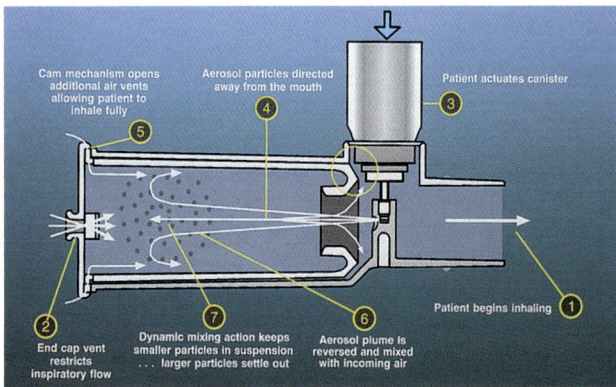

Figure 15-6 How the Optihaler works. (Reprinted with permission from Respironics, Inc. and its affiliates. Respironics, Asthma, and Allergy Products, Cedar Grove, NJ).

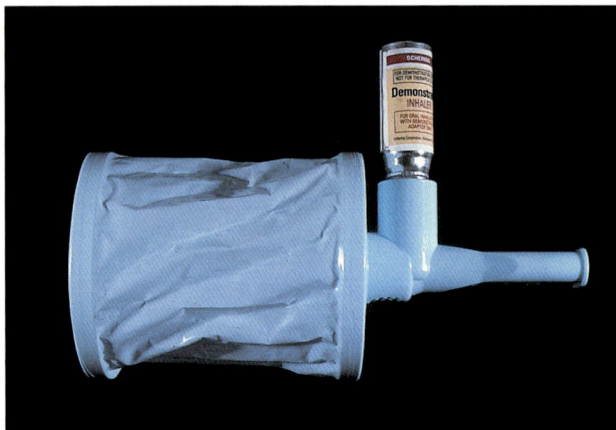

Figure 15-7 The InspirEase collapsible chamber device shown with attached canister.

C. Tips for Use of Spacer Devices

1. Actuate only one puff of medication at a time into the spacer.
2. Take a deep, slow breath after the medication is introduced into spacer. It is not necessary to actuate the MDI and inhale at the same instant.
3. Do not wait more than 2 seconds before inhaling from the spacer.
4. Hold your breath for about 10 seconds after inhaling.

REFERENCE

1. Lee H, Evans HE: Evaluation of inhalation aids of metered dose inhalers in asthmatic children. Chest 1987;91:366–369.

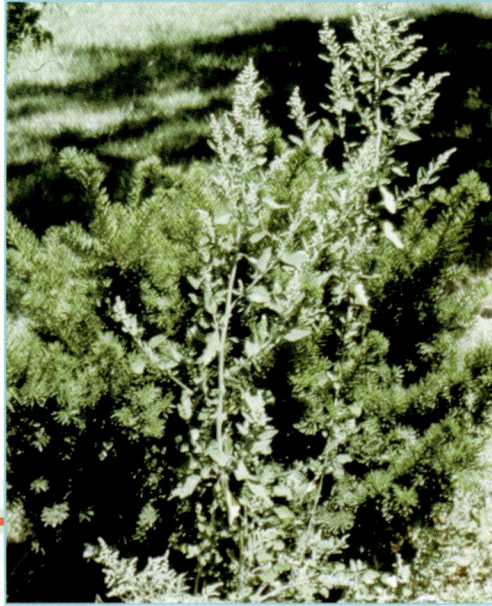

Lambs Quarter *Courtesy of Hollister-Stier Laboratory*

CHAPTER 16
Pulmonary Function Testing

Sheldon L. Spector and Ricardo A. Tan

I. Spirometry

A. Technique

Full computerized spirometry should be performed in all asthmatics to obtain the most accurate picture of lung function. The proper technique is crucial in obtaining reliable results. A skilled technician should be able to demonstrate the proper technique and guide the subject in taking a full inspiration and making a forceful and prolonged exhalation. The subject should exhale for at least 6 seconds. The maneuver should be performed at least three times, and the highest value utilized for clinical correlation. Spirometry may be performed with the subject sitting or standing, but consistency is important.[1]

B. FEV$_1$ (Forced Expiratory Volume in 1 Second)

1. The diagnosis of asthma can be confirmed by demonstrating an increase in FEV$_1$ of 12% or more from baseline after an inhaled β_2-agonist treatment. The American Thoracic Society designates a 12% increase from baseline FEV$_1$ and an absolute change of 200 mL as a positive bronchodilator response.[2] The American College of Chest Physicians considers an at least 15% increase from baseline FEV$_1$ after bronchodilator treatment to be significant.[3]

2. FEV$_1$ reflects the volume expired in the first second of forced vital capacity (FVC), expressed in liters, and is the most widely used measure of airflow for the diagnosis of asthma. FEV$_1$ is largely effort dependent and requires a full, forceful effort from the subject to truly reflect airflow limitation. The effort-dependent portion of the FVC reflects the state of the large airways, the contraction of the expiratory muscles, and the elastic recoil of the lungs.[4]

3. FEV$_1$ correlates with peak flow volume measurements.

4. FEV$_1$ is important in assessing the severity of an acute exacerbation as well as in classifying severity for the purpose of managing chronic asthma with a stepwise approach.

C. Vital Capacity and Forced Vital Capacity

Vital capacity (VC) is the maximum amount of air that can be exhaled after maximum inspiration. It is also commonly referred to as the "slow" vital capacity, to distinguish it from FVC, which is the maximum amount of air exhaled after a forceful expiration. FVC is felt to be more reflective of airflow limitation. Both VC and FVC are expressed in liters. FEV_1, $FEF_{25\%-75\%}$, and PEFR are all derived from FVC.

D. FEV_1/FVC Ratio

The ratio of FEV_1 to FVC can assist in classifying lung disease as obstructive or restrictive. In obstructive disease, airflow limitation causes a diminished FEV_1 while FVC may remain normal, causing a lowered FEV_1/FVC ratio. In restrictive disease, the FVC is diminished due to poor lung expansion. FEV_1 is usually proportionally decreased, leading to a normal or elevated FEV_1/FVC ratio. Although this ratio is helpful, the most reliable indicator of restrictive problems is *total lung capacity* (TLC).

Care must be taken in interpreting ratios when there is a poor expiratory effort. The ratio of a truly low FEV_1 and a low FVC from a suboptimal effort could be falsely normal in a patient with airway obstruction. The FEV_1/FVC ratio should also be interpreted in light of the individual FEV_1 and FVC results. Healthy athletes can sometimes have normal or elevated FEV_1 and a low FEV_1/FVC ratio.[2]

E. $FEF_{25\%-75\%}$ (Forced Expiratory Flow Rate in 25%–75% of Expired Volume)

$FEF_{25\%-75\%}$, also known as the maximum midexpiratory flow rate (MMFR), reflects the average flow rate in the middle portion, or 25% to 75%, of the volume expired and is expressed in liters per second. It is mostly effort independent and has been widely used to reflect the state of the smaller airways. It is not as reproducible or as sensitive as FEV_1. Since $FEF_{25\%-75\%}$ is calculated from the slope of the midportion of the volume-time curve of FVC, a shortened expiration in severe airway obstruction may actually cause $FEF_{25\%-75\%}$ to be falsely elevated.[4]

F. MVV (Maximal Voluntary Ventilation)

Maximal voluntary ventilation (MVV) is the maximum amount of air that can be moved voluntarily in 1 minute. It is very effort dependent and is measured by having the subject breathe rapidly and fully for about 30 seconds. The maximum volume moved over any 15 seconds is expressed in liters per minute. MVV is useful in evaluating preoperative lung function, weaning from mechanical ventilation, evaluating respiratory muscle function, and assessing exercise tolerance.

G. Flow-Volume Curves

1. The flow-volume curve or loop is a recording of the relationship between flow and volume during maximum expiration followed by maximum inspiration. It is very helpful in diagnosing or evaluating conditions such as asthma or upper airway obstruc-
tion, which display characteristic patterns in the flow-volume loop. The first part of the expiratory curve is effort dependent and depends largely on the pressure exerted by the expiratory muscles and the elastic recoil of the lung. The downward-sloping part of the curve is largely effort independent and is determined mainly by the elastic recoil of the lung and upstream resistance such as from bronchoconstriction, making it a more significant reflection of airflow limitation. The inspiratory part of the loop is more sensitive to central airway obstruction.

2. The characteristic pattern in asthma will show an increased concavity in the downward curve of the expiratory part of the flow-volume loop. This is also seen in emphysema.

3. Extrathoracic airway obstruction, such as vocal cord dysfunction, produces a recognizable pattern that helps identify patients misdiagnosed as having asthma. The inspiratory loop will have a characteristic flattened appearance that is due to the collapse of the upper airway during inhalation from negative pressure inside the airway.

II. Lung Volumes

Measurement of lung volumes provides important information for evaluating lung function in patients with complicated conditions such as mixed obstructive and restrictive disease. Tidal volume (VT), vital capacity (VC), expiratory reserve volume (ERV), and inspiratory capacity (IC) can be measured by spirometry. Residual volume (RV) and functional residual capacity (FRC) can be measured indirectly only with more complicated procedures, such as body plethysmography or gas dilution techniques such as helium dilution and nitrogen washout. These procedures are usually available only in research and hospital-based facilities. VC is the maximum amount that can be exhaled after maximum inspiration. VT is the amount inhaled and exhaled during quiet breathing. RV is the amount of air remaining in the lung after the end of maximum expiration, and FRC is the amount of air remaining after normal expiration. Both FRC and RV are increased in asthma. ERV is the additional amount that can be expelled after a normal expiration. IC is the maximum amount of air that can be inspired after normal expiration. Total lung capacity (TLC) is the sum of RV and VC. VC can also be computed as the sum of IC and ERV. Several sets of predicted values for TLC and RV have been derived from different studies, but only the Crapo study, based on studies of nonsmoking adults, conforms to the American Thoracic Society's standards for spirometry.[5]

TABLE 16-1

FEV₁ Predicted Normal Values for Males 18–50 Years Old

Age (years)	Height (inches)															
	54	55	56	57	58	59	60	61	62	63	64	65	66	67	68	69
18	3.05	3.15	3.26	3.36	3.47	3.58	3.68	3.79	3.89	4.00	4.10	4.21	4.31	4.42	4.52	4.63
19	3.02	3.13	3.24	3.34	3.45	3.55	3.66	3.76	3.87	3.97	4.08	4.18	4.29	4.39	4.50	4.60
20	3.00	3.11	3.21	3.32	3.42	3.53	3.63	3.74	3.84	3.95	4.05	4.16	4.26	4.37	4.47	4.58
21	2.98	3.08	3.19	3.29	3.40	3.50	3.61	3.71	3.82	3.92	4.03	4.13	4.24	4.34	4.45	4.55
22	2.95	3.06	3.16	3.27	3.37	3.48	3.58	3.69	3.79	3.90	4.00	4.11	4.21	4.32	4.42	4.53
23	2.93	3.03	3.14	3.24	3.35	3.45	3.56	3.66	3.77	3.87	3.98	4.08	4.19	4.29	4.40	4.50
24	2.90	3.01	3.11	3.22	3.32	3.43	3.53	3.64	3.74	3.85	3.95	4.06	4.16	4.27	4.38	4.48
25	2.88	2.98	3.09	3.19	3.30	3.40	3.51	3.61	3.72	3.82	3.93	4.04	4.14	4.25	4.35	4.46
26	2.85	2.96	3.06	3.17	3.27	3.38	3.48	3.59	3.70	3.80	3.91	4.01	4.12	4.22	4.33	4.43
27	2.83	2.93	3.04	3.15	3.25	3.36	3.46	3.57	3.67	3.78	3.88	3.99	4.09	4.20	4.30	4.41
28	2.81	2.91	3.02	3.12	3.23	3.33	3.44	3.54	3.65	3.75	3.86	3.96	4.07	4.17	4.28	4.38
29	2.78	2.89	2.99	3.10	3.20	3.31	3.41	3.52	3.62	3.73	3.83	3.94	4.04	4.15	4.25	4.36
30	2.76	2.86	2.97	3.07	3.18	3.28	3.39	3.49	3.60	3.70	3.81	3.91	4.02	4.12	4.23	4.33
31	2.73	2.84	2.94	3.05	3.15	3.26	3.36	3.47	3.57	3.68	3.78	3.89	3.99	4.10	4.20	4.31
32	2.71	2.81	2.92	3.02	3.13	3.23	3.34	3.44	3.55	3.65	3.76	3.86	3.97	4.07	4.18	4.28
33	2.68	2.79	2.89	3.00	3.10	3.21	3.31	3.42	3.52	3.63	3.73	3.84	3.95	4.05	4.16	4.26
34	2.66	2.76	2.87	2.97	3.08	3.18	3.29	3.39	3.50	3.61	3.71	3.82	3.92	4.03	4.13	4.24
35	2.63	2.74	2.84	2.95	3.06	3.16	3.27	3.37	3.48	3.58	3.69	3.79	3.90	4.00	4.11	4.21
36	2.61	2.72	2.82	2.93	3.03	3.14	3.24	3.35	3.45	3.56	3.66	3.77	3.87	3.98	4.08	4.19
37	2.59	2.69	2.80	2.90	3.01	3.11	3.22	3.32	3.43	3.53	3.64	3.74	3.85	3.95	4.06	4.16
38	2.56	2.67	2.77	2.88	2.98	3.09	3.19	3.30	3.40	3.51	3.61	3.72	3.82	3.93	4.03	4.14
39	2.54	2.64	2.75	2.85	2.96	3.06	3.17	3.27	3.38	3.48	3.59	3.69	3.80	3.90	4.01	4.11
40	2.51	2.62	2.72	2.83	2.93	3.04	3.14	3.25	3.35	3.46	3.56	3.67	3.77	3.88	3.98	4.09
41	2.49	2.59	2.70	2.80	2.91	3.01	3.12	3.22	3.33	3.43	3.54	3.64	3.75	3.86	3.96	4.07
42	2.46	2.57	2.67	2.78	2.88	2.99	3.09	3.20	3.30	3.41	3.52	3.62	3.73	3.83	3.94	4.04
43	2.44	2.54	2.65	2.75	2.86	2.97	3.07	3.18	3.28	3.39	3.49	3.60	3.70	3.81	3.91	4.02
44	2.41	2.52	2.63	2.73	2.84	2.94	3.05	3.15	3.26	3.36	3.47	3.57	3.66	3.78	3.89	3.99
45	2.39	2.50	2.60	2.71	2.81	2.92	3.02	3.13	3.23	3.34	3.44	3.55	3.65	3.76	3.86	3.97
46	2.37	2.47	2.58	2.68	2.79	2.89	3.00	3.10	3.21	3.31	3.42	3.52	3.63	3.73	3.84	3.94
47	2.34	2.45	2.55	2.66	2.76	2.87	2.97	3.08	3.18	3.29	3.39	3.50	3.60	3.71	3.81	3.92
48	2.32	2.42	2.53	2.63	2.74	2.84	2.95	3.05	3.16	3.26	3.37	3.47	3.58	3.68	3.79	3.89
49	2.29	2.40	2.50	2.61	2.71	2.82	2.92	3.03	3.13	3.24	3.34	3.45	3.55	3.66	3.77	3.87
50	2.27	2.37	2.48	2.58	2.69	2.79	2.90	3.00	3.11	3.21	3.32	3.43	3.53	3.64	3.74	3.85

From Crapo RO, Morris AH, Gardner RM: Reference spirometric values using techniques and equipment that meet ATS recommendations. Am Rev Respir Dis 1981;123:659–664. Reproduced with permission.

III. Reference Values

A. Numerous studies have been done to determine reference values for spirometry and pulmonary function testing. However, there is no one set of values that can be universally applied to all populations. The American Thoracic Society has extensively reviewed and listed all the studies and their strengths and limitations.[2] Because of variability among individuals and populations, the society recommends that practitioners become familiar

70	71	72	73	74	75	76	77	78	79	80	81	82	83	84	85
4.73	4.84	4.94	5.05	5.15	5.26	5.36	5.47	5.57	5.68	5.78	5.89	5.99	6.10	6.20	6.31
4.71	4.81	4.92	5.02	5.13	5.23	5.34	5.44	5.55	5.65	5.76	5.86	5.97	6.07	6.18	6.28
4.68	4.79	4.89	5.00	5.10	5.21	5.31	5.42	5.52	5.63	5.73	5.84	5.94	6.05	6.16	6.26
4.66	4.76	4.87	4.97	5.08	5.18	5.29	5.39	5.50	5.60	5.71	5.82	5.92	6.03	6.13	6.24
4.63	4.74	4.84	4.95	5.05	5.16	5.27	5.37	5.48	5.58	5.69	5.79	5.90	6.00	6.11	6.21
4.61	4.71	4.82	4.93	5.03	5.14	5.24	5.35	5.45	5.56	5.66	5.77	5.87	5.98	6.08	6.19
4.59	4.69	4.80	4.90	5.01	5.11	5.22	5.32	5.43	5.53	5.64	5.74	5.85	5.95	6.06	6.16
4.56	4.67	4.77	4.88	4.98	5.09	5.19	5.30	5.40	5.51	5.61	5.72	5.82	5.93	6.03	6.14
4.54	4.64	4.75	4.85	4.96	5.06	5.17	5.27	5.38	5.48	5.59	5.69	5.80	5.90	6.01	6.11
4.51	4.62	4.72	4.83	4.93	5.04	5.14	5.25	5.35	5.46	5.56	5.67	5.77	5.88	5.98	6.09
4.49	4.59	4.70	4.80	4.91	5.01	5.12	5.22	5.33	5.43	5.54	5.64	5.75	5.85	5.96	6.07
4.46	4.57	4.67	4.78	4.88	4.99	5.09	5.20	5.30	5.41	5.51	5.62	5.73	5.83	5.94	6.04
4.44	4.54	4.65	4.75	4.86	4.96	5.07	5.18	5.28	5.39	5.49	5.60	5.70	5.81	5.91	6.02
4.41	4.52	4.62	4.73	4.84	4.94	5.05	5.15	5.26	5.36	5.47	5.57	5.68	5.78	5.89	5.99
4.39	4.50	4.60	4.71	4.81	4.92	5.02	5.13	5.23	5.34	5.44	5.55	5.65	5.76	5.86	5.97
4.37	4.47	4.58	4.68	4.79	4.89	5.00	5.10	5.21	5.31	5.42	5.52	5.63	5.73	5.84	5.94
4.34	4.45	4.55	4.66	4.76	4.87	4.97	5.08	5.18	5.29	5.39	5.50	5.60	5.71	5.81	5.92
4.32	4.42	4.53	4.63	4.74	4.84	4.95	5.05	5.16	5.26	5.37	5.47	5.58	5.68	5.79	5.89
4.29	4.40	4.50	4.61	4.71	4.82	4.92	5.03	5.13	5.24	5.34	5.45	5.55	5.66	5.76	5.87
4.27	4.37	4.48	4.58	4.69	4.79	4.90	5.00	5.11	5.21	5.32	5.42	5.53	5.64	5.74	5.85
4.24	4.35	4.45	4.56	4.66	4.77	4.87	4.98	5.08	5.19	5.30	5.40	5.51	5.61	5.72	5.82
4.22	4.32	4.43	4.53	4.64	4.75	4.85	4.96	5.06	5.17	5.27	5.38	5.48	5.59	5.69	5.80
4.19	4.30	4.41	4.51	4.62	4.72	4.83	4.93	5.04	5.14	5.25	5.35	5.46	5.56	5.67	5.77
4.17	4.28	4.38	4.49	4.59	4.70	4.80	4.91	5.01	5.12	5.22	5.33	5.43	5.54	5.64	5.75
4.15	4.25	4.36	4.46	4.57	4.67	4.78	4.88	4.99	5.09	5.20	5.30	5.41	5.51	5.62	5.72
4.12	4.23	4.33	4.44	4.54	4.65	4.75	4.86	4.96	5.07	5.17	5.28	5.38	5.49	5.59	5.70
4.10	4.20	4.31	4.41	4.52	4.62	4.73	4.83	4.94	5.04	5.15	5.25	5.36	5.46	5.57	5.67
4.07	4.18	4.28	4.39	4.49	4.60	4.70	4.81	4.91	5.02	5.12	5.23	5.33	5.44	5.55	5.65
4.05	4.15	4.26	4.36	4.47	4.57	4.68	4.78	4.88	4.99	5.10	5.21	5.31	5.42	5.52	5.63
4.02	4.13	4.23	4.34	4.44	4.55	4.66	4.76	4.87	4.97	5.08	5.18	5.29	5.39	5.50	5.60
4.00	4.10	4.21	4.32	4.42	4.53	4.63	4.74	4.84	4.95	5.05	5.16	5.26	5.37	5.47	5.58
3.98	4.08	4.18	4.29	4.40	4.50	4.61	4.71	4.82	4.92	5.03	5.13	5.24	5.34	5.45	5.55
3.95	4.06	4.16	4.27	4.37	4.48	4.58	4.69	4.79	4.90	5.00	5.11	5.21	5.32	5.42	5.53

with the applicability and limitations of different sets of published reference values. If a computerized spirometer is being used, clinicians should know which set of reference values has been programmed in order to designate results as normal, elevated, or decreased. Most reference tables list age and height as variables and have separate tables for men and women. Race, past, and present health are also important variables. Among the studies often used for predicted values are those done by Crapo et al.[6] (Tables 16-1 and 16-2) and Dockery

TABLE 16-2

FEV₁ Predicted Normal Values for Females 18–50 Years Old

		54	55	56	57	58	59	Height (inches) 60	61	62	63	64	65	66	67	68	69
	18	2.65	2.74	2.83	2.91	3.00	3.09	3.18	3.26	3.35	3.44	3.52	3.61	3.70	3.78	3.87	3.96
	19	2.63	2.72	2.80	2.89	2.98	3.06	3.15	3.24	3.32	3.41	3.50	3.58	3.67	3.76	3.84	3.93
	20	2.60	2.69	2.78	2.86	2.95	3.04	3.12	3.21	3.30	3.38	3.47	3.56	3.65	3.73	3.82	3.91
	21	2.58	2.66	2.75	2.84	2.92	3.01	3.10	3.19	3.27	3.36	3.45	3.53	3.62	3.71	3.79	3.88
	22	2.55	2.64	2.73	2.81	2.90	2.99	3.07	3.16	3.25	3.33	3.42	3.51	3.59	3.68	3.77	3.85
	23	2.53	2.61	2.70	2.79	2.87	2.96	3.05	3.13	3.22	3.31	3.40	3.48	3.57	3.66	3.74	3.83
	24	2.50	2.59	2.67	2.76	2.85	2.94	3.02	3.11	3.20	3.28	3.37	3.46	3.54	3.63	3.72	3.80
	25	2.48	2.56	2.65	2.74	2.82	2.91	3.00	3.08	3.17	3.26	3.34	3.43	3.52	3.60	3.69	3.78
	26	2.45	2.54	2.62	2.71	2.80	2.88	2.97	3.06	3.14	3.23	3.32	3.41	3.49	3.58	3.67	3.75
	27	2.42	2.51	2.60	2.68	2.77	2.86	2.95	3.03	3.12	3.21	3.29	3.38	3.47	3.55	3.64	3.73
	28	2.40	2.49	2.57	2.66	2.75	2.83	2.92	3.01	3.09	3.18	3.27	3.35	3.44	3.53	3.62	3.70
	29	2.37	2.46	2.55	2.63	2.72	2.81	2.89	2.98	3.07	3.16	3.24	3.33	3.42	3.50	3.59	3.68
	30	2.35	2.43	2.52	2.61	2.70	2.78	2.87	2.96	3.04	3.13	3.22	3.30	3.38	3.48	3.56	3.65
	31	2.32	2.41	2.50	2.58	2.67	2.76	2.84	2.93	3.02	3.10	3.19	3.28	3.36	3.45	3.54	3.63
	32	2.30	2.38	2.47	2.56	2.64	2.73	2.82	2.90	2.99	3.08	3.17	3.26	3.34	3.43	3.51	3.60
	33	2.27	2.36	2.45	2.53	2.62	2.71	2.79	2.88	2.97	3.05	3.14	3.23	3.31	3.40	3.49	3.57
	34	2.25	2.33	2.42	2.51	2.59	2.68	2.77	2.85	2.94	3.03	3.11	3.20	3.29	3.38	3.46	3.55
	35	2.22	2.31	2.39	2.48	2.57	2.65	2.74	2.83	2.92	3.00	3.09	3.18	3.26	3.35	3.44	3.52
	36	2.19	2.28	2.37	2.46	2.54	2.63	2.72	2.80	2.89	2.98	3.06	3.15	3.24	3.32	3.41	3.50
	37	2.17	2.26	2.34	2.43	2.52	2.60	2.69	2.78	2.86	2.95	3.04	3.12	3.21	3.30	3.39	3.47
	38	2.14	2.23	2.32	2.40	2.49	2.58	2.67	2.75	2.84	2.93	3.01	3.10	3.19	3.27	3.36	3.45
	39	2.12	2.21	2.29	2.38	2.47	2.55	2.64	2.73	2.81	2.90	2.99	3.07	3.16	3.25	3.33	3.42
	40	2.09	2.18	2.27	2.35	2.44	2.53	2.61	2.70	2.79	2.87	2.96	3.05	3.14	3.22	3.31	3.40
	41	2.07	2.15	2.24	2.33	2.41	2.50	2.59	2.68	2.76	2.85	2.94	3.02	3.11	3.20	3.28	3.37
	42	2.04	2.13	2.22	2.30	2.39	2.48	2.56	2.65	2.74	2.82	2.91	3.00	3.08	3.17	3.26	3.34
	43	2.02	2.10	2.19	2.28	2.36	2.45	2.54	2.62	2.71	2.80	2.89	2.97	3.06	3.15	3.23	3.32
	44	1.99	2.08	2.16	2.25	2.34	2.43	2.51	2.60	2.69	2.77	2.86	2.95	3.03	3.12	3.21	3.29
	45	1.97	2.05	2.14	2.23	2.31	2.40	2.49	2.57	2.66	2.75	2.83	2.92	3.01	3.09	3.18	3.27
	46	1.94	2.03	2.11	2.20	2.29	2.37	2.46	2.55	2.63	2.72	2.81	2.90	2.98	3.07	3.16	3.24
	47	1.91	2.00	2.09	2.17	2.26	2.35	2.44	2.52	2.61	2.70	2.78	2.87	2.96	3.04	3.13	3.22
	48	1.89	1.98	2.06	2.15	2.24	2.32	2.41	2.50	2.58	2.67	2.76	2.84	2.93	3.02	3.11	3.19
	49	1.86	1.95	2.04	2.12	2.21	2.30	2.38	2.47	2.56	2.65	2.73	2.82	2.91	2.99	3.08	3.17
	50	1.84	1.92	2.01	2.10	2.19	2.27	2.36	2.45	2.53	2.62	2.71	2.79	2.88	2.97	3.05	3.14

Age (years) (vertical label)

From Crapo RO, Morris AH, Gardner RM: Reference spirometric values using techniques and equipment that meet ATS recommendations. Am Rev Respir Dis 1981;123:659–664. Reproduced with permission.

et al.,[7] both of which were done on nonsmoking white men and women. For children, the Polgar table of predicted normal values is often used (Table 16-3).

B. Race is an important variable that practitioners tend to overlook. In general, nonwhite populations show lower values for lung volumes. A correction factor of 0.88 is used when reference values established in white populations are used for black Americans.[8]

C. The varying ranges for predicted "normal" values makes it imperative for the practitioner to correlate all pulmonary

70	71	72	73	74	75	76	77	78	79	80	81	82	83	84	85
4.04	4.13	4.22	4.30	4.39	4.48	4.56	4.65	4.74	4.83	4.91	5.00	5.09	5.17	5.26	5.35
4.02	4.11	4.19	4.28	4.37	4.45	4.54	4.63	4.71	4.80	4.89	4.97	5.06	5.15	5.23	5.32
3.99	4.08	4.17	4.25	4.34	4.43	4.51	4.60	4.69	4.77	4.86	4.95	5.04	5.12	5.21	5.30
3.97	4.05	4.14	4.23	4.31	4.40	4.49	4.58	4.66	4.75	4.84	4.92	5.01	5.10	5.18	5.27
3.94	4.03	4.12	4.20	4.29	4.38	4.46	4.55	4.64	4.72	4.81	4.90	4.98	5.07	5.16	5.24
3.92	4.00	4.09	4.18	4.26	4.35	4.44	4.52	4.61	4.70	4.78	4.87	4.96	5.05	5.13	5.22
3.89	3.98	4.06	4.15	4.24	4.33	4.41	4.50	4.59	4.67	4.76	4.85	4.93	5.02	5.11	5.19
3.87	3.95	4.04	4.13	4.21	4.30	4.39	4.47	4.56	4.65	4.73	4.82	4.91	4.99	5.08	5.17
3.84	3.93	4.01	4.10	4.19	4.27	4.36	4.45	4.53	4.62	4.71	4.80	4.88	4.97	5.06	5.14
3.81	3.90	3.99	4.07	4.16	4.25	4.34	4.42	4.51	4.60	4.68	4.77	4.86	4.94	5.03	5.12
3.79	3.88	3.96	4.05	4.14	4.22	4.31	4.40	4.48	4.57	4.66	4.74	4.83	4.92	5.00	5.09
3.76	3.85	3.94	4.02	4.11	4.20	4.28	4.37	4.46	4.55	4.63	4.72	4.81	4.89	4.98	5.07
3.74	3.82	3.91	4.00	4.09	4.17	4.26	4.35	4.43	4.52	4.61	4.69	4.78	4.87	4.95	5.04
3.71	3.80	3.89	3.97	4.06	4.15	4.23	4.32	4.41	4.49	4.58	4.67	4.75	4.84	4.93	5.02
3.69	3.77	3.86	3.95	4.03	4.12	4.21	4.29	4.38	4.47	4.56	4.64	4.73	4.82	4.90	4.99
3.66	3.75	3.83	3.92	4.01	4.10	4.18	4.27	4.36	4.44	4.53	4.62	4.70	4.79	4.88	4.96
3.64	3.72	3.81	3.90	3.98	4.07	4.16	4.24	4.33	4.42	4.50	4.59	4.68	4.77	4.85	4.94
3.61	3.70	3.78	3.87	3.96	4.04	4.13	4.22	4.31	4.39	4.48	4.57	4.65	4.74	4.83	4.91
3.58	3.67	3.76	3.85	3.93	4.02	4.11	4.19	4.28	4.37	4.45	4.54	4.63	4.71	4.80	4.89
3.56	3.65	3.73	3.82	3.91	3.99	4.08	4.17	4.25	4.34	4.43	4.51	4.60	4.69	4.78	4.86
3.53	3.62	3.71	3.79	3.88	3.97	4.05	4.14	4.23	4.32	4.40	4.49	4.58	4.66	4.75	4.84
3.51	3.60	3.68	3.77	3.86	3.94	4.03	4.12	4.20	4.29	4.38	4.46	4.55	4.64	4.72	4.81
3.48	3.57	3.66	3.74	3.83	3.92	4.00	4.09	4.18	4.26	4.35	4.44	4.53	4.61	4.70	4.79
3.46	3.54	3.63	3.72	3.80	3.89	3.98	4.07	4.15	4.24	4.33	4.41	4.50	4.59	4.67	4.76
3.43	3.52	3.61	3.69	3.78	3.87	3.95	4.04	4.13	4.21	4.30	4.39	4.47	4.56	4.65	4.73
3.41	3.49	3.58	3.67	3.75	3.84	3.93	4.01	4.10	4.19	4.27	4.36	4.45	4.54	4.62	4.71
3.38	3.47	3.55	3.64	3.73	3.82	3.90	3.99	4.08	4.16	4.25	4.34	4.42	4.51	4.60	4.68
3.36	3.44	3.53	3.62	3.70	3.79	3.88	3.96	4.05	4.14	4.22	4.31	4.40	4.48	4.57	4.66
3.33	3.42	3.50	3.59	3.68	3.76	3.85	3.94	4.02	4.11	4.20	4.29	4.37	4.46	4.55	4.63
3.30	3.39	3.48	3.56	3.65	3.74	3.83	3.91	4.00	4.09	4.17	4.26	4.35	4.43	4.52	4.61
3.26	3.37	3.45	3.54	3.63	3.71	3.80	3.89	3.97	4.06	4.15	4.23	4.32	4.41	4.49	4.58
3.25	3.34	3.43	3.51	3.60	3.69	3.77	3.86	3.95	4.04	4.12	4.21	4.30	4.38	4.47	4.56
3.23	3.31	3.40	3.49	3.58	3.66	3.75	3.84	3.92	4.01	4.10	4.16	4.27	4.36	4.44	4.53

function test results with other clinical findings in individual patients. The patient's age, size, sex, and ethnic origin should all be considered. The American Thoracic Society recommends *not* using 80% of predicted as the lower limit of normal for pulmonary function test results because it applies only to persons with average characteristics and may result in the classification of healthy persons as abnormal.[2] Following changes in a patient's spirometry values over time is the best way to evaluate that person's status at any point in time.

TABLE 16-3

FEV_1 Predicted Normal Values for Males and Females 4–17 Years Old

Height (cm)	*Pred. FEV_1*	*Height (cm)*	*Pred. FEV_1*	*Height (cm)*	*Pred. FEV_1*
90	0.62	127	1.63	164	3.34
91	0.64	128	1.67	165	3.40
92	0.66	129	1.71	166	3.46
93	0.68	130	1.74	167	3.51
94	0.70	131	1.78	168	3.57
95	0.72	132	1.82	169	3.63
96	0.75	133	1.86	170	3.69
97	0.77	134	1.90	171	3.75
98	0.79	135	1.94	172	3.82
99	0.81	136	1.98	173	3.88
100	0.84	137	2.02	174	3.94
101	0.86	138	2.06	175	4.01
102	0.88	139	2.10	176	4.07
103	0.91	140	2.14	177	4.14
104	0.93	141	2.19	178	4.20
105	0.96	142	2.23	179	4.27
106	0.98	143	2.28	180	4.33
107	1.01	144	2.32	181	4.40
108	1.04	145	2.37	182	4.47
109	1.06	146	2.41	183	4.54
110	1.09	147	2.46	184	4.61
111	1.12	148	2.51	185	4.68
112	1.15	149	2.55	186	4.75
113	1.18	150	2.60	187	4.82
114	1.21	151	2.65	188	4.90
115	1.24	152	2.70	189	4.97
116	1.27	153	2.75	190	5.04
117	1.30	154	2.80	191	5.12
118	1.33	155	2.85	192	5.19
119	1.36	156	2.90	193	5.27
120	1.39	157	2.96	194	5.35
121	1.43	158	3.01	195	5.42
122	1.46	159	3.06	196	5.50
123	1.49	160	3.12	197	5.58
124	1.53	161	3.17	198	5.66
125	1.56	162	3.23	199	5.74
126	1.60	163	3.28	200	5.82

From Polgar G, Promodhat V: Pulmonary Function Testing in Children: Techniques and Standards, p 272. Philadelphia: WB Saunders, 1971. Reproduced with permission.

REFERENCES

1. American Thoracic Society: Standardization of spirometry: 1994 update. Am J Respir Crit Care Med 1995;152:1107–1136.
2. American Thoracic Society: Lung function testing: Selection of reference values and interpretive strategies. Am Rev Respir Dis 1991;144:1202–1218.
3. American College of Chest Physicians: Committee report: Criteria for the assessment of reversibility in airways obstruction. Report of the Committee on Emphysema. Chest 1974;65:552–553.
4. McFadden ER Jr: Pulmonary structure, physiology, and clinical correlates in asthma. In Middleton E Jr, et al (eds): Allergy: Principles and Practice, 4th ed, pp 672–693. St. Louis: Mosby, 1993.
5. Crapo RO, Morris AH, Clayton PD, Nixon CR: Lung volumes

in healthy nonsmoking adults. Bull Eur Physiopathol Respir 1982;18:419–425.

6. Crapo RO, Morris AH, Gardner RM: Reference spirometric values using techniques and equipment that meet ATS recommendations. Am Rev Respir Dis 1981;123:659–664.

7. Dockery DW, Ware JH, Ferris BG Jr, et al: Distribution of forced expiratory volume in one second and forced vital capacity in healthy, white, adult never-smokers in six US cities. Am Rev Respir Dis 1985;131:511–520.

8. Rossiter CE, Weill H: Ethnic differences in lung function: Evidence for proportional differences. Int J Epidemiol 1974;3:55–61.

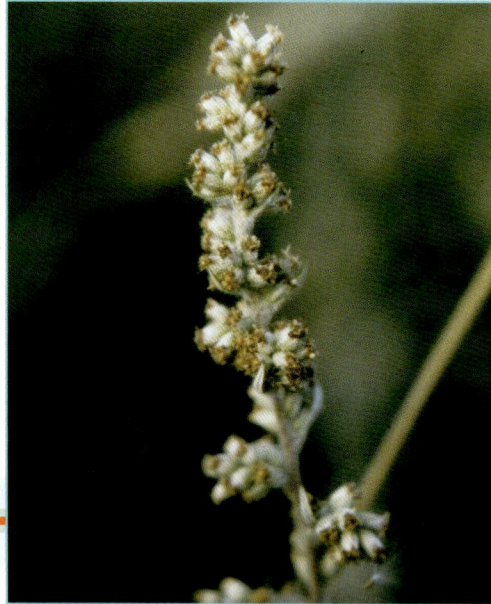

CHAPTER 17
Bronchial Challenge
Sheldon L. Spector and Ricardo A. Tan

I. Bronchial Challenge Testing or Bronchoprovocation

A. Nonspecific Bronchial Challenge

1. If a patient has normal spirometry values but asthma is still suspected, a bronchial challenge can be performed.[1] The patient is exposed to progressively increasing doses of a bronchonconstrictor substance, usually methacholine or histamine, with a positive response being a reduction in FEV_1 (forced expiratory volume in 1 second) from baseline. The responses elicited with methacholine or histamine are usually short-lived and therefore ideal for testing. The response to provocation is measured by the concentration (PC_{20} FEV_1) or cumulative dose (PD_{20} FEV_1) of methacholine or histamine required to decrease the subject's baseline FEV_1 by 20%. The concentration is expressed in milligrams per milliliter (mg/mL), while the cumulative dose is expressed in cumulative μmoles or cumulative breath units. Each breath unit is equivalent to one breath of a 1 mg/mL concentration.[2] Because approximately 85%–100% of asthmatics will have a PC_{20} FEV_1 of 8 mg/mL or less of methacholine or histamine,[3,4] this is generally considered the cutoff point for a positive challenge test.

2. Nonisotonic aerosols cause change in airway osmolarity leading to bronchoconstriction and can be used for nonspecific bronchial challenges. Water in hypotonic or hypertonic saline solutions of 2.7%, 3.6% and 4.5% NaCl is commonly used. This test is especially helpful for clinicians who prefer to use nonpharmacologic alternatives for evaluating airway hyperresponsiveness. Bronchoprovocation with nonisotonic aerosols is cheap, easy to perform, and relatively free of side effects.[5]

3. If asthma symptoms appear to be triggered only by exercise, a challenge utilizing exercise on a treadmill or cycle ergometer may be performed.

4. Hyperventilation testing is an alternative for patients unable to do the exercise procedure.[6]

B. Specific Bronchial Challenge Testing

Specific challenges are currently performed only in hospital or research facilities with appropriate equipment.[7] Specialized inhalation chambers where exposure to test substances can be rigorously controlled are utilized for challenge testing. Challenge with environmental allergens (e.g., pollen, animal dander) is an important tool for research into mechanisms of inflammation and inflammatory mediators, identification of new allergens, evaluation of the response to immunotherapy, and assessment of the efficacy of new therapeutic agents, among others. Testing for occupational allergens such as wood dusts or resins may be important for diagnosing occupational asthma.

REFERENCES

1. Tan RA, Spector SL: Lung disease. In Kemp SF, Lockey RF (eds): Diagnostic Testing of Allergic Disease, pp 175–197. New York: Marcel Dekker, 2000.
2. Fish JE: Bronchial challenge testing. In Middleton E Jr, et al (eds): Allergy: Principles and Practice, 4th ed, pp 613–627. St. Louis: Mosby, 1993.
3. Cockcroft DW, Killian DN, Mellon JJA, et al: Bronchial reactivity to inhaled histamine: A method and clinical survey. Clin Allergy 1977;7:235.
4. Hopp RJ, Bewtra AK, Nair NM, et al: Specificity and sensitivity of methacholine inhalation challenge in normal and asthmatic children. J Allergy Clin Immunol 1984;74:154.
5. Anderson SD, Smith CM, Rodwell LT, du Toit JI, Riedler J, Robertson CF: The use of nonisotonic aerosols for evaluating bronchial hyperresponsiveness. In Spector SL (ed): Provocative Testing in Clinical Practice, pp 249–278. New York: Marcel Dekker, 1995.
6. Tan RA, Spector SL: Asthma and exercise. In Weisman IM, Zeballos RJ (eds): Clinical Exercise Testing. Prog Respir Res 2002;32:205–216.
7. Spector SL: Allergen inhalation challenges. In Spector SL (ed): Provocative Testing in Clinical Practice, pp 325–368. New York: Marcel Dekker, 1995.

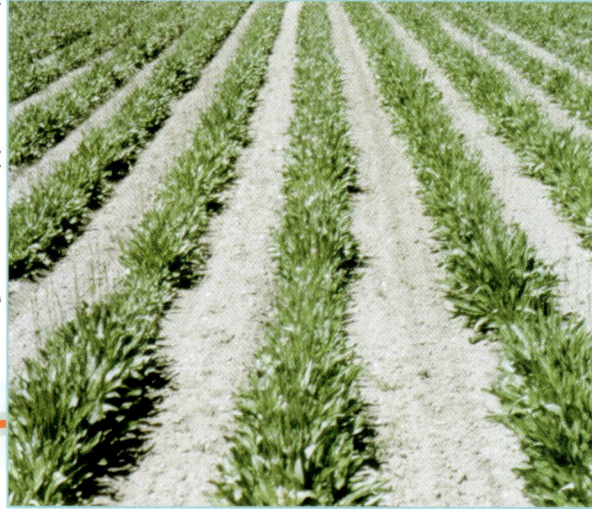

CHAPTER 18
Peak Flow Monitoring

Guillermo R. Mendoza

I. Introduction

Peak expiratory flow rates are important airway measurements for asthma screening and diagnosis at a population level, for assessing disease severity and instability at a patient level, and as part of a comprehensive self-management program. The relationship between peak flow levels, peak flow variability, and the clinical presentation of asthma is complex, but many studies have demonstrated significant correlations. There are advantages and limitations to the use of peak flow rates in everyday clinical practice.

II. Home Monitoring: A Quick Start

The merits of using peak flowmeters may seem self-evident, but getting patients to use them at home can be a challenge. Without reinforcement from the provider, meters can end up neglected when they could be helping the patient avoid the common pitfalls of asthma self-management.

To get the biggest bang for the peak flow buck, keep it simple: Don't make the patient check peak flows without a specific purpose, and never ask the patient to do something you wouldn't be able to do.

Which Peak Flowmeter? Does It Make a Difference?

1. There are a dozen or so different kinds of peak flowmeters available today (Fig. 18-1). Most of them are internally consistent, reliable, and capable of improving your patients' care.[1] An important cautionary note: Few of them agree with each other or with any spirometer you are likely to use, so stick with one brand of meter for both office and home use. To make the meters extra helpful, pick a meter that has useful built-in features, such as green, yellow, and red zone markers that can be coordinated with the patient's self-care plan.

2. Presumably you will be using the same meters for different patients, so you will need to use a meter with a disposable mouthpiece. All things being equal, pick a meter that is commonly used by asthma specialists in your community.

3. While doing a correct peak flow requires scarcely more than a "see one, do one, teach one" technique, all members of your staff need to be "peak flow certified" or you will be recording haphazard data. Describing the technique to most patients doesn't work as well as demonstrating the correct technique.

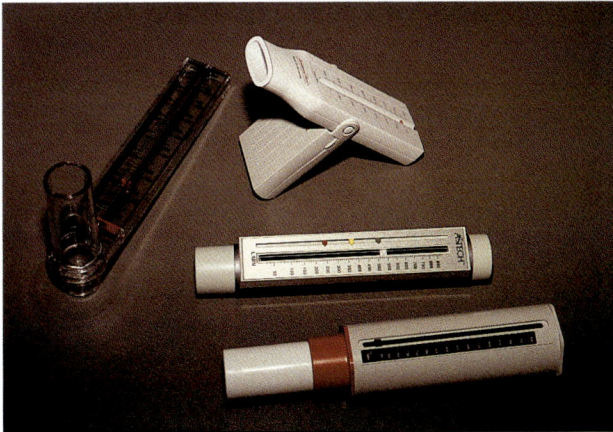

Figure 18-1 Sample of peak flowmeters.

4. We generally ask the patient to blow several times before picking the best effort.
   a. The best effort is almost never the first effort, especially for new patients, so expect the need for practice. An inadequate effort may confound the interpretation of a postbronchodilator improvement: Did the peak flow improve due to the bronchodilator, or did the patient simply figure out how to blow correctly?
   b. As your staff gains experience, they may want to record a few observations along with the actual best peak flow, such as whether or not the patient coughs with each effort or whether the peak flow values seem to drift down with repeated efforts. Both of these features are common in patients with less than stable asthma (Box 18-1).

III. Phase 1: Establishing Baseline Best Peak Flow and Best Peak Flow Variability

A. The "One-Minute" Approach

This approach is not generally recommended unless you are content to do peak flow screening because the added information from a postbronchodilator peak flow can be invaluable. There is a wide range of predicted peak flow values for any given sex, height, and age (Fig. 18-2). An asymptomatic patient with a 90% of predicted best peak flow may end up blowing 110% post bronchodilator and 120% after a 4-week trial of an inhaled steroid. Consider the consequences if the patient were to return with mild symptoms and 75% of predicted peak flow. This might appear to be only a mild deviation from an apparent best of 90%, whereas in reality it represents a significant drop from 120%.

B. The "20-Minute" Approach

The prebronchodilator peak flow is recorded and the patient is given two or three puffs of a short-acting β-agonist (SABA) or a nebulized dose of the same SABA. Waiting 30–60 minutes before rechecking the peak flow may be ideal but is impractical. Twenty minutes is a good compromise. A 10%–15% improvement in peak flow is usually considered significant.

1. Because the peak flow may rise and fall 10%–20% in a diurnal circadian pattern over 24 hours, the clinician must be careful when interpreting the significance of a postbronchodilator peak flow improvement.
2. An early morning peak flow of 90% that improves 10% post bronchodilator is normal. However, a 10% midday improvement is suspicious because the early morning peak flow was probably considerably lower than 90% and the daily peak flow variability could easily exceed 10%–20%.

C. The Weekend Approach

For one reason or another, you may feel that your office assessment was inadvertently confounded by inadequate practice or suspect technique, or that the patient may have used a SABA shortly before the appointment. Perhaps the implications of the office assessment were too unexpected to make a potentially controversial change in asthma medications. At times like this, it may be reasonable to defer changing plans until you have more data. The patient can come back and try again, or you can ask the patient to take a meter home to measure peak flows. A weekend or more of peak flow monitoring may clear up any doubt about the baseline best peak flow and typical day-to-day peak flow variability.

D. Getting the Right Peak Flow Data from Home

1. To make a good assessment, ideally one should have peak-to-trough variability data. The best time to check

---

BOX 18-1

How to Use the Peak Flowmeter

1. Insert mouthpiece on peak flowmeter if used by more than one patient.
2. Place measuring indicator at the bottom of the scale.
3. Inhale as deeply as possible and place lips with a tight seal around mouthpiece.
4. Exhale as hard and as fast as possible. This should raise the measuring indicator up the scale.
5. Take note of the measurement, time, and date.
6. Repeat this procedure three times and record the best result.

A.

Men

75
72
69
66
63
Ht. (ins.)

Standard deviation men = 48 litres/min.
Standard deviation women = 42 litres/min.

Women

69
66
63
60
57
Ht. (ins.)

In men, values of PEF up to 100 litres/min. less than predicted and in women less than 85 litres/min. less than predicted, are within normal limits

PEF L/min.

Age in Years

B.

Peak Flow Rate (L/min.)

+95%

MEAN

−95%

Height (cm)

C.

Predicted Average Peak Expiratory Flow for Normal Males
(liters per minute)

Age	Height				
	60"	65"	70"	75"	80"
20	554	602	649	693	740
25	543	590	636	679	725
30	532	577	622	664	710
35	521	565	609	651	695
40	509	552	596	636	680
45	498	540	583	622	665
50	486	527	569	607	649
55	475	515	556	593	634
60	463	502	542	578	618
65	452	490	529	564	603
70	440	477	515	550	587

D.

Predicted Average Peak Expiratory Flow for Normal Females
(liters per minute)

Age	Height				
	55"	60"	65"	70"	75"
20	390	423	460	496	529
25	385	418	454	490	523
30	380	413	448	483	516
35	375	408	442	476	509
40	370	402	436	470	502
45	365	397	430	464	495
50	360	391	424	457	488
55	355	386	418	451	482
60	350	380	412	445	475
65	345	375	406	439	468
70	340	369	400	432	461

E.

Predicted Average Peak Expiratory Flow for Normal Children and Adolescents
(liters per minute)

Ht. (in.)	Males and Females	Ht. (in.)	Males and Females
43	147	56	320
44	160	57	334
45	173	58	347
46	187	59	360
47	200	60	373
48	214	61	387
49	227	62	400
50	240	63	413
51	254	64	427
52	267	65	440
53	280	66	454
54	293	67	467
55	307		

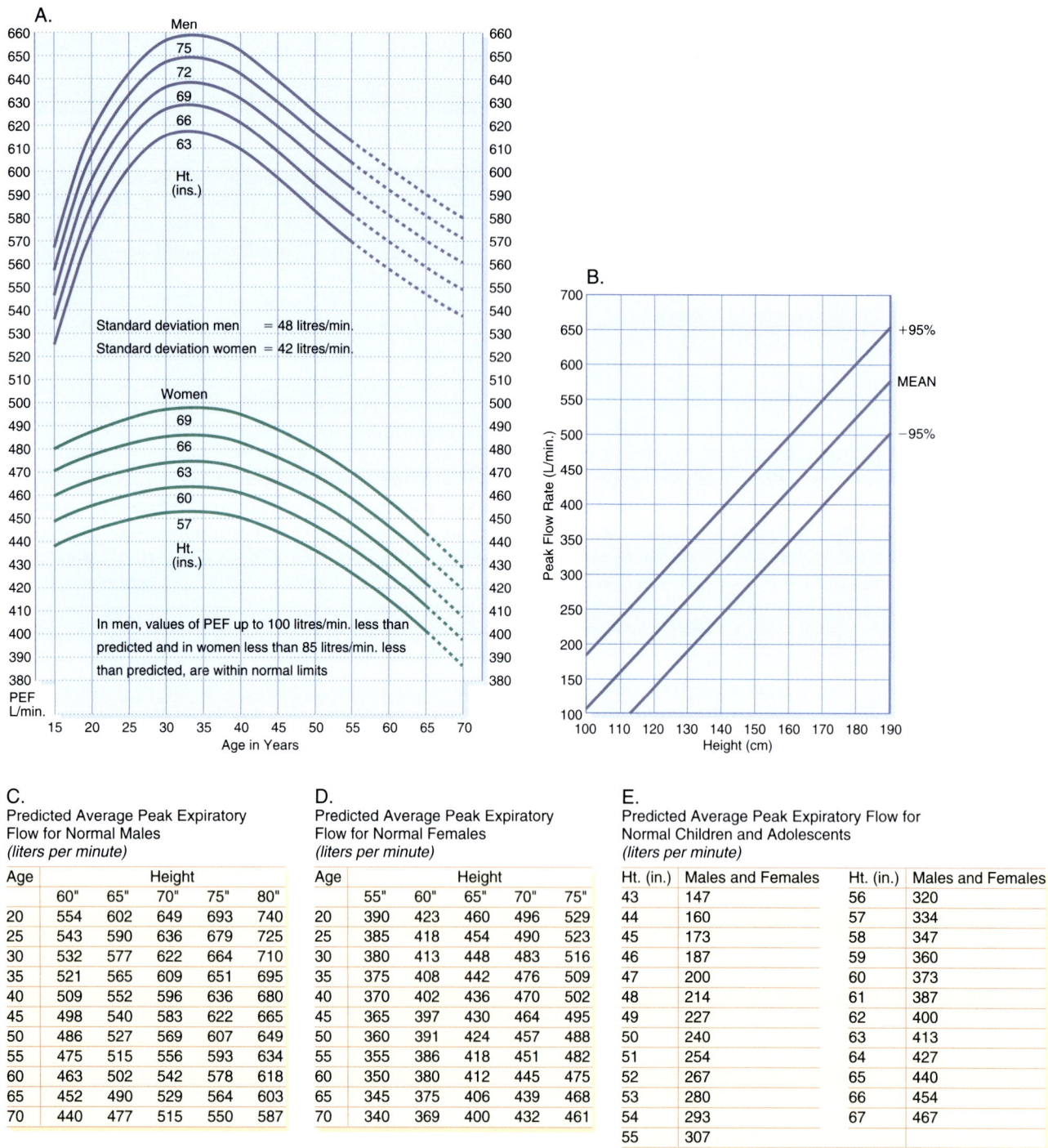

Figure 18-2 **A–E**, Average predicted peak expiratory flow values. *Note*: These tables are averages and are based on tests with a large number of people. An individual's PEFR may vary widely. Further, many individuals' PEFR values are consistently higher or lower than the average values. It is recommended that PEFR objectives for therapy be based on each individual's "personal best," which is established after a period of PEFR monitoring while the individual is under effective treatment. (**A**, Adapted from Nunn AJ, Gregg L: Brit Med J 1989;298:1068–1070. **B**, Godfrey S, et al: Brit J Dis Chest 1970;64:15–24. **C & D**, Leiner GC, et al: Expiratory peak flow rate. Standard values for nomal subjects. Use as a clinical test of ventilatory function. Am Rev Respr Dis 1963;88:644. **E**, Polger G, Promedhas V: Pulmonary Function Testing in Children: Techniques and Standards. Philadelphia: WB Saunders, 1971.)

a trough level is in the early morning, around break-fast time—obviously before any SABA is taken.

2. The second best time to check trough values is at bedtime, but for many patients the evening trough doesn't begin to develop until after the patient falls asleep.

3. Midday peak flows may occur anytime between lunchtime and late afternoon.

IV. Phase 2: Using Peak Flow to Determine the Best Starting Dose for the Unstable Patient

The clinical parameters of mild, moderate, and severe asthma are helpful when planning the starting dose of an anti-inflammatory medication (see Chapter 2, Asthma). If there is disparity between the clinical and peak flow estimate of severity, err on the side of labeling the patient with more severe asthma. For example, if the clinical history suggests mild asthma but the peak flow dips are consistent with moderate persistent asthma, treat the patient as having moderate asthma. Even if all criteria point to the same level of severity, it is customary to start therapy with comparatively high doses of inhaled anti-inflammatory (IAI) medications. When the asthma is stable, the IAIs can be stepped down.

Low and Unresponsive Peak Flows

The new or rarely seen patient with a low prebron-chodilator peak flow that does *not* improve after bron-chodilator use poses a challenging diagnostic dilemma.

1. Is the obstruction due to stubborn bronchospasm, severe airway inflammation, or long-term airway remodeling?

2. Most instances of bronchospasm will respond to aggressive doses of a SABA. One to two months of an aggressive dose of an IAI, perhaps fortified with a short burst of oral corticosteroids, should reverse airway swelling due to inflammation. The determination of irreversible airway damage is a process of elimination.

3. In compliant patients with generally stable asthma, the gradual development of a low and nonrespon-sive peak flow is almost always due to a bacterial infection, more commonly sinusitis than a lower respiratory infection in children and younger adults. This "pearl" is especially valuable when the clinical diagnosis of sinusitis is equivocal. Not uncommonly the sinusitis will induce a low peak flow unrespon-sive even to stepped-up doses of IAI medications or even a burst of oral corticosteroids.

4. On the flip side, a patient may describe a lingering upper respiratory tract infection that was probably viral when it started but with time begins to look like bacterial sinusitis. In such cases, we tend to err on the side of stepping up the IAIs and *not* using antibiotics if the low peak flow *improves significantly* after bronchodilator use. This simple strategy has greatly helped us to be more selective in the use of IAIs versus antibiotics in various upper respiratory tract infection scenarios.

V. Phase 3: Getting the Unstable Patient Back to Normal

You have decided on a medication plan, but is this the right time to give the patient a written peak flow–based self-care plan? Wait a few weeks. You may still not know the patient's best peak flow, and in 3–6 weeks you may decide to step down the IAI medications.

A. At this stage the patient needs to concentrate on adher-ing to the new asthma medications and checking whether the peak flow variability is returning to normal. "Return-ing to normal" means no symptoms or need for SABAs more than once a week, and the best peak flow should hover between 80% and 100%, preferably 90%–100%, on most days.

B. Before the patient goes home with a new plan, we make sure a follow-up visit is scheduled in 3–6 weeks. A mid-course reassessment of symptoms and peak flow can be scheduled over the phone a week or so after the initial visit. If the peak flow hypervariability has not yet improved, this is an opportune time to consider inten-sifying the IAIs.

C. Even if the peak flow stabilizes quickly, it is advisa-ble to have the patient return for a clinic visit for repeat spirometry to make sure the FEV_1 has returned to normal. Usually what is good for the low peak flow is good for the low FEV_1, but not always.

A persistent small airway obstruction may require additional time to heal, or we may decide to step up the patient's IAI medications. This cycle of medication titra-tion and follow-up continues until the patient is deemed stable.

VI. Phase 4: Keeping the Stable Patient from Backsliding

The patient is now stable. This is the ideal time to start a peak flow–based self-management plan. A green/yellow/red zone strategy with color-coded graphs and peak flowmeters works well to simplify the concept of stable versus unstable peak flows (Fig. 18-3). The written

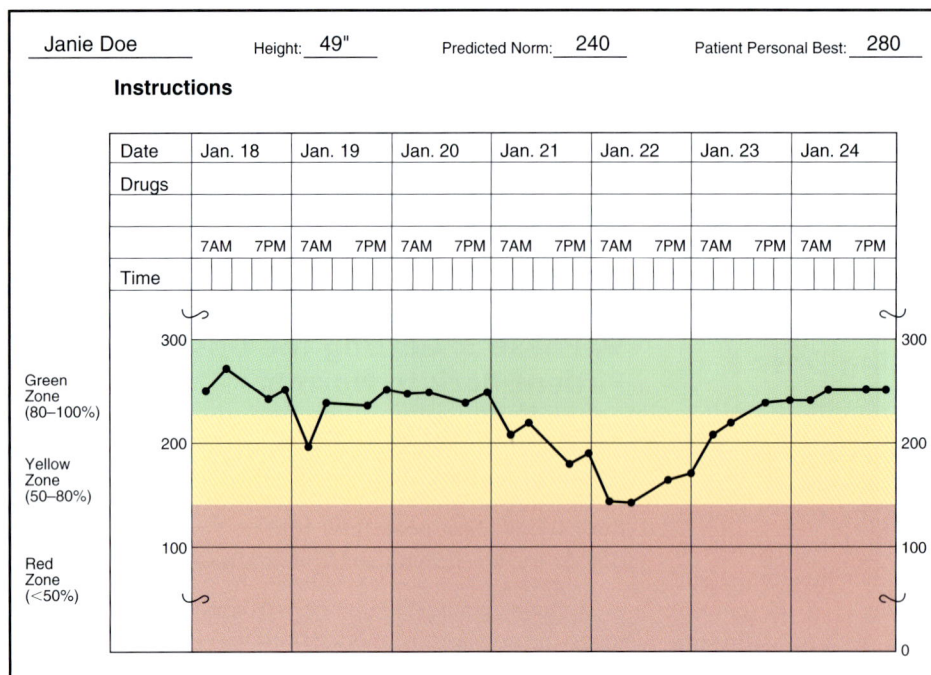

Figure 18-3 Typical daily record depicting daily peak flow measurements using the traffic light measuring system. (From National Heart, Lung and Blood Institute. Expert Panel Report 2. Guidelines for the Diagnosis and Management of Asthma. National Asthma Education and Prevention Program, 1997. NIH Publication 97-4051. Bethesda, MD: NIH, 1997.)

plans can be simple or complex (Fig. 18-4). The provider is encouraged to customize a plan that feels comfortable.

A. The green/yellow/red zone strategy is inherently simple: The patient needs to keep the peak flow consistently in the green zone.

1. If the prebronchodilator peak flow dips significantly into the yellow zone, the management plan needs to specify how much to step up the dose of the baseline IAI.

2. If the peak flow drops into the red zone, the patient needs to self-start a burst of oral steroids. Moreover, the plan should remind the patient when he or she should call for advice or seek urgent care.

B. If the patient is truly stable, checking peak flows on a regular basis can be both boring and counterproductive. This is a time when meters tend to disappear and gather dust. Instead, encourage the patient to replace daily peak flow monitoring with periodic spot checks. Rehearse "what-if" scenarios so that the patient can become selectively vigilant when the asthma begins to relapse—for example, at the onset of colds or during the early days of a new allergy season.

C. The key operative strategy is reinforcement. If the patient calls on the telephone for help but doesn't mention recent peak flows, ask for them. If the patient hasn't checked a peak flow, insist on having the patient check the peak flow, even if it means waiting on the phone or having the patient call back.

1. Emphasize the need for objective data before making critical decisions about medications. Nothing reduces the patient's motivation for checking peak flows faster than offering advice that is based purely on clinical symptoms—even if your clinical judgment proves to be correct.

VII. Peak Flow 101

A. For a comprehensive review of the physiologic basis for the use of peak flow in both the office and home, for cutoffs in values between asthmatics and nonasthmatics, as well as details about daily measurements and timing of observations, the reader should refer to a comprehensive review by Harold Nelson.[2]

B. The importance of objective measures of airflow for assessing asthma, both in the office and at home, is underscored by the inherent limitations of auscultation, the increased risk of patients with blunted perception of dyspnea (POD) for near-fatal asthma, and the high frequency of patients with aberrant POD.

A 2-year study identified 41% of patients with abnormal perception of asthma—15% with high POD and 26% with low POD—compared with normal subjects.[3]

NAME | MR # | DATE | MD | MD OFFICE PHONE

- Use of your daily peak flow/symptom diary will give you better control of your asthma.
- **MY PERSONAL BEST PEAK FLOW READING =** ____
- If your peak flow is less than 80% of your personal best, check your peak flow 2-3 TIMES A DAY and follow the self-management plan below as indicated.
- Always **use a spacer with your inhalers.**
- At the *start* of a *cold,* follow your SELF-MANAGEMENT PLAN in the YELLOW ZONE and monitor your peak flow carefully.
- During your *"asthma season,"* monitor your peak flow carefully and anticipate the need to step up to your YELLOW ZONE plan.

ZONE	ACTION
GREEN ZONE: THIS IS YOUR DAILY PLAN. ABOVE 80% ____ (OPTIMALLY 90% ____). Able to do usual activities. Sleeping all night. Your asthma bothers you less than twice a week.	Controller: Azmacort®/Flovent®/Pulmicort® ____ puffs ____ times/day. Reliever: Albuterol®: **Take only if needed** for asthma symptoms. 2 or ____ puffs 20 min. before exercise or every ____ hours **as needed** for asthma symptoms. (Your reliever should NOT be used regularly when you are in the green zone.) Other: ____ mg or puffs every ____ hours or ____ times/day. Other: ____ mg or puffs every ____ hours or ____ times/day.
YELLOW ZONE: INCREASE IN SYMPTOMS. ALSO USE AT THE **START OF A COLD** AND CONTINUE FOR ____ DAYS. RANGE 50% ____ TO 80% ____. Increased asthma symptoms—including waking at night. Usual activities somewhat limited. Increased cough, chest tightness, or wheezing. Peak flow does not return to the green zone after a few doses of the bronchodilator.	**Consider what may be causing your flare-up (e.g., infection, heartburn, allergies, smoke, etc.) and treat the problem.** Increase fluid intake. Increase Controller: Azmacort®/Flovent®/Pulmicort® to ____ puffs ____ times/day. Increase Reliever: Albuterol® to ____ puffs every ____ hours until back into the green zone. Then use as needed. Other: ____ mg or puffs every ____ hours or ____ times/day. ☐ Same as green zone Other: ____ mg or puffs every ____ hours or ____ times/day. ☐ Same as green zone If you are **not improving after 2-3 days and your Peak Flow remains below 65%** ____, use the Yellow Zone controller dose for at least 2-3 weeks and begin **Prednisone/Medrol® dose as in the red zone.** ☐ *CALL THE NUMBER AT THE TOP OF THIS FORM OR* ☐
RED ZONE: MEDICAL ALERT. BELOW 50% ____ **before** Reliever. Asthma medications have not reduced symptoms. Peak flow reading stays low. Very short of breath. Usual activities severely limited. Persistent cough, wheeze, and/or waking up several times at night due to asthma.	Immediately begin Prednisone/Medrol® dose ____ mg ____ **times/day.** Increase Reliever: Albuterol® 4-6 puffs or nebulizer every 10-20 minutes up to 3 times only. **Then** ____ **puffs every** ____ **hours.** Controller: Azmacort®/Flovent®/Pulmicort® ____ puffs Other: ____ mg or puffs every ____ hours or ____ times/day. ☐ Same as green zone Other: ____ mg or puffs every ____ hours or ____ times/day. ☐ Same as green zone ☐ *CALL THE NUMBER AT THE TOP OF THIS FORM OR* ☐ *If not significantly improved, go to the EMERGENCY ROOM. Have a plan for getting Emergency Care QUICKLY.* ALWAYS CARRY A RELIEVER MEDICATION WITH YOU.
DANGER SIGNS: **Difficulty walking/talking due to shortness of breath.** **Unable to catch breath or struggling to breathe.**	**GO TO THE EMERGENCY ROOM OR CALL *911* NOW.**

Figure 18-4 Asthma self-management plan for adults used by Kaiser Permanente. (From the Permanente Medical Group, Inc., Asthma Self-Management Plan [ADULTS] © 2001, used with permission.)

203

C. Recent controlled clinical trials comparing symptom and peak flow monitoring continue to yield conflicting results, possibly reflecting differences in study design, age, ethnicity, and socioeconomic status. The appropriateness of self-management decisions was studied in a pharmacist-based study of 110 patients over the age of 6 years who were assigned to either symptom monitoring or PEFR monitoring.

1. The average monthly frequency of appropriate responses was higher for patients using PEFR than symptom monitoring.
2. Inappropriate use of medications was higher in patients with symptom monitoring, and these patients also tended to underestimate the severity of their asthma.[4]
3. Six to 12-year-old children (n = 113) were evaluated for symptom evaluation, PEFR at time of symptoms, and daily PEFR monitoring. Children who used PEFR meters when symptomatic had a lower severity score, fewer symptom days, and less health care utilization than children in the other two groups.
4. The results were partially dependent on ethnicity and socioeconomic status—with minority children and poor children showing the greatest improvement.[5]
5. A prospective randomized trial of 134 adults with moderate asthma and normal POD were managed with symptom or peak flow monitoring and followed for 12 months. There were significant improvements in hospitalization rate, emergency department visits, days off from school or work and PD_{20} histamine values, but there were no between-group differences.[6]

D. National and international asthma guidelines stipulate the need for spirometry in patients with persistent asthma. However, reimbursement and logistical access barriers continue to inhibit widespread use of spirometry, and unfortunately, most patients are never evaluated for FVC, FEV_1, or $FEF_{25\%-75\%}$ during any stage of their care.

E. Despite the fact that peak flowmeters measure airflow through large but not small airways, peak flow remains a useful surrogate for FEV_1 for diagnosis. Meters are inexpensive and easy to use, which makes them a practical way to measure airway function.

F. Reversible airflow obstruction occurs when the airway is compromised either by bronchospasm or by inflammation (or both). At its mildest level of severity, asthma is primarily characterized by exaggerated diurnal oscillations in peak flow. This circadian peak flow variability (low in the morning and high at midday) is less than 20% both in subjects *without* asthma and in asthmatics in optimal control.

G. When the diagnosis of asthma is unclear, a 24-hour peak flow variation greater than 20% is diagnostic of unsta-

ble asthma. For many patients, peak flow variability greater than 10% is associated with asthma symptoms. The range of peak flow variation in stable asthmatics can vary from 10% to 20%, levels that may be indistinguishable from those in subjects *without* asthma.

VIII. Symptom-Based Management versus Peak Flow–Based Self-Care

A. Symptom-based asthma management works well enough to allow many patients to self-medicate and avoid most adverse events. Unfortunately, patients vary widely in their ability to discriminate and perceive symptoms and to know when to start or step up medications.

B. About one-fourth of patients have a significantly low POD and tend to underreport symptoms. These patients are prone to undermedicate themselves and are at greater risk for adverse events than patients with normal POD.

About one-fifth of patients are high-POD patients and may feel tight when their peak flows are close to normal. That means that about 50% of asthmatics are reasonably aware of their symptoms and capable of making symptom-based management work well on a consistent basis.

C. Unfortunately, it is not easy to identify low- or high-POD patients a priori because misperception of symptoms often goes unrecorded. Consequently, most discoveries of low- or high-POD problems occur serendipitously during routine follow-up visits or during impending crises when it is evident that the patient made one or more mistakes (e.g., delayed a step-up because the patient felt comfortable and didn't bother to check peak flows).

D. The major physiologic basis for peak flow monitoring is the relationship between peak flow variability and the likelihood of an impending asthmatic exacerbation. Patients with stable asthma tend to have normal or near normal peak flow variability, just like subjects without asthma. When variability significantly exceeds a normal range, airways become unstable, prompting the need for more aggressive management.

E. Although there are many inherent study design limitations in various studies testing the value of written plans based on symptoms or peak flow, a Cochrane review of 25 studies concluded that written actions significantly benefited a number of different self-management programs.[7]

1. The 2002 Executive Summary of the National Asthma Education and Prevention Program Expert Panel Report concurs:

"It is the opinion of the Expert Panel that the use of written action plans as part of an overall effort to educate patients in self-management is recommended, especially for patients with moderate or severe persistent asthma and patients with a history of severe exacerbations."

2. The Executive Summary also concludes that

"peak flow monitoring for patients with moderate or severe persistent asthma should be considered because it may enhance clinician-patient communication and may increase patient and caregiver awareness of the disease status and control."

F. At Kaiser Permanente, written action plans with both symptom and peak flow monitoring have been systematically incorporated as an important tool within a comprehensive toolbox containing a variety of self-management educational strategies (see Fig. 18-3). The learning curves for peak flow monitoring for both providers and patients vary considerably, and full mastery may require years of gradual event-by-event learning.

G. Successful action plans may be written or provided orally. Each form has self-evident advantages and disadvantages. Unintentional sabotage of peak flow–driven plans can occur in all clinical settings, and consistent reinforcement is the operative strategy. Written plans need not be limited to handouts. Prescription labels for asthma medications can be linked to specific peak flow values (e.g., prednisone, 20 mg, one tablet twice daily for 5 days if peak flow <240). Peak flowmeters are now commonly color-coded to coincide with written plans.

H. Establishing the patient's best peak flow is a fundamental necessity for home monitoring. No less significant is the need to know the patient's best peak flow variability, which may range from 5% to 20%.

1. For screening, a value of 80% of predicted is the traditional cutoff between normal and asthmatic peak flows. However, the cutoff between normal and abnormal peak flow variability is less easily normed.
2. If the patient is accustomed to a 5%–10% peak flow variability on a good day, written plans that cue a yellow zone backup plan only if the peak flow dips below 80% will put the patient at risk for a belated intervention.
3. For some patients, a green/yellow cutoff of 90% may be unrealistic. Trial and error may best determine whether a patient will benefit from a 90% or 80% green/yellow zone transition.

I. Having established the best ever peak flow and best possible peak flow variability, a written home monitoring plan should establish simple rules for stepping up medications when the peak flow dips to different levels.

1. A green/yellow/red zone strategy reinforces the need to recognize separate but interlinked medication plans

when the patient's peak flow variability is normal, moderately abnormal, or severely abnormal.

2. The boundaries between green/yellow and yellow/red can be individualized to some degree and the final numbers can be rounded off for the sake of simplicity. We customarily use 50% or 60% of best peak flow as the boundary between the yellow and red zones. Subject to trial and error, the green/yellow boundary is set somewhere between 80% and 90%.

J. The medication rules for each zone need to be validated for each patient and periodically reviewed from time to time. Rapidly growing children will outgrow their best peak flow, and outdated self-care plans can contribute to delayed interventions.

K. The simplicity of a green/yellow/red zone-based system of self-care belies the complexity of the underlying decision making that the patient must gradually master.

1. The frequency for checking peak flows varies according to the patient's overall stability. Daily peak flow checks are critical when the patient's asthma is first assessed, is unstable, or is likely to become unstable, such as at the onset of the pollen season or the beginning of a viral upper respiratory tract infection. At other times, when the asthma is stable, periodic, once or twice weekly spot checks may suffice.
2. A yellow zone peak flow dip cues the need to step up the dose of an anti-inflammatory medication. However, the patient also needs to understand the optimal time course for the backup plan to kick in—or risk worsening if the step-up is not effective and further interventions are delayed. If the step-up is effective, the patient also needs to know when it is advisable to resume the green zone plan. As important as these concepts are, it is not easy to incorporate all of them into a written plan.
3. Given the prevalence of low-POD asthmatics, it may be said that asthma "attacks" develop gradually but are noticed suddenly.
4. Yellow zone peak flows usually improve after only a few days of starting or stepping up inhaled corticosteroids. Long-standing yellow zone peak flows (present for months or years of undertreatment) may not respond to bronchodilators, suggesting significant airway inflammation or even possible irreversible airway remodeling.
5. Fifty percent red zone dips need to be carefully defined as a prebronchodilator assessment. Otherwise patients may mistakenly defer a burst of oral corticosteroids because the postbronchodilator peak flow falls into the yellow zone. Life-threatening asthma attacks are almost avoidable if the steroid burst is

started within a few hours of the first yellow/red transition. Semi-acute red zone dips that don't improve significantly within 1–2 days of starting a burst of steroids should prompt the consideration of occult sinusitis.

L. Unintentional errors by patients, providers, or medical staff can critically undermine the appropriateness of office and home decision making.

1. The patient's personal best peak flow may never have been determined, and the difference between the yet-to-be-determined best value and the predicted value may be significant.
2. In the absence of readily documented best peak flows in the medical record, patients may recall inaccurate or outdated best peak flow values.
3. Peak flowmeters may be accompanied by nomograms based on published data from other brands of meters, introducing the risk of significant errors in the assessment of stability.
4. Lack of peak flow education may result in providers failing to interpret the significance of low peak flow values.
5. Asthma affects large and small airways and not always symmetrically. Monitoring FEV_1 in the office is no less important than tracking peak flow trends at home.

M. Fortunately, once these pitfalls are overcome, the patient can make most asthma self-management decisions with appropriate mentoring by the asthma care provider. With time, most critical decisions can be mentored over the phone, with selective office-based follow-up for atypical or very severe exacerbations. Routine follow-up visits offer valuable opportunities to monitor the patient's self-care skills, seasonal changes in asthma, and monitor small airway obstruction with office spirometery.

IX. Keeping Things in Perspective: The Cycle of Asthma Care

A. Assessment

In practice, we tend to treat reversible peak flows with lower doses of IAI medications than we treat airways that are more inflamed and do not respond to a SABA. The exception to this rule is a low peak flow that approaches or dips just below 50%. These dips get treated with several days of oral corticosteroids, *regardless* of the postbronchodilator improvement.

B. Getting the Patient Back to Normal

There are many pitfalls and barriers to getting back to normal: underassessment of severity with accompanying undertreatment, noncompliance, premature resumption of a green zone strategy, and untreated occult sinusuitis, to name a few.

It is imperative to document that the unstable patient actually gets back to normal by validating the return of normal peak flow variability with home monitoring and arranging for an office follow-up visit to ascertain small airway recovery.

C. Keeping the Patient Stable

For almost all patients, daily peak flow checks are *not* a realistic strategy 365 days a year. Instead, we try encouraging selective vigilance and random spot checks.

1. Early morning peak flow checks can detect the earliest sign of peak flow hypervariability.
2. Midday checks are not suitable for routine surveillance monitoring since abnormal early morning peak flow dips may self-correct by midday.

D. Keeping the Peak Flow Normal

In theory, making sure the peak flow stays normal should be the easiest step of the self-regulatory cycle. However, in practice this is the most common stage for self-sabotage. Stable patients tend to have an unerring belief that they will "know" when it is time to resume peak flow monitoring. They forget to check peak flow values when they feel well—only to discover that their perception of dyspnea is faulty, with attendant "sudden and unexpectedly" low peak flow crashes.

For low-POD patients with arguably the greatest need for self-monitoring, the learning curve for home monitoring can be long and slow but, with perseverance, ultimately successful.

REFERENCES

1. Jackson AC: Accuracy, reproducibility, and variability of portable peak flowmeters. Chest 1995;107:648–651.
2. Nelson HS: Asthma guidelines and outcomes. In Middleton E Jr, et al (eds): Allergy: Principles and Practice, pp 930–933. St. Louis: Mosby; 1998.
3. Magadle R, Berar-Yanay N, Weiner P: The risk of hospitalization and near-fatal and fatal asthma in relation to the perception of dyspnea. Chest 2002;121:329–333.
4. Bheekie A, Syce JA, Weinberg EG: Peak expiratory flow rate and symptom self-monitoring of asthma initiated from community pharmacies. J Clin Pharm Ther 2001;4:287–296.
5. Yoos HL, Kitzman H, McMullen A, et al: Symptom monitoring in childhood asthma: A randomized clinical trial comparing peak expiratory flow rate with symptom monitoring. Ann Allergy Asthma Immunol 2002;88:283–291.
6. Adams RJ, Boath K, Homan S, et al: A randomized trial of peak-flow and symptom-based action plans in adults with moderate-to-severe asthma. Respirology 2001;6:297–304.
7. Gibson PG, Coughlan J, Wilson AJ, et al: Self-management education and regular practitioner review for adults with asthma (Cochrane Review). The Cochrane Library, Issue 4, 2002. Oxford, U.K.: Update Software.

Black Walnut *Courtesy of Hollister-Stier Laboratory*

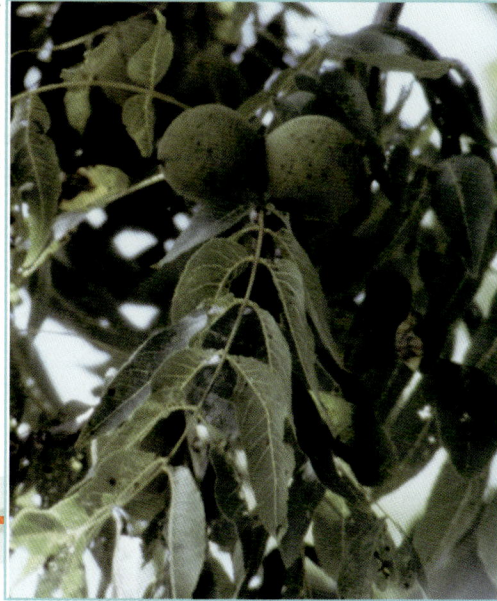

CHAPTER 19
Rhinolaryngoscopy

Etan C. Milgrom

I. Introduction

Flexible fiber-optic rhinolaryngoscopy is a safe, convenient, and effective procedure for examining the upper airway. Anatomical structures (Fig. 19-1 and Box. 19-1) that normally cannot be viewed with the usual nasal and oral specula can be easily identified using the direct rhinolaryngoscope. The vocal cords, larynx, pharynx, and surrounding structures can be more readily and comfortably visualized than with indirect mirrors or rigid telescopes. This relatively simple technique gives the well-trained clinician a whole new perspective and approach to the diagnosis and management of upper airway pathology.

II. Indications

A. For a primary care clinician, probably the most important role of flexible rhinolaryngoscopy is in screening for and identifying cancers of the head and neck.

1. Specifically, this would include patients who have a significant history of smoking and who complain of chronic or recurrent hoarseness and persistent unexplained unilateral nosopharyngeal pain.

2. Other symptoms that might suggest cancer include hemoptysis, dysphagia, odynophagia, malaise, and unexplained weight loss.

B. From an allergic perspective, the most common indications for rhinolaryngoscopy include chronic sinusitis, sinus discomfort, chronic postnasal drip, chronic rhinitis, and nasal obstruction of unknown etiology. These and other indications are listed in Box 19-2.

III. Contraindications

A. Although the procedure is relatively easy to perform and free of complications or contraindications, several potential risks should be kept in mind and addressed with patients before the procedure is performed.

1. Special attention should be paid to patients with an acute illness, adverse reactions to decongestants or topical anesthetics, blood dyscrasias, or other chronic debilitating illnesses.

2. As with any procedure, aside from the required appropriate history taking and preprocedural head and neck examination, informed consent needs to be obtained.

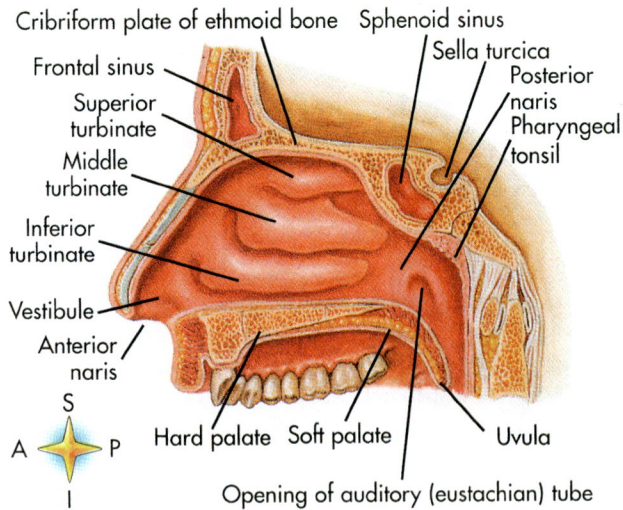

A

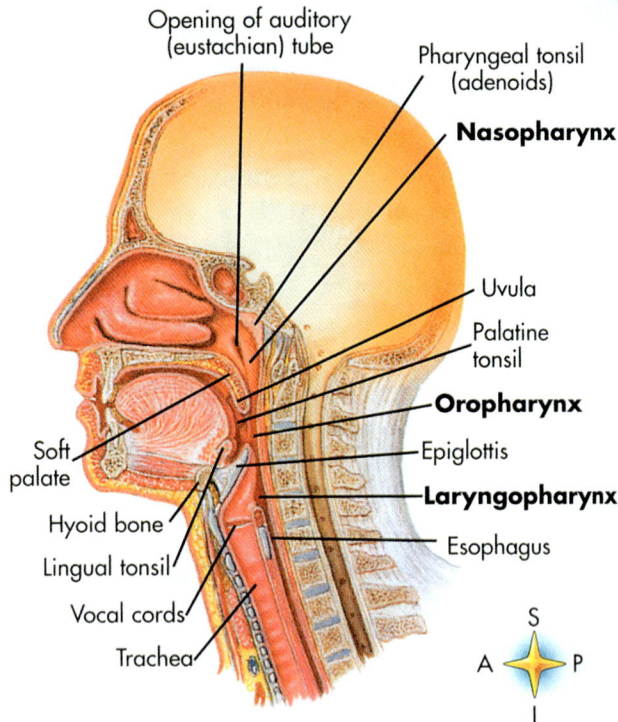

B

Figure 19-1 **A**, Schematic cross-section of the nasal cavity. **B**, Schematic cross-section of the pharynx. (From Thibodeau G, Patton K: Anthony's Textbook of Anatomy and Physiology, 16th ed. St. Louis: Mosby, 1999. Reproduced with permission.)

3. Side effects and complications need to be carefully explained to patients.

B. Furthermore, proper patient education materials should be given to and discussed with all patients undergoing this procedure (see Patient Education section).

1. ***Contraindications***
   a. Acute epiglottitis
   b. Impending airway obstruction

c. Blood dyscrasias
d. Hypersensitivity to topical anesthetics

2. ***Complications***
   a. Adverse reactions to decongestants and anesthetics
   b. Sneezing and coughing
   c. Gagging
   d. Bleeding

BOX 19-1

Normal Anatomic Structures of Importance in the Upper Airway

Nasal fossa (see Fig. 19-1A)
Septum and nasal floor (Fig. 19-2)
Turbinates
  Inferior
  Middle (Fig. 19-3)
  Superior (Fig. 19-4)
  Supreme
Sinus orifices
  Frontal
  Anterior ethmoidal
  Maxillary
  Posterior ethmoidal
  Sphenoidal
Nasolacrimal duct

Nasopharynx, superior oropharynx
(see Fig. 19-1B)
Eustachian orifice, torus tubarius (Figs. 19-5 and 19-6)
Rosenmueller's fossa (Fig. 19-7)
Adenoids
Pharyngeal wall
Soft palate
Uvula (Fig. 19-8)

Inferior oropharynx, oropharynx, hypopharynx (see Fig. 19-1B)
Posterior tongue (Fig. 19-9)
Lingular tonsil (Fig. 19-10)
Pharyngeal wall
Vallecula (see Fig. 19-9)
Piriform sinuses (Fig. 19-11)
Glottic structures
  Larynx (Fig. 19-12)
  Epiglottis (see Fig. 19-9)
  True and false vocal cords (Figs. 19-13 and 19-14)
  Arytenoids, para-arytenoid structures
  Subglottis
  Trachea (Fig. 19-15)

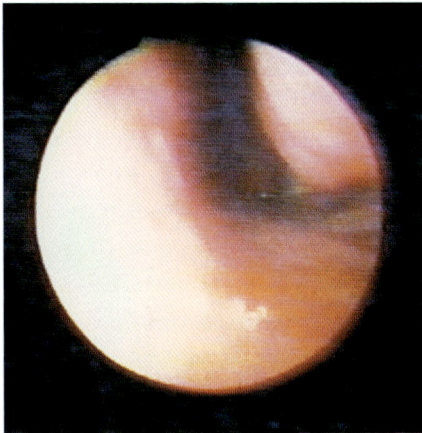

Figure 19-2 In this view, the nasal floor appears below, the left middle turbinate at the upper right, and the nasal septum to the left. (From Welch Allyn. Reproduced with permission ©2003.)

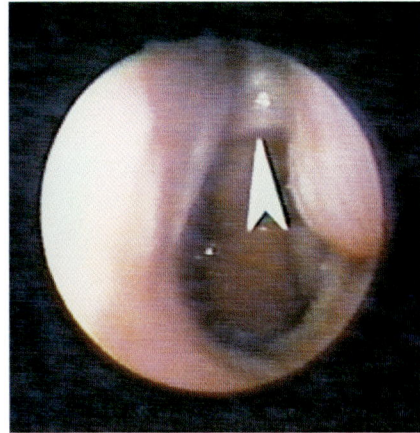

Figure 19-3 Arrow points to the choana, the opening to the pharynx. (From Welch Allyn. Reproduced with permission ©2003.)

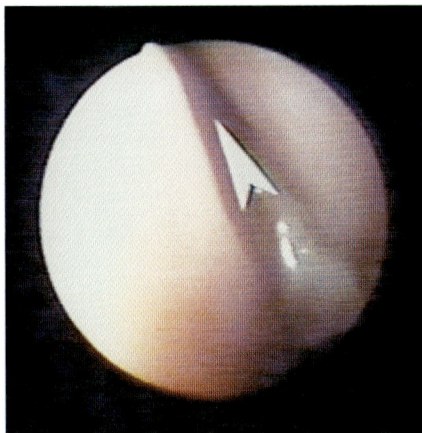

Figure 19-4 Arrow points to sphenoethmoid recess. (From Welch Allyn. Reproduced with permission ©2003.)

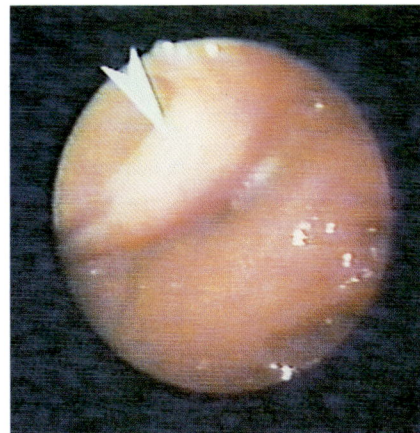

Figure 19-5 Arrow points to torus tubarius. Just to the right are Rosenmueller's fossa and the adenoidal pad. (From Welch Allyn. Reproduced with permission ©2003.)

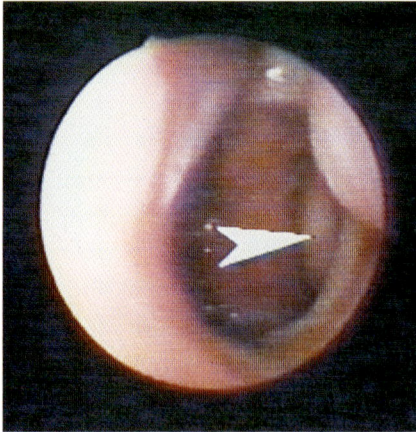

Figure 19-6 Arrow points to the left torus tubarius from a different angle as the scope enters the nasal cavity and passes under the inferior turbinate. In the upper right corner is the tip of the left middle turbinate. (From Welch Allyn. Reproduced with permission ©2003.)

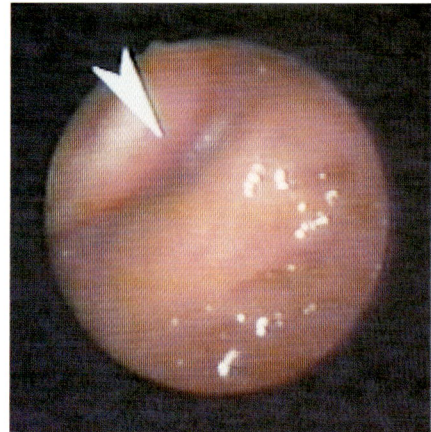

Figure 19-7 Arrow points to Rosenmueller's fossa. Pharyngeal tumors most commonly originate in this recess. (From Welch Allyn. Reproduced with permission ©2003.)

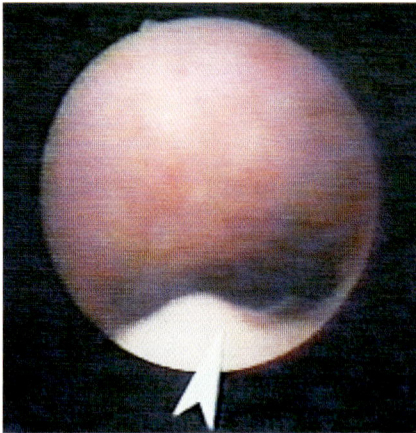

Figure 19-8 Arrow points to the uvula. This is the first structure seen as the tip of the scope is deflected downward after entering the posterior pharynx. (From Welch Allyn. Reproduced with permission ©2003.)

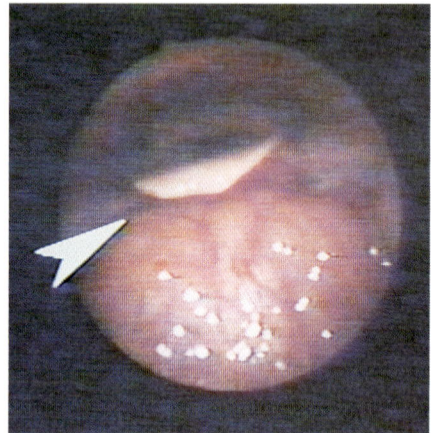

Figure 19-9 Arrow points to base of the tongue and the epiglottis. The space between these two structures is called the valeculla. (From Welch Allyn. Reproduced with permission ©2003.)

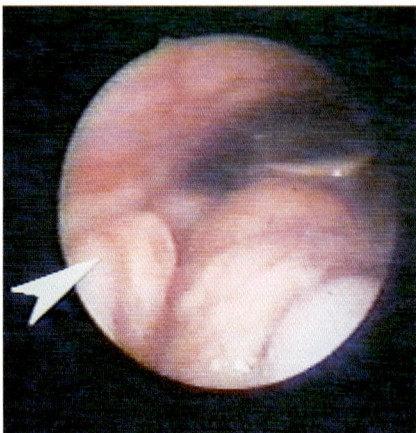

Figure 19-10 Arrow points to the lingular tonsil. (From Welch Allyn. Reproduced with permission ©2003.)

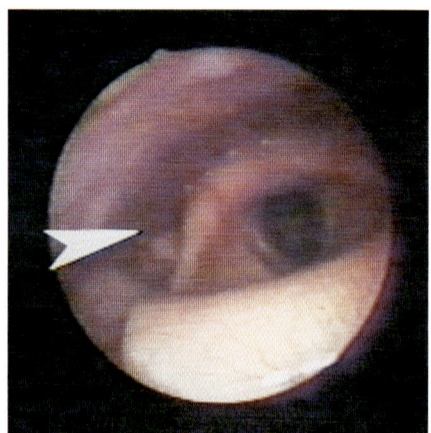

Figure 19-11 Arrow points to the right piriform sinus. (From Welch Allyn. Reproduced with permission ©2003.)

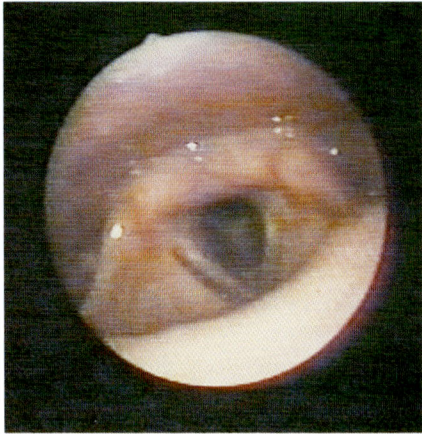

Figure 19-12 Full view of the larynx. (From Welch Allyn. Reproduced with permission ©2003.)

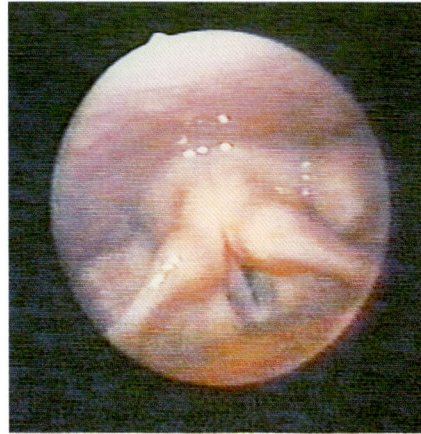

Figure 19-14 View of the larynx during phonation, which allows the vocal cords to come together. (From Welch Allyn. Reproduced with permission ©2003.)

   e. Laryngospasm
   f. Reflex hypertension
   g. Vasovagal hypotension

IV. Required Instrumentation and Anesthesia

A. Ephedrine 1% or oxymetazoline (Afrin) or 0.05% Neosynephrine or 0.5% cocaine in spray dispenser.

B. Lidocaine 4% (mixed in nasalcrom or nasal steroid sprayer in a 1 : 1 dilution becomes a 2% lidocaine mixture) (benzodiazepines and narcotics not necessary).

C. Viscous lidocaine to apply to scope for lubrication and topical anesthesia (optional).

D. Fiber-optic rhinolaryngoscope (Fig. 19-16) with appropriate light source.

V. Procedure

A. Before undergoing any procedure it is important to discuss with patients indications and complications of the procedure prior to obtaining a signed consent.

  1. The first step in the procedure should include a routine speculum examination to identify the most accessible and patent nasal passage.
  2. This should be followed by applying two sprays of ephedrine 1% to each nostril to induce vasoconstriction, followed by two sprays of lidocaine 2%–4% spray to each nostril for topical anesthesia.
  3. Viscous lidocaine 2% can be applied to the scope for lubrication and additional anesthesia, although this is optional. Some patients who are very relaxed and have a naturally patent nasal passage do not need any anesthetic at all.

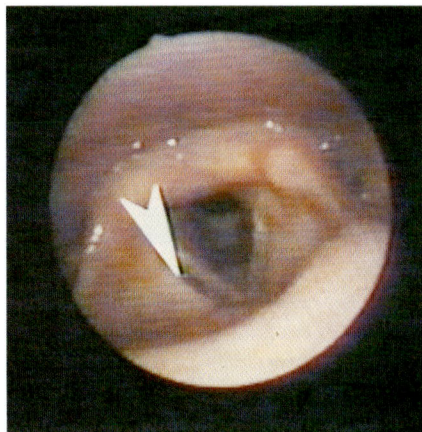

Figure 19-13 Arrow points to the false vocal cords. (From Welch Allyn. Reproduced with permission ©2003.)

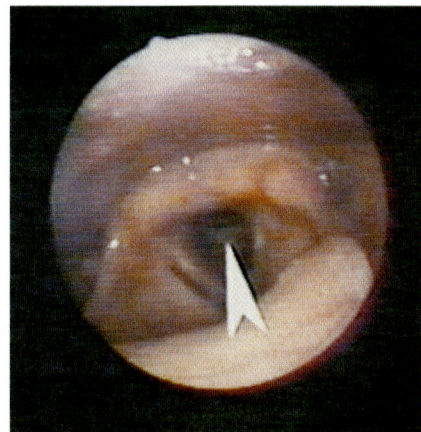

Figure 19-15 Arrow points to tracheal ring. (From Welch Allyn. Reproduced with permission ©2003.)

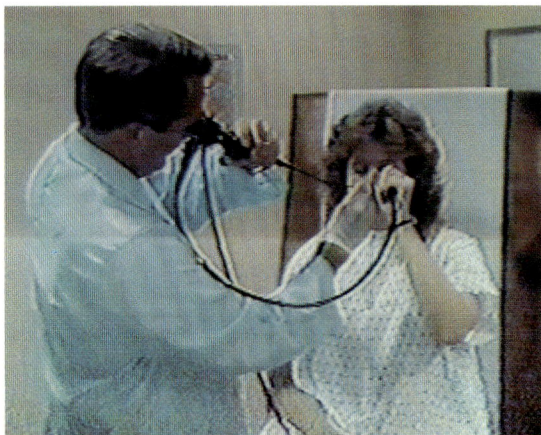

Figure 19-16 Patient in correct sitting position being examined by a physician with a fiber-optic rhinolaryngoscope. The patient is also watching the progress of the procedure with the aid of an accessory teaching scope. (From Welch Allyn. Reproduced with permission ©2003.)

4. The patient should be placed in the sitting position with the head leaning against a head rest to avoid sudden jolting away from rhinolaryngoscope during the procedure (see Fig. 19-16).

5. If there is a video hookup with the scope, the patient can be positioned facing the screen in order to view the anatomy during the examination (see Fig. 19-16). Patients may prefer not to see the examination and therefore should be asked whether they desire such a setup.

6. Patients should be told not to swallow during the procedure but reassured that if they swallow, it will not harm them. It is also advantageous to have patients breathe through their mouth rather than their nose during the procedure because nasal breathing is more likely to fog up the scope.

7. The scope should rest in the clinician's hand on the angle between the index finger and thumb so that the first finger is free to manipulate the angulation tip on the scope (Fig. 19-17). The fifth finger of the clinician's other hand rests gently against the patient's face, with the thumb, index, and second digit helping to guide the scope through the nasal passage.

8. The hand touching the face should control the movement of the tip of the scope through the nasal passage and should maintain contact with the patient's face throughout the course of the procedure.

9. It is recommended to advance the scope to its end point, then observe anatomy and structures methodically as the scope is withdrawn. However, this is not required for good results, and in fact, many clin-

icians prefer to observe the anatomy as the scope is placed in the nares.

10. It is paramount to advance the scope along the floor of the cavity below the turbinate and avoid making contact with the scope against the nasal septum because this will cause discomfort to the patient. Additional effort should be made to avoid touching the scope against the pharynx because this might induce the gag reflex, which will make the examination more difficult for both the patient and the physician.

11. Advance the scope along the posterior pharyngeal wall (without touching it) over the uvula until the larynx is in full view. The angulation tip should be pushed forward to move the scope tip inferiorly (see Fig. 19-17) until the larynx is in full view. This is the end of the scope insertion and where careful examination begins. As the laryngeal structures are observed, the clinician should ask the patient to phonate (say, "eee") to observe vocal cord mobility.

12. As the scope is withdrawn to the level of the posterior pharynx, the clinician observing the torus tubarius on the ipsilateral side can observe the contralateral torus tubarius as well. This is accomplished by deflecting the tip of the scope downward and rotating the hand holding the head of the scope (Fig. 19-18) in the ipsilateral direction.

13. Another scope manipulation is required once the scope is withdrawn proximal to the choana. At this point the tip of the scope should be deflected upward in order to observe the superior sphenoethmoid structures (Fig. 19-19).

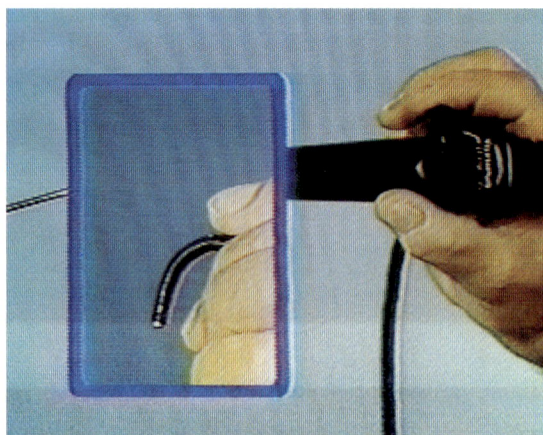

Figure 19-17 Rhinolaryngoscope correctly positioned in the examiner's hand, cradled between the first finger and thumb. Note downward deflection of the tip of the scope. (From Welch Allyn. Reproduced with permission ©2003.)

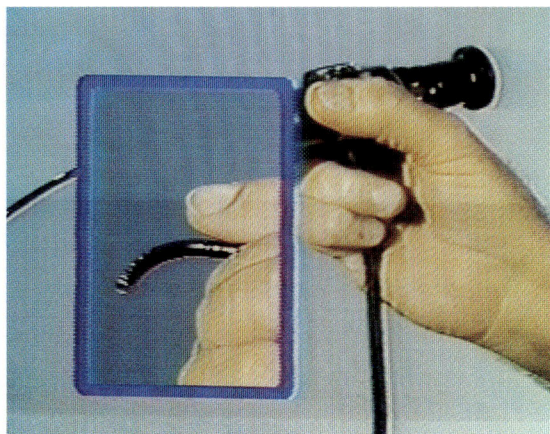

Figure 19-18 The rhinolaryngoscope is manipulated to view anatomical structures on the contralateral side during the examination of the pharynx. (From Welch Allyn. Reproduced with permission ©2003.)

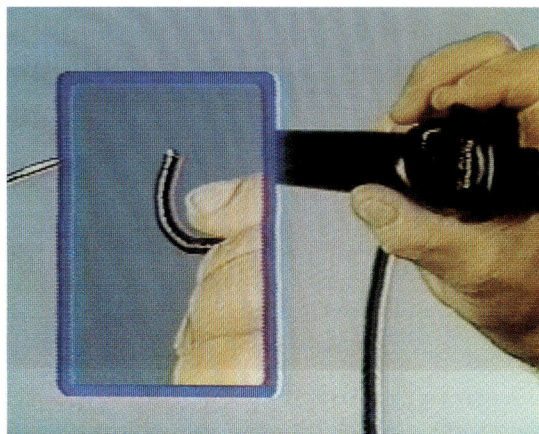

Figure 19-19 During the examination of the sphenoethmoid recess, the tip of the scope is deflected upward. (From Welch Allyn. Reproduced with permission ©2003.)

14. Refer to the CD provided with this text, which contains a video segment on the rhinolaryngoscopy procedure.

VI. Cleaning the Scope

At the end of the procedure, the scope must be properly cleaned. Most scopes come with cleansing guidelines. These guidelines generally include wiping with soap and water, 70% isopropyl alcohol, as well as inserting the scope into sporicidin-like solutions for a minimum of 10 minutes.

VII. Interpreting and Recording the Results

Rhinolaryngoscopy is not hard to perform. The difficult part is developing the skill and experience to differentiate normal anatomy (see Box 19-1 and Fig. 19-1) from abnormal pathology (Box 19-3; see CD provided with this text for video of abnormal pathology.)

In addition to identifying abnormal structures, the clinician should pay special attention to the color, appearance, mobility, and function of each pertinent structure (e.g., vocal cords), and to any abnormal exudates, which may help identify pathology (e.g., sinusitis, gastroesophageal reflux). If polyps are present, their nature and extent should be characterized, especially if treatment is anticipated. Refer to the CD provided with this text, which includes a short video segment on how to perform the direct rhinolaryngoscopic exam.

Proper procedural documentation is crucial, not only for medical-legal reasons, but for appropriate chart record-ing, follow-up, and patient care. Box 19-4 shows one format for documenting the procedure.

VIII. Patient Education[1]

A. What Is Rhinolaryngoscopy?

Direct fiber-optic rhinopharyngolaryngoscopy is a method for examining the nose and throat from the inside with a flexible, thin fiber-optic scope. Usual methods, which involve using a light source and a tongue blade, allow examination only of the anterior part of the nose and the back of the throat above the tongue. Indirect rhinolargoscopy involves placing a tiny mirror in the back of the throat and angling the mirror toward the larynx (voice box) to view the internal anatomy. This technique often stimulates the gag reflex, which is uncomfortable for the

---

BOX 19-3

Common Pathologies of the Nose, Ear, Pharynx, and Larynx

Nasal polyp (Fig. 19-20)
Upper respiratory and sinus infection (Fig. 19-21)
Deviated septum (Fig. 19-22)
Vocal cord paralysis (Fig. 19-23)
Carcinoma of the vocal cords (Fig. 19-24)
Adenoid stellate scar (Fig. 19-25)
Interior of maxillary sinus (Fig. 19-26)
Perforated tympanic membrane (Fig. 19-27)
Enlarged adenoidal tissue (Fig. 19-28)

BOX 19-4

Medical Report for Fiber-optic Nasolaryngoscopy

Patient's name_____

        Date_____

Patient's age_____ Sex M_____ F_____   Examining physician_____

Medical record number_____

        Assistant_____

Indication for procedure (circle those that apply):

(*ICD-9 Codes in Parentheses*)

1. Chronic hoarseness (476.0)
2. Chronic postnasal drip (477.8)
3. Chronic rhinitis (472.0)
4. Chronic sinusitis (473.0)
5. Foreign body, possible (478.79*)
6. Nasal bleeding (784.7)
7. Nasal polyp(s) (471.0)

    8. Obstruction (478.79*)
    9. Suspected tumor (235.6)
  10. Surveillance, cancer (V10.21)
  11. Vocal cord polyp (478.4)
  12. Chronic cough (491.0)
  13. Other_____

         _____

Billing requires report.

Medications used (circle those that apply):

1. Phenylephrine (spray or drops)
2. Cocaine, 4–10%
3. Lidocaine 2% gargle
4. Diazepam premedication

  5. Lidocaine spray
  6. Analgesic premedication
  7. Nothing used
  8. Other_____

    _____

    _____

Examined (place check mark beside those that apply):

One nostril_____ Both nostrils_____ Oral route_____ All_____

Findings (circle those that apply and identify location [i.e., left or right]):

1. Normal examination
2. Acute inflammation
3. Angiodysplasia
4. Bleeding site
5. Chronic rhinitis
6. Chronic sinusitis
7. Foreign body

    8. Malignancy
    9. Polyp
  10. Vocal cord lesion
  11. Obstruction
  12. Vocal cord paralysis
  13. Mucosa abnormal, nonspecific
  14. Mass (describe)_____

Procedure time (time scope was in patient)_____(minutes)

Any complications? No_____ Yes_____ If yes, please describe

_____

_____

Diagnosis after procedure_____

Patient tolerance_____

Examination performed as above.

_____, M.D.

From Curry RW Jr: Flexible fiberoptic nasolaryngoscopy. Fam Pract Recertification 1990;12(6):21–36. Reproduced with permission.

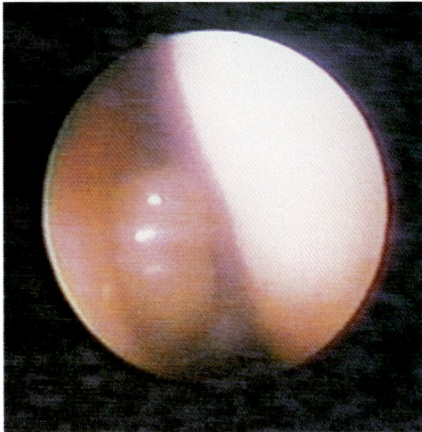

Figure 19-20 Nasal polyp. (From Welch Allyn. Reproduced with permission ©2003.)

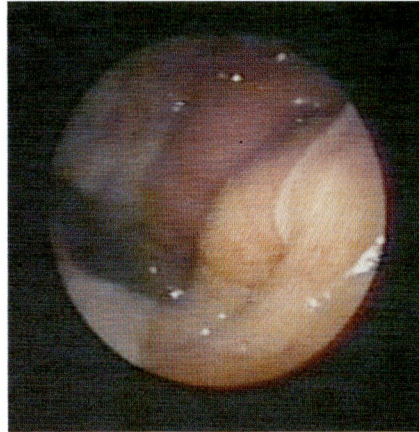

Figure 19-21 Upper respiratory infection with exudative pus dripping into the torus tubarius from the sinus ostia. (From Welch Allyn. Reproduced with permission ©2003.)

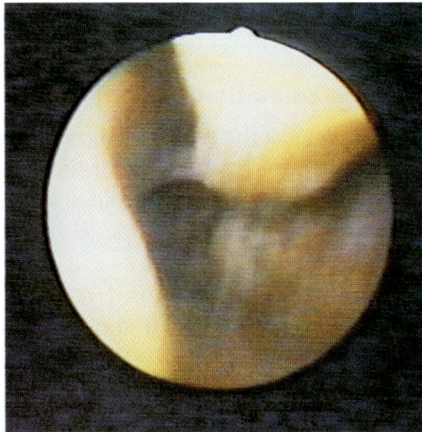

Figure 19-22 Deviated septum. (From Welch Allyn. Reproduced with permission ©2003.)

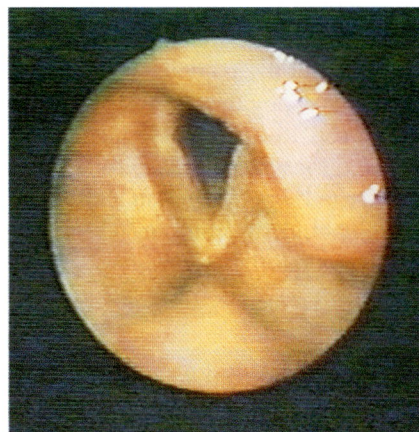

Figure 19-23 Vocal cord paralysis. Note left vocal cord is stuck in the closed position. (From Welch Allyn. Reproduced with permission ©2003.)

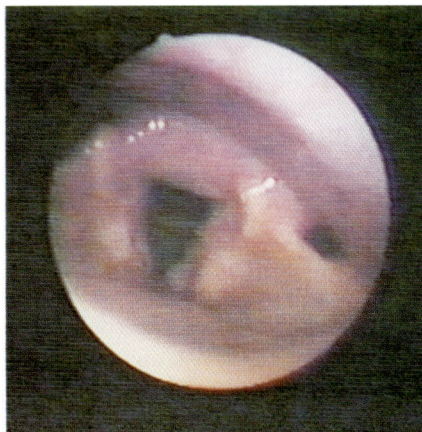

Figure 19-24 Vocal cord carcinoma. Early detection is crucial for a good therapeutic outcome. (From Welch Allyn. Reproduced with permission ©2003.)

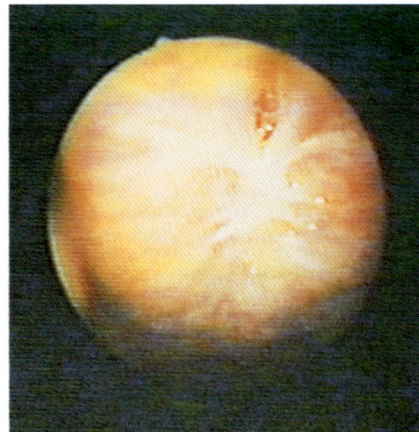

Figure 19-25 Stellate scar after an adenoidectomy. (From Welch Allyn. Reproduced with permission ©2003.)

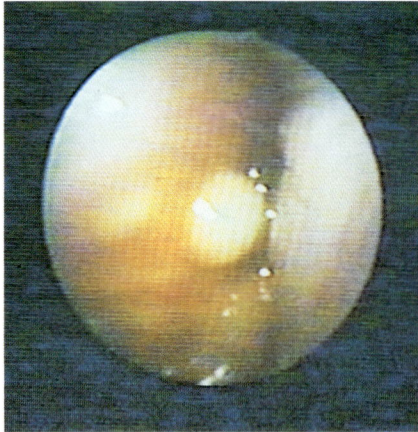

Figure 19-26 Mucous cyst inside sinus cavity that was visualized through antral window created by surgical procedure. (From Welch Allyn. Reproduced with permission ©2003.)

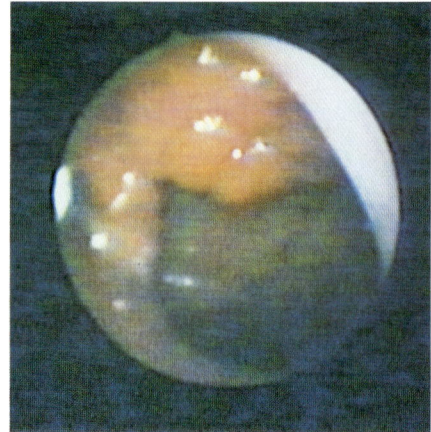

Figure 19-28 Enlarged adenoidal pad causing upper airway obstruction. (From Welch Allyn. Reproduced with permission ©2003.)

patient. In direct fiber-optic rhinolaryngoscopy the scope is inserted through the anesthetized nose, which is much more comfortable for the patient.

In rhinolaryngoscopy, the physician can examine most of the inside of the nose, the eustachian tube openings, the adenoids and tonsils, the throat, and the vocal cords. The procedure can be performed in children and adults. Small children should sit on a parent's lap. If the child is extremely uncomfortable and the examination is absolutely necessary, sedation can be provided, but this is rarely necessary.

B. What Is a Rhinoscope?

The rhinoscope is a small, flexible plastic tube with fiber-optics for viewing the airway. The rhinoscope can be attached to a television camera so that the patient and

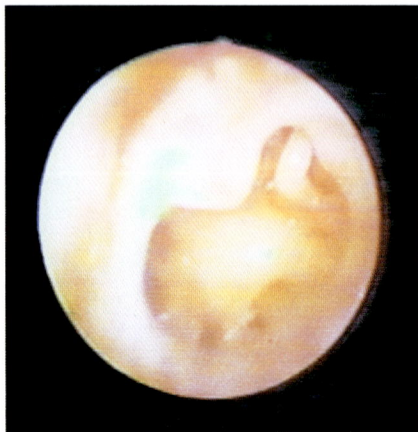

Figure 19-27 Perforated tympanic membrane visualized with a pediatric rhinolaryngoscope through the external ear canal. (From Welch Allyn. Reproduced with permission ©2003.)

physician can view the procedure while it is in progress, and to provide a permanent record of the examination.

C. What Is the Examination Like?

1. First, we decongest the nose with a nose spray, such as NeoSynephrine. Then a local anesthetic nose spray is sprayed in the nostril. We also place a topical anesthetic gel on the tip of the scope to help minimize any discomfort.
2. As the scope enters your nose, you will feel the presence of the scope, but it shouldn't hurt if the examination is performed properly.
3. Certain parts of the nasal examination can cause a pressure sensation if you have tight nasal passages. The pressure sensation can be painful. Be sure to tell the physician if you feel any pain during the procedure.
4. During the examination of the nose, it is helpful if you breathe through your mouth, so the scope does not fog up.
5. It is OK to cough or swallow during the examination, but it is preferable if you can avoid any movement.
6. Sometimes the local anesthetic drips down the back of the nose and numbs the back of the throat. This sensation may feel uncomfortable, but it only lasts a few minutes.
7. The entire procedure should take no more than 10–15 minutes. The physician can review the entire examination with you if it was recorded on videotape. Please don't hesitate to ask any questions throughout the process.

D. What If Something Is Wrong?

Should we find any abnormality that is not likely to respond to medication, or if we have questions about your examination, we will refer you to an ear, nose, and throat specialist.

REFERENCES

1. Selner JC: Concepts and clinical application of fiberoptic examination of the upper airway. Clin Rev Allergy 1988:6:303–320.
2. Curry RW Jr: Flexible fiberoptic nasolaryngoscopy. Family Pract Recert 1990;12(6):21–36.

OTHER SUGGESTED READING

Corey GA, Hocutt JE, Rodney WM: Preliminary study of rhinolaryngoscopy by family physicians. Family Med 1988;20:252–265.

DeWitt DE: Fiberoptic rhinolaryngoscopy in primary care. Postgrad Med 1988;84:85.

Milgrom EC: Rhinolaryngoscopy. In Rakel RE (ed): Manual of Medical Practice, 2nd ed. Philadelphia: WB Saunders, 2002.

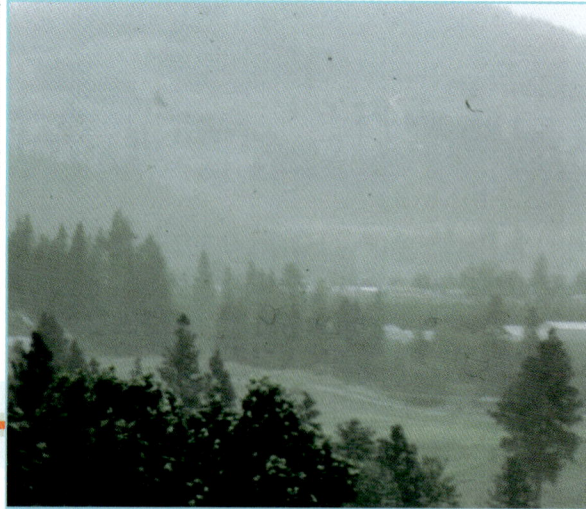

Pine Blooming *Courtesy of Hollister-Stier Laboratory*

CHAPTER 20

Allergen Patch Testing
Etan C. Milgrom

I. Introduction

Contact allergen patch testing is a simple, objective method for identifying allergic triggers in the environment that cause contact dermatitis. Box 20-1 lists different allergen categories of specific allergen triggers. Identifying the specific allergic trigger can help patients take appropriate steps to avoid exposure to the allergic agent that is causing their skin ailment. This procedure can also be used in the diagnostic workup of several diseases, including atopic dermatitis, seborrheic dermatitis, dyshydrotic eczema, stasis dermatitis, and psoriasis.[1–4]

II. Indications for Contact Allergy Patch Testing[2–4]

A. Eczema that is recalcitrant to therapy

B. Persistent and recurring eczema

C. Any suspected contact dermatitis

D. Hand eczema especially with dorsal presentation

E. Unusual presentation and location of eczema

F. Facial eczema, excluding seborrheic dermatitis

G. Foot and leg eczema

H. Perianal and perineal eczema

I. Chronic otitis externa

J. Discoid eczema

K. Atypical forms of eczema

III. Contraindications[3,4]

A. Do not apply to irritated, inflamed skin.

B. Do not apply if systemic and/or severe local reactions are known occur with any of the allergen testing components.

IV. Warnings[3,4]

A. Itching and burning sensation are common occurrences with contact allergen testing.

B. Medications may be necessary to alleviate symptoms.

C. On rare occasions it may be necessary to remove allergen patch tests earlier than expected due to severe reactions such as bullous eruptions, ulceration, and pronounced dermatitis.

BOX 20-1

Allergen Categories

Food
Nickel sulfate
Fragrance mix
Balsam of Peru

Rubber products
Carba mix
Black rubber mix
Mercaptobenzothiazole
Mercapto mix
Thiuram mix
p-Phenylenediamine

Cosmetics
Wool alcohol
Fragrance
Paraben
Cl + Me-isothiazolinone
Colophony
Balsam of Peru
Quaternium-15

Formaldehyde
p-Phenylenediamine
Thimerosal

Pharmaceuticals
Wool alcohol
Colophony
Balsam of Peru
Neomycin
Parabens
Thimerosal
Caine mix
Ethylenediamine
Cl + Me-isothiazolinone
Fragrance mix (topicals)
Quaternium-15

Clothing, shoes, jewelry
Nickel sulfate
Potassium dichromate
p-Phenylenediamine

Formaldehyde
Cobalt
p-tert-Butylphenol
  formaldehyde
Carba mix
Black rubber mix
Mercapto mix
Mercaptobenzothiazole
Thiuram

Cleaning products
Wool alcohol
Colophony
Formaldehyde
Epoxy resin
p-tert-Butylphenol
  formaldehyde
Fragrance mix

Manufacturing
Wool alcohol

Chromium salts
Colophony
Epoxy resins
Ethylenediamine
Cobalt
p-tert-Butylphenol
  formaldehyde
Cl + Me-isothiazolinone
Quaternium-15
Formaldehyde
p-Phenylenediamine
Nickel
Carba mix
Black rubber mix
Mercapto mix
Mercaptobenzothiazole
Thiuram

From Allerderm Laboratories, Inc. Reproduced with permission.

D. Contact sensitization may occur 7 days after testing without prior reactions.

E. Hyperpigmentation may occur at the test site during healing and usually resolves within 2–5 weeks.

V. Precautions[3,4]

A. Tanning or sunbathing prior to testing may interfere with interpretations of results.

B. Apply only to healthy skin that is free of disease or irritation.

C. Oral or topical steroids may inhibit the test results and should be avoided for 2 weeks prior to testing.

VI. Application of Patch Test Allergens[2,4]

A. The T.R.U.E. TEST allergen patch test comes in ready-to-use test panels, which are convenient to use and require no mixing or measuring (Boxes 20-2 and 20-3).

B. Ready-to-use test panels (Boxes 20-4 and 20-5) can be applied directly to nonhairy healthy skin, preferably on the patient's upper back. The outer surface of the upper arm may be used alternatively.

C. Hairy surfaces may need to be shaved prior to application.

D. Peel open the packaging and remove the test panel.

E. Remove the protective plastic covering without touching the testing substance.

F. Apply the test panel to a clean, flat test site and make sure each testing antigen is in direct contact with the skin (Fig. 20-1).

G. Label panels with pen marks to help identify positive and negative reactions.

H. Repeat the process with other test panels as needed. (see Chapter 4, Fig. 4-13).

I. Test panels should be kept dry for a minimum of 48 hours and removed at that time. A first reading should be performed at this time to identify any irritant reaction.

J. Results can be interpreted during a second reading anywhere between 72 and 96 hours after patch test application. The second reading is essential to differentiate allergic from irritant reactions.

VII. Interpretation of Results[2–4]

A. The allergen patch test should be read at 48 hours and 72–96 hours after application of the patch test material.

B. Some materials produce late reactions 4–5 days after application (neomycin sulfate and *p*-phenylenediamine) and may cause a black discoloration that may last up to 4 weeks.

BOX 20-2

T.R.U.E Test Composition

Allergens evenly incorporated in a hydrophilic gel.
No chance for cross reactivity.
Allergen dehydrated, then placed on flexible occlusive polyester backing.
TEWL and perspiration rehydrate allergen for quick penetration.
Numbered allergens are placed on surgical tape.
For accurate reading every time.
Uncoated polyester patch (negative control).
Useful for comparator in the interpretation of doubtful or minimal reactions.

From Allerderm Laboratories, Inc. Used with permission.

BOX 20-3

Unique Attributes of T.R.U.E. Test

Ready-to-use patch test system
Zero prep time
Lot-to-lot consistency
Consistent results with each patient
Standard consistent location
No staff mistakes when prepping tests
Dehydrated allergens
No cross-contamination or spills
Optimal dose of allergen
Reduced chance for false negative/false positive result

From Allerderm Laboratories, Inc. Used with permission.

BOX 20-4

T.R.U.E. Test Allergens—A

Nickel sulfate	Paraben mix
Wool alcohols	Negative control
Neomycin sulfate	Balsam of Peru
Potassium dichromate	Ethylenediamine dihydrochloride
Caine mix	
Fragrance mix	Cobalt dichloride
Colophony	

From Allerderm Laboratories, Inc. Used with permission.

BOX 20-5

T.R.U.E. Test Allergens—B

p-tert-Butylphenol formaldehyde resin	Mercaptobenzothiazole
	p-Phenylenediamine
Epoxy resin	(PPD)
Carba mix	Formaldehyde
Black rubber mix	Mercapto mix
Cl + Me-sothiazolinone	Thimerosal
Quaternium-15	Thiuram mix

From Allerderm Laboratories, Inc. Used with permission.

C. An identification template is provided with the T.R.U.E. TEST system that helps correlate the skin reactions with the appropriate antigen. Marks on the skin should correspond to the notches on the template.

D. The degree of reactivity is based on a method recommended by the International Dermatitis Research Group (Fig. 20-2). Note that the degree of reactivity is based on erythema, infiltration, and papular and vesicular patterns.

E. True positives are usually graded +++ or ++. As in skin testing, any true positive patch test result should correlate with a history of recent exposure to that particular antigen. Figure 20-3 exhibits a standard collection form for proper recording of test results.

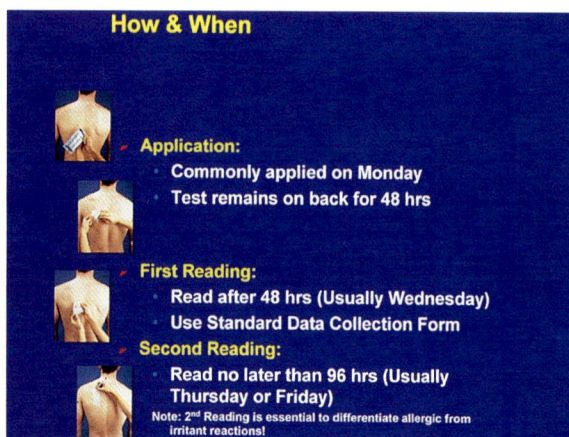

Figure 20-1 Method of applying T.R.U.E. TEST allergen patch test in ready-to-use test panels. (From Allerderm Laboratories, Inc. Reproduced with permission.)

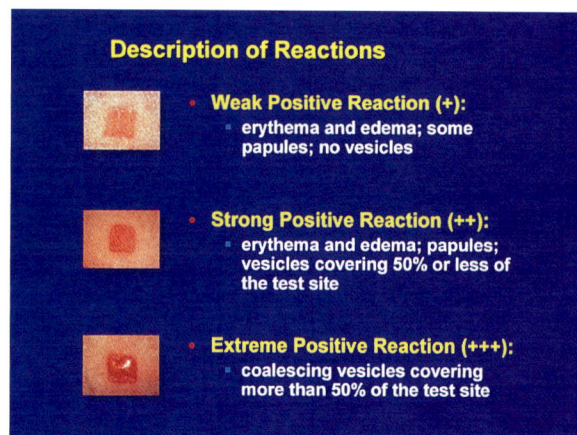

Figure 20-2 Assessment of degree of reactivity to allergen patch testing. (From Allerderm Laboratories, Inc. Reproduced with permission.)

Shade Involved Site

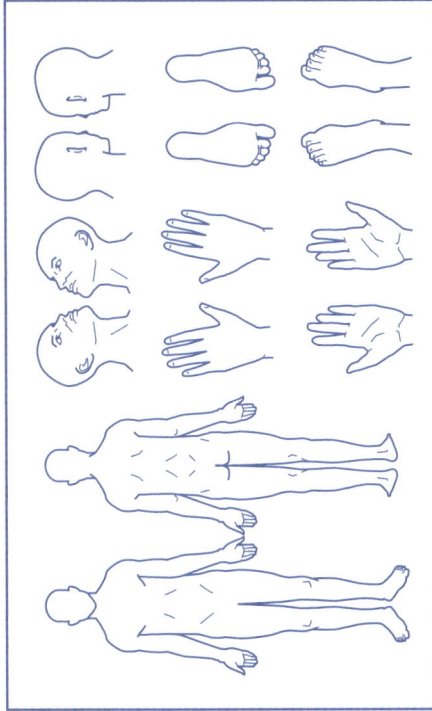

Patient _____ Age _____ Sex (M/F) _____ Race _____

Chart No _____

Physician _____

Address _____ Phone No. _____

City _____ State _____ Zip _____

Lot No. _____

Date Applied

| Date | 1st Reading |
| Date | 2nd Reading |

PANEL 1.1

1 = Nickel Sulfate
1st _____
2nd _____

2 = Wool Alcohols
1st _____
2nd _____

3 = Neomycin Sulfate
1st _____
2nd _____

4 = Potassium Dichromate
1st _____
2nd _____

5 = Caine Mix
1st _____
2nd _____

6 = Fragrance Mix
1st _____
2nd _____

7 = Colophony
1st _____
2nd _____

8 = Paraben Mix
1st _____
2nd _____

9 = Negative Control
1st _____
2nd _____

10 = Balsam of Peru
1st _____
2nd _____

11 = Ethylenediamine Dihydrochloride
1st _____
2nd _____

12 = Cobalt Dichloride
1st _____
2nd _____

PANEL 2.1

13 = p-tert Butylphenol Formaldehyde Resin
1st _____
2nd _____

14 = Epoxy Resin
1st _____
2nd _____

15 = Carba Mix
1st _____
2nd _____

16 = Black Rubber Mix
1st _____
2nd _____

17 = Cl+ Me– Isothiazolinone
1st _____
2nd _____

18 = Quaternium –15
1st _____

19 = Mercaptobenzo-thiazole
1st _____
2nd _____

20 = p-Phenylene-diamine
1st _____
2nd _____

21 = Formaldehyde
1st _____
2nd _____

22 = Mercapto Mix
1st _____
2nd _____

23 = Thimerosal
1st _____
2nd _____

24 = Thiuram Mix
1st _____
2nd _____

Positive Reactions

Allergen No.

Clinical Relevance

Present	Past	Unknown

Comments

Patch Test Appearance Codes For 1st and 2nd Reading:

1 = Weak (nonvesicular) Reaction: erythema, infiltration, possibly papules (+)

2 = Strong (edematous and vesicular) Reaction: erythema, edema, papules, and vesicles (++)

3 = Extreme (spreading, bulous, ulcerative) Reaction (+++)

4 = Doubtful Reaction, macular erythema only (?)

5 = Irritant Reaction (IR)

6 = Negative Reaction (–)

Figure 20-3 Standard data collection form used with the T.R.U.E. TEST allergen patch test system for proper recording of test results. (From Allerderm Laboratories, Inc. Reproduced with permission.)

221

Description of Reactions

- **Irritant Reaction (IR):**
  - fine wrinkling follicular papules; irregular and patchy pustules, confined to the test site; reactions fade within 48 hrs. (allergic reactions continue to develop)

- **Doubtful Reaction (?) or Negative Reaction (-):**
  - faint spotty erythema or homogenous erythema covering only a portion of the test site; some edema, no lesions

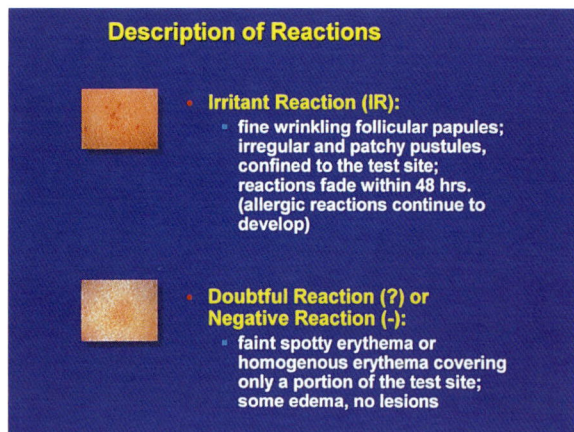

Figure 20-4 Irritant and true negative reactions to allergen patch testing. (From Allerderm Laboratories, Inc. Reproduced with permission.)

F. True negative reactions (25%–60%) are usually graded + and below and can help narrow the scope of clinical investigation.

G. False positive reactions (10%) may be caused by a strong positive reaction to an adjacent positive reaction, irritable skin, aged material or faulty storage, and acute dermatitis. False positive irritant reactions most commonly occur with metals and mixes.

H. False negative results can occur from poor application of the patch test antigen, ingestion or application of steroid medication within 2 weeks of the testing, and when test results are interpreted less than 72 hours after the initial application of the patch test material.

I. Irritant reactions usually appear within 48 hours after application of the patch test material and are more eczematous than vesicular (Fig. 20-4).

J. If the 23 T.R.U.E. TEST allergens are not sufficient for proper diagnosis, there are more than 300 allergens available, especially personal care products, through the use of Finn Chamber, which is the gold standard of patch testing.[5]

REFERENCES

1. Mydlarski PR, Katz AM, Sauder DN: Allergic contact dermatitis. In Middleton E Jr, et al (eds): Allergy Principles and Practice, 5th ed, pp 1135–1147. St. Louis: Mosby, 1998.
2. Werfel T, Kapp A: Atopic dermatitis and allergic contact dermatitis. In Holgate ST, Church MK, Lichtenstein LM (eds): Allergy, 2nd ed, pp 122–125. St. Louis: Mosby, 2001.
3. Allerderm Laboratories: Full Prescribing Information for T.R.U.E. TEST (Allergen Patch Test). Allerderm Laboratories, Petaluma, CA, May 2001.
4. Allerderm Laboratories: Reference Manual, Allergen Patch Test T.R.U.E. TEST. Allerderm Laboratories, Petaluma, CA, May 2001.
5. Trolab Patch Test Allergens—Omniderm. Hudson, Canada: Finn Chamber Products, 2001 (www.finnchambers.com).

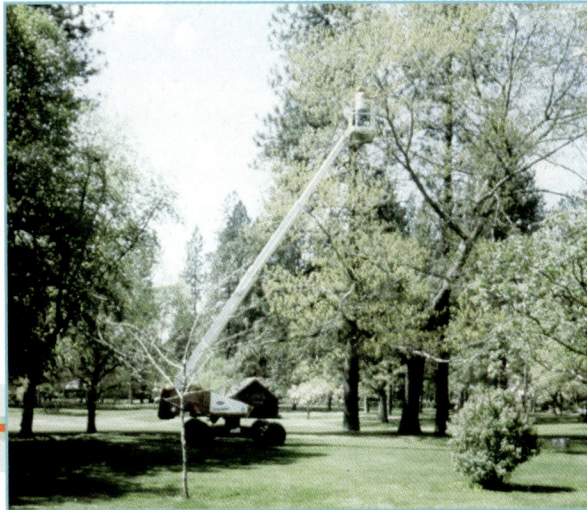

Red Oak (collecting) *Courtesy of Hollister-Stier Laboratory*

CHAPTER 21
Unconventional Allergy Practices

Abba I. Terr

I. Introduction

Allergic diseases are effectively managed by using methods of diagnosis and treatment based on sound scientific principles and validated by proper clinical trials. Unfortunately, there are a number of unconventional and unproved procedures, theories, and practices derived from anecdotal observations. These are either untested or have failed proper clinical trials; they should not be confused with *experimental* procedures of new and promising methods of diagnosis and treatment undergoing legitimate clinical trials.

II. Unconventional Theories of Allergy (Box 21-1)

Some of the theories on which unproven allergy practices rely are based on outmoded concepts of immunology and inflammation. Others invoke mechanisms, such as toxicity, that are not relevant to allergy, or they incorrectly attribute certain physical or psychiatric conditions to allergy.

A. Allergic Toxemia

The allergic toxemia theory postulates that allergens are inherently toxic and that subjective symptoms without

pathology can be attributed to allergy. In fact, allergens are not toxins, and allergic illnesses are inflammatory and not toxic in their pathogenesis. Proponents of allergic toxemia usually give this diagnosis to patients with multiple vague complaints, such as fatigue, anxiety, cognitive difficulties with memory and concentration, and a variety of physically unexplained pains and other bodily discomforts.

1. The "allergens" implicated are usually foods, food additives, drugs, drug additives, chemical pollutants, yeasts, and fungi. This syndrome has also been referred to as the *allergic tension fatigue syndrome*[1] and sometimes as *cerebral allergy*.[2] No definitive controlled studies justify the existence of such a syndrome.
2. The allergic toxemia concept has also been applied to certain recognized psychiatric conditions, especially food colors and preservatives as a cause of attention deficit disorder (ADD) in children[3] and wheat as a cause of adult schizophrenia.[4,5]

B. Environmental Illness

Environmental illness, also called *multiple chemical sensitivities* and more recently *idiopathic environmental*

BOX 21-1

BOX 21-1

Unconventional Theory of Allergy

Allergic toxemia
Environmental allergies
   Multiple chemical sensitivity
   Idiopathic environmental intolerance
Chronic fatigue immune dysfunction syndrome (CFIDS)
Candida hypersensitivity syndrome
Delayed food allergy
Atmospheric mold sensitivity

intolerances,[6] is a form of allergic toxemia which attributes many symptoms to numerous common everyday environmental chemicals, especially pesticides, solvents, perfumes, new carpets, plastic materials, new clothing, and virtually any synthetic chemical or commercial product with an odor.[7–10]

1. Occasionally, electromagnetic fields generated by nearby electric power lines or household appliances and dental amalgams are implicated. No specific physical examination finding or laboratory abnormality is required for the diagnosis.[11,12] Because there is no characteristic history either, the diagnosis usually depends on one or more of the unproven methods described later, even though there are no diagnostic criteria for this condition using these tests.[13,14] The practice based on these ideas is known as *clinical ecology.*[15]

2. The condition is said to be an acquired disease caused by the large-scale release into the environment of synthetic industrial chemicals in recent years. It is characterized by wide-ranging symptomatology subjectively triggered by exposure to numerous environmental "chemicals."[16] Theories to explain the illness include failure of adaptation, allergy, autoimmunity, immunotoxicity, neurotoxicity, or some combination of these.[17–19] There is no experimental support for any of these theories.[20]

3. The prevailing opinion of those who have independently evaluated the clinical conditions of the patients is that the symptoms allegedly triggered by chemical exposure cannot be reproduced in controlled trials[21] and are best explained by psychiatric mechanisms.[22–27]

C. Chronic Fatigue Immune Dysfunction Syndrome

Chronic fatigue immune dysfunction syndrome (CFIDS) is indistinguishable from environmental illness, chronic fatigue syndrome, and other controversial subjective conditions. There is no evidence, however, that these patients have an immune system abnormality.

D. *Candida* Hypersensitivity Syndrome

This syndrome is a variant of "environmental illness." Proponents of this concept state that *Candida albicans,* a commensal organism in the gastrointestinal tract and vagina, is the cause of behavioral and emotional diseases and a variety of physical illnesses and symptomatic states.[28,29]

Antibiotics, corticosteroids, birth control pills, and pregnancy are said to make the patient susceptible to the condition. The diagnosis is made from the history only, and a rotary diversified diet with avoidance of sugar, yeast, and mold, along with antifungal drugs and vitamin and mineral supplements, is recommended as treatment.

A *Candida*-producing immunotoxin has been proposed as the cause, although no such chemical has yet been identified and characterized.

E. Delayed Food Allergy

Delayed food allergy is diagnosed especially in children with symptomatic complaints and behavior problems. Symptoms reportedly occurring hours, days, or even weeks after food ingestion are accepted as diagnostic, contrary to double-blind studies, which fail to confirm the existence of delayed food allergy. Fatigue and many other symptoms ascribed to delayed food allergy are common in some children without a specific illness and are more likely caused by psychological or social factors.

1. Multiple foods are often implicated, because elimination diets rarely have a sustained therapeutic benefit, leading to the progressive elimination of additional foods.

2. In contrast, IgE-mediated allergic responses to foods begin less than 2 hours after ingestion, and severe reactions, including anaphylaxis, may start within minutes. To date, no unequivocal food hypersensitivities have been shown to involve IgG or IgM antibodies, immune complexes, immune cytolysis, or systemic T-cell-dependent inflammation. The delayed food allergy concept depends on the patient's self-report of symptoms, often supplemented with untested or unproved diagnostic methods.

F. Atmospheric Mold Sensitivity

Atmospheric mold sensitivity is a recently emerging concept applied to a variety of subjective complaints or illnesses in persons living in homes or working in buildings that have sustained water damage from flooding or excessive humidity promoting indoor mold growth.

1. The diagnosis in these cases rests on the presence of low levels of antifungal antibodies in serum. However, the concentrations of these antibodies have not yet been shown to be different from those found in healthy persons. As in the case of

"environmental illness," a combined toxicity/hypersensitivity theory is often invoked.

2. This should not be confused with allergic diseases caused by fungal allergy, especially asthma, some cases of hypersensitivity pneumonitis, allergic bronchopulmonary aspergillosis, and allergic fungal sinusitis. These can be identified by localized symptomatology and objective physical findings, functional and/or imaging studies that confirm pathology, and the presence of the relevant immune response by the patient.

III. Unconventional Diagnostic Methods *(Box 21-2)*

The procedures included in this category are not based on sound scientific principles, and they have not been shown by proper controlled clinical trials to be capable of assisting in the diagnosis for any condition. Some are ineffective for allergy diagnosis, although they may be useful in certain nonallergic conditions. Others are not diagnostic of any disease.

A. Nonimmunologic Tests That Are Inappropriate for Allergy Diagnosis

1. The *cytotoxic test,* also known as the leukocytotoxic test or Bryan's test, consists of applying a drop of the patient's blood to a microscope slide containing a minute quantity of a food or drug.[30,31]
   a. The unstained blood sample is then inspected microscopically for alterations in the morphology of the leukocytes, supposedly indicating

---

BOX 21-2

Unconventional Diagnostic Methods

Nonimmunologic tests that are inappropriate for allergy diagnosis
Cytotoxic test
Provocation–neutralization
Electrodermal diagnosis
Applied kinesiology
Serial end-point titration
Pulse test
Quantitation of environmental chemicals

Immunologic tests that are inappropriate in allergy diagnosis
Serum IgG antibodies
Total serum immunoglobulin levels
Lymphocyte subset counts
Lymphocyte functional tests
Circulating immune complexes
Quantitation of cytokines

---

allergy to the food or drug. Assessment of leukocyte morphology is subjective. The procedure has not been standardized for time of incubation, pH, osmolarity, temperature, or other conditions. In practice, a sample of the patient's blood is tested to a panel of a hundred or more individual foods. The *antigen leukocyte cellular antibody test* (ALCAT) is the same procedure utilizing electronic instrumentation for blood cell identification and computerized data analysis.[32]
   b. The test is based on the theory that allergy results in "toxicity" to leukocytes. There are no known allergic diseases caused by leukocyte cytotoxicity from foods, either directly or immunologically. Several controlled clinical trials have shown that the cytotoxic test is not reproducible, and it does not correlate with objective clinical evidence of food allergy.[33,34] Furthermore, no form of immunologic cytotoxicity, whether mediated by complement activation, cytotoxic T-cells, or natural killer (NK) cells, has ever been shown to be diagnosed by these leukocyte cytotoxicity procedures.

2. *Provocation-neutralization* consists of "testing" the patient with a small amount of a substance by either injection or sublingual drop.[35] The occurrence of any symptoms or sensations over a period of 10 minutes is taken as indication that the test is "positive," regardless of whether the same symptom occurs in the patient's illness. The test is repeated using the same substance at lower concentrations until the patient reports having no symptom, at which point the allergy (i.e., the symptom) is said to be "neutralized."[35,36] The neutralizing dose of the substance is then prescribed as treatment.
   a. There are no standardized criteria for a positive test; these are at the discretion of the tester. Negative controls are not included. The procedure is claimed by its proponents to diagnose allergy to foods,[37] inhalant allergens, and environmental chemicals. It is also used to diagnose allergy to hormones and microorganisms, particularly *Candida albicans.*
   b. Modern concepts of immunologic disease provide no rationale or plausible theory for the presumed provocation of subjective symptoms and their immediate neutralization under the conditions used in this procedure. Published reports yield conflicting results. They include subjects with varying clinical manifestations, different testing methods, and variable criteria for a positive test, reflecting the unstandardized and subjective nature of provocation–neutralization. The only rigorous, properly controlled study showed that

food extracts were indistinguishable from placebo in double-blind testing.[38]

    c. This procedure should not be confused with controlled provocation by inhalation of suspected allergens using objective measures of a response, nor should it be confused with double-blind placebo-controlled food allergy testing.[39] For certain unusual clinical presentations and for research purposes, inhalation provocation is an accepted method of testing an asthmatic response to an aeroallergen by monitoring with spirometry or plethysmography. A similar technique for studying rhinitis measures objective changes in nasal airway resistance. A double-blind placebo-controlled oral food allergen challenge can assess self-reported symptoms or exacerbations of respiratory, skin, and gastrointestinal reactions.

3. *Electrodermal diagnosis* employs a device to measure the electrical resistance of the skin while the patient holds a container of food.[40,41] A change in the galvanic resistance of the skin at certain acupuncture points is used to diagnose allergy to that food. This procedure is without any rational basis, and there have been no studies to support its use. The equipment used in electrodermal allergy testing is not approved for use as a medical device in the United States by the Food and Drug Administration.

4. *Applied kinesiology* is a practice based on an unscientific concept that a variety of diseases, especially allergy, cause a reduction in the strength of skeletal muscle while the patient holds or contacts a container of the food.[42]

    a. Muscle strength testing is performed subjectively. There is no experimental proof of either the diagnostic efficacy of the procedure or validation of the theory. Testing of infants is done by surrogate testing of a parent or unrelated relative while carrying the infant or holding the child's hand.

    b. Proponents of applied kinesiology use such mystical terms as "energy field" and "liver stress" to explain the results.

5. The *serial end-point titration* (Rinkel) method employs 5-fold serial increasing intradermal concentrations of allergen for testing suspected atopic allergy.[43–45]

    a. The end point, defined as the concentration of allergen used in testing which initiates a progressive increase in wheal diameter of 2 mm or more, is used to indicate both a safe dose to initiate immunotherapy and by calculation (usually 25–50 times greater) the "optimal" maintenance dose for treatment.

    b. Trials of the efficacy of this method for immunotherapy dosing showed that it is too conservative in estimating a safe starting dose and not capable of determining an "optimal" dose for treatment.[46,47]

6. The *pulse test* measures the pulse rate of the patient before and after food ingestion. An increase or decrease (or both) is said to indicate food allergy. There is no theory to explain such a phenomenon, and there are no clinical studies to support its use.[48]

7. *Quantitation of environmental chemicals* in samples of whole blood, erythrocytes, serum, urine, fat, or hair is used to diagnose environmental illness. The usual ones tested are organic solvents, other hydrocarbons, and pesticides. Quantitative analysis of metals, foods, drugs, vitamins, amino acids, and allergens is also used by some practitioners.

    a. Such testing is based on unsupported theories that these substances can be toxic to the immune system, leading to a state of subjective sensitivity to the environment and the presence of environmental chemicals within the body.

    b. Under some circumstances, it may be acceptable and appropriate to detect toxic quantities of a suspected chemical where poisoning is suspected, but the presence of such chemicals in the body has never been shown to be relevant to hypersensitivity diseases.

B. Immunologic Tests That Are Inappropriate in Allergy Diagnosis

Clinical laboratories offer tests for detecting serum concentrations of immunoglobulins, specific antibodies, complement components, circulating immune complexes, and blood levels of lymphocyte subsets. These are valuable tests for diagnosing a variety of diseases. Except for detecting and quantitating serum levels of IgE antibodies to allergens, they do not relate to the clinical evaluation of allergic disease.

1. *Serum IgG antibodies* to inhalant, food, or other allergens have no diagnostic value for atopic disease, but they may be helpful in some cases of serum sickness, hypersensitivity pneumonitis, or allergic pulmonary aspergillosis. Concentrations of the causative antibodies in the latter two conditions are high enough that standard procedures, such as the precipitin-in-gel reaction, are sufficiently sensitive for diagnosis.

    a. Very low levels of specific IgG antibody to injected allergens are induced during the course of allergen immunotherapy for atopic disease. Although referred to as "blocking antibodies," their protective role in injection therapy of atopic respiratory disease is uncertain.

b. The radioallergosorbent test (RAST) or the enzyme-linked immunosorbent assay (ELISA) detect and quantitate antibody of any isotype (immunoglobulin class) at extremely low concentrations in serum. Therefore, they can be used as an alternative to the immediate wheal/erythema skin test for diagnosing IgE-mediated atopic or anaphylactic allergic diseases. RAST or ELISA can also detect similarly low concentrations of specific antibodies of other immunoglobulin classes, such as IgG, but IgG antibodies to foods and molds can be found in normal serum in the very low concentrations detected by these tests.[49,50] Some clinicians erroneously attribute diagnostic significance to these antibodies in atopy, and others claim that IgG antibodies to foods and molds cause a variety of nonspecific symptoms.

2. *Total serum immunoglobulin levels* are significantly low in the various immunoglobulin deficiency diseases.[51] Polyclonal increases in serum immunoglobulins occur in some chronic infections and autoimmune diseases. Monoclonal hyperproduction characterizes multiple myeloma and Waldenström's macroglobulinemia.

   Total serum IgE is generally higher in atopic patients than in nonatopic controls, especially in some patients with atopic dermatitis, but the total serum IgE is not a useful "screen" for atopy, because a significant number of atopic patients have levels that fall within the normal range.

   Furthermore, these levels give no information about antibody specificity. In allergic bronchopulmonary aspergillosis, the total serum IgE level has prognostic significance because it correlates with disease activity.[52]

3. *Lymphocyte subset counts* are useful in diagnosis of lymphocyte cellular immunodeficiencies and lymphocytic leukemias, but they are not abnormal in allergy. The "normal range" for many of the subsets of lymphocytes is wide, and the circulating levels fluctuate considerably under normal circumstances.

4. *Lymphocyte functional tests* using mitogens (phytohemagglutinin, pokeweed mitogen, concanavalin A) can be helpful in the diagnosis of cellular immunodeficiencies, but the tests are normal in allergy.

5. *Circulating immune complexes* can be analyzed by several methods, and they may be present in the serum of patients with vasculitis.

   Some medical laboratories offer a test to detect and quantitate circulating immune complexes containing food antigens (*food immune complex assay* [FICA]), and some clinicians use the presence of such complexes as evidence for allergy to that food.

Immune complexes containing food antigens (not necessarily allergens) circulate in the blood of normal children and adults following ingestion of the food.[53–55] This is especially common in some patients with either intestinal malabsorption or atopy.

However, there is no known pathogenic role for food immune complexes in causing food allergy or any other human disease, so the test is not diagnostic. Patients with IgA deficiency may have high circulating concentrations of immune complexes to bovine albumin, but the pathophysiologic role of these complexes is unknown.[56]

6. *Quantitation of cytokines* and their cellular *receptors* is offered by many clinical laboratories, but there is no support for their use in allergy diagnosis or for "environmental illness."

IV. Unconventional Treatment Methods

Effective management of allergic disease is an individualized program of allergen avoidance, medications, and allergen immunotherapy, based on an accurate and specific diagnosis. Monitoring treatment should be part of the program.

This section discusses systems of medical practice and specific treatments that are ineffective or inappropriate for allergy, even though some are widely used and may result in temporary symptomatic improvement or sense of well-being because of a placebo effect. They are generally based on incorrect theories of allergy and allergic disease, unproved methods of allergy testing, and observations based on case reports and anecdotes.

The controversial practices and treatments described here have either failed critical tests of efficacy and safety, or they have not been evaluated because of the lack of any compelling reason to do so.

A. Controversial Practice Systems (Box 21-3)

Traditional Chinese medicine, acupuncture, homeopathy, naturopathy, and chiropractic are only a few of the many practices that claim to diagnose and treat diseases and to promote health and a sense of well-being. These are commonly referred to as complementary or alternative medicine. They are popular today in spite of their lack

BOX 21-3

Unconventional Practice Systems

Acupuncture
Herbal therapy
Homeopathic remedies
Detoxification

of any basis in medical science or clinical evidence to support their theories or practices. A few of the more common practices offering treatment for allergy will be mentioned here.

1. *Acupuncture* has been used for centuries to treat a wide range of diseases by the insertion of needles at defined points on the body with some presumed relationship to a particular organ or disease. It is used exclusively by some practitioners, and by others as an adjunct to other treatment measures.
   a. Although the prevalence of its use for allergy is unknown, many patients have tried acupuncture at some time for relief of asthma, allergic rhinitis, and allergic dermatoses.
   b. It is also used by patients who believe that other symptoms or medical problems are allergic.
   c. In spite of reports of short-term efficacy, there are no definitive studies that document superiority of acupuncture over standard therapy for either symptomatic or long-term improvement of allergic disease.

2. *Herbal therapy* is used by many patients in the belief that herbs are a more natural, safer, and more effective treatment than is drug therapy. This is a component of many alternative practices. A particular herb may or may not have pharmacologically active components, but no single herbal preparation has demonstrated therapeutic activity superior to medications available today for treating any allergic disease.

3. *Homeopathic remedies* are based on the unproved principle of "like treats like," i.e., that an agent that supposedly causes a disease is also therapeutic for that disease if given in infinitesimally small amounts. This presumes that the disease etiology is known and identifiable as a particular substance.
   a. Homeopathy consists of orally administered "remedies," which are extracts of natural products, including plants, animal organs, and insects. The extracts are serially diluted through a process of "succussion," which is simply the violent shaking of a container of diluted extract on the theory that the remedy molecule impresses a mirror image of itself upon water molecules in solution.
   b. The remedies are given in vanishingly small amounts. How these putative altered molecules treat the disease is purely speculative. Homeopathists also prescribe "natural" hormones from animals, in the form of extracts of endocrine glands, including adrenal cortex, thyroid, thymus, pancreas, and spleen.
   c. The practice of homeopathy has a superficial resemblance to allergen immunotherapy, and

homeopathic practitioners offer their remedies for the treatment of allergy.
   d. The procedure also can be incorrectly likened to infectious disease immunization. However, immunizations for allergy or infection have documented therapeutic benefits deriving from the induction of specific protective immune responses. There is no evidence that homeopathic remedies have therapeutic effect for any disease, including allergy.

4. *Detoxification* is the treatment prescribed by certain physicians who ascribe to the theory of immunotoxicity as a cause of allergic disease.
   a. This is an unproven theory underlying the concept of "multiple chemical sensitivities," also called "idiopathic environmental intolerance," whereby certain people are believed to react to common environmental items, especially those that can be detected by odor. The symptoms of this condition are numerous but entirely subjective.
   b. In this concept, lipid-soluble environmental chemicals are believed to be stored in body fat for long periods. Reducing the "body burden" of foreign chemicals is supposedly achieved through a formalized program of exercise followed by a sauna to induce sweating. Body fluids are replenished by drinking water. Sodium, potassium, calcium, magnesium, and vitamin supplements are also administered.
   c. High-dose niacin therapy is used to induce erythema. Four "essential oils" (soy, walnut, peanut, and safflower) are given, allegedly to displace fat-soluble chemical contaminants. This procedure takes about 5 hours and is repeated daily for 20 days or longer.[57]
   d. The idea that increased circulation, vasodilation, and oral ingestion of vegetable oils can mobilize "toxins" from fat into sweat is unproven, and there are no studies showing that the method is safe.

B. Controversial Diets

Avoidance is the only reliable method for treating food allergy. Although any food is potentially allergenic, food allergy in adults is relatively uncommon, and each patient is usually sensitive to one or at most a few foods. Food allergy is more common among allergic infants and small children. Except for very rare cases, effective avoidance therapy does not require an extensive elimination diet, and adequate food substitutes are readily available.

1. The unsubstantiated concept of multiple food allergies causing vague subjective symptoms, behavioral problems, and emotional illness leads to the unnecessary restriction of large numbers of foods,

usually based on unproven testing procedures such as provocation-neutralization, the cytotoxic test, and testing for IgG food antibodies.

2. A diet based on faulty testing often results in further unnecessary food restrictions because the underlying condition, whether physical or psychological, is not addressed properly.

3. The *rotary diversified diet* is often recommended to limit but not totally restrict foods by eating each food on a 5-day rotation cycle.
   a. The rotary diet is also recommended by some practitioners who believe that many foods are toxic or that excessive exposure to a food makes it allergenic. The latter has no scientific basis.
   b. Elimination of specific food items such as sugar, wheat, corn, red meats and all additives is usually recommended, whether or not the patient has experienced any adverse effects from them.

4. *Dietary supplements* are sometimes recommended for symptomatic relief or cure of allergies, based on an unsubstantiated theory that deficiency of these substances causes allergy, or that they have immune-enhancing properties.
   a. Vitamins, minerals, amino acids, anti-oxidants, or a combination of these are the usual supplements prescribed in many controversial allergy practices.
   b. Although oxidative tissue damage is inherent in any inflammatory disease, including allergy, there is no evidence that ingestion of anti-oxidants such as vitamins C or E or glutathione enhances the normal activity of endogenous antioxidants.

C. Environmental Chemical Avoidance

1. Conventional allergy management emphasizes avoidance of allergens where possible, based on accurate identification of specific allergic sensitivities. An effective program should not cause unnecessary lifestyle restrictions.

2. In contrast, excessive avoidance therapy is a feature of many controversial forms of allergy practice, usually because of unreliable diagnostic tests that supposedly "uncover" allergies. Extreme environmental chemical avoidance for patients with so-called multiple chemical sensitivities may lead to major lifestyle changes to avoid any possible exposure to synthetic products and items that can be detected by odor.[7]
   a. Patients often wear masks in public, live in stripped-down homes or trailers, and avoid wearing synthetic clothing. Some of them live in isolated communities.
   b. Avoiding electromagnetic radiation and removal of dental amalgams is often advised. These

patients usually have chronic vague symptoms without physical or laboratory evidence of disease.

3. No scientifically valid study testing the effectiveness and safety of such extreme environmental avoidance therapy has yet been undertaken. On the contrary, there are many anecdotal reports of serious iatrogenic disability resulting from extreme "chemical" restrictions.

D. Immunologic Manipulation

1. Allergic diseases arise from an inappropriate response by the immune system to environmental allergens in certain genetically susceptible individuals. In theory it might be possible to modify the immune system therapeutically to remove the specific allergic sensitivity without disturbing other necessary immune functions.

2. Immunostimulating drugs, therapeutic monoclonal antibodies to certain components of the immune system, and immunoregulatory cytokines are currently being exploited for treatment of other immune-mediated diseases, particularly autoimmunity, and for cancer. Therapeutic gamma globulin injections are standard treatment for documented IgG antibody deficiency, and they are effective in idiopathic thrombocytopenic purpura and Kawasaki disease by an uncertain mechanism. Some practitioners recommend these treatments for allergy, but until effectiveness is shown by proper double-blind studies, they should be considered experimental.

3. At this time no form of immune system manipulation for allergic disease is available as standard therapy. Removal of IgE with monoclonal anti-IgE antibody for treatment of atopic disease, especially asthma, has undergone clinical trials with reported partial success, but it remains experimental at this time.

E. Controversial Forms of Immunotherapy

1. Specific allergen immunotherapy is the established treatment for selected patients with respiratory atopic allergy and Hymenoptera venom anaphylaxis. A number of controlled clinical trials validate its use.
   a. The effect is allergen-specific and is accompanied by a treatment-induced immune response.
   b. The specific allergens and dosage necessary to optimize efficacy and safety must be tailored to the individual patient, so standardized protocols are of limited value.
   c. The usual procedures consist of perennial subcutaneous injections beginning with progressively increasing quantities of allergen that culminate in a program of stable high doses of allergen maintained for a period of several years.

2. Numerous properly controlled studies document the efficacy of allergen immunotherapy. There are no known long-term adverse consequences, and the immediate side effects and dangers are known and can be minimized when the treatment is used properly. There is a clear need to find ways to enhance its effectiveness and perhaps extend its use to conditions such as food anaphylaxis and to reduce the risk of life-threatening systemic reactions, cost and inconvenience. These will require rigorous controlled clinical trials.

3. Alternative routes of administration of allergen have been sought for many years to avoid the discomfort and the life-threatening systemic reactions of subcutaneous treatment. They include nasal insufflation, bronchial inhalation, oral ingestion and sublingual absorption.

4. Efforts have also been made to alter the allergen used in immunotherapy to improve efficacy and lessen the chance of adverse reactions.
   a. Allergen modification by denaturing the molecule with phenol or polymerizing with glutaraldehyde has not proved to be advantageous in treatment.
   b. Recently, injections of peptide epitopes rather than the intact protein allergen have been tried for the purpose of inducing specific T-cell anergy, but the clinical results of controlled trials have not been promising, and adverse reactions in some patients require further investigation.
   c. The use of adjuvants such as pyridine or aqueous/lipid allergen suspensions have also been tried, but they have not improved on the standard subcutaneous injections of aqueous extracts.

5. ***Immunotherapies*** (Box 21-4)
   a. *Neutralization* (symptom-relieving) therapy assumes that exposure to a particular dose of allergen induces an immediate relief of ongoing allergic symptoms.[58] The so-called neutralizing dose is based on provocation-neutralization testing. The allergen is self-administered by the patient intradermally, subcutaneously, or sublingually.[35] It has been prescribed for use whenever the patient perceives an ongoing allergic reaction, routinely several times a day, or as a prophylactic measure in anticipation of expected allergen exposure.

      1) Physicians who prescribe neutralization therapy do so to treat a wide range of illnesses and symptomatology. These include recognized allergic diseases, rheumatologic diseases, viral and other infections, premenstrual discomfort, and functional somatic syndromes. "Neutralizing" allergy is done not only with extracts of commonly recognized inhalant allergens, but also with environmental chemicals, vaccines, hormones, histamine, foods, drugs, and many other substances.[17]

      2) There is no rational mechanism or immunologic theory that could account for immediate symptom neutralization of allergic disease. In practice, the symptoms that are provoked and cleared in this way are subjective, nonspecific, and not consistent with the symptoms that are widely recognized as being allergic.

      3) Most of the published studies of this form of therapy are either anecdotal or inadequate. One double-blind placebo-controlled clinical trial, however, showed that prompt symptom provocation and neutralization cannot be distinguished from placebo responses,[38] and therefore they occur only because of an expectation of a particular response.[59]

      4) This form of therapy must not be confused with conventional allergen immunotherapy for atopy or anaphylaxis, in which the well-validated therapeutic response is determined not by immediate symptom relief but rather by an overall attenuation of the disease.

   b. *Serial end-point titration* (the Rinkel method) refers to the use of quantitative skin testing to determine dosages of allergen for both initiating and optimizing injection treatment of allergic disease. This is described previously. Clinical trials of immunotherapy using the "end-point" dosage method have shown that it is almost always too low, so that treatment leads to therapy that is ultimately no more effective than placebo.

      If the patient fails to improve as expected, retesting to establish a new end point is done,

---

BOX 21-4

Controversial Forms of Immunotherapy

Neutralization
Serial end-point titration
Enzyme-potentiated desensitization
Oral immunotherapy
Sublingual drop therapy
Bronchial inhalation
Local nasal immunotherapy
Injection of food extracts
Autogenous urine injection

but there are no studies to assess the clinical validity of this recommendation.

c. *Enzyme-potentiated desensitization* (EPD) was first proposed in the 1970s from experiments in sensitized rodents which showed a partial protection from anaphylactic challenge when the enzyme β-glucuronidase was added to the allergen. At that time, a few patients with hay fever were treated in a similar fashion and reported improvement.[60]

  1) A small group of practitioners have recently revived the practice, which consists of injecting an exceedingly low dose of allergen, approximately equivalent to that delivered in a standard prick test, pre-mixed with β-glucuronidase in an amount that is a small fraction of that normally found in the body.

  2) Typically, a single preseasonal intradermal injection is given to patients with seasonal pollen allergies, or every 2 to 6 months for those with perennial symptoms. Allergens include inhalants, foods, and environmental chemicals, and it is recommended for seasonal and perennial allergic rhinitis, asthma, nasal polyposis, sinusitis, eczema, anaphylactic food allergy, urticaria, ulcerative colitis, irritable bowel syndrome, rheumatoid arthritis, migraine headaches, petit mal seizures, chronic fatigue syndrome, "immune dysfunction syndrome," food-induced depression and anxiety, and childhood hyperactivity believed to be caused by ingestion of certain foods.

  3) Patients must avoid common food allergens, food additives, all medications for 3 days before and 3 weeks after each injection, and environmental exposure to allergens for 24 hours before and 48 hours after the injection.

  4) They must consume a special "EPD diet" for 24 hours before and 48 hours after the injection, and they must take specific vitamins and minerals.

  5) The injection is given only during the first 2 weeks of the menstrual cycle, and not during pregnancy or within 5 days of an upper respiratory infection. The patient must avoid scented products or ointments near the injection site, heat, stress, environmental chemicals, smoke, air conditioning, newsprint, and photocopiers.

  6) Efficacy is believed to be enhanced by taking zinc, folic acid, vitamins A and B_6, and magnesium either orally or intravenously for several days before the injection.

  7) A temporary return of the allergic symptoms for which the patient is being treated is considered a favorable sign that the treatment will be effective.

  8) Recent controlled short-term clinical trials describe improved symptoms of allergic rhinitis or asthma, but objective measures of disease activity are either absent or not measured. Specific antibody responses are variable and conflicting. No trial has compared EPD treatment with the allergen alone or the enzyme alone. There is no information about possible chemical or biological alteration of the allergen when mixed with the enzyme.[61,62]

  9) A single controlled trial using food extracts reportedly improved tolerance to foods believed to cause hyperactive behavior in children.

d. *Oral immunotherapy* to avoid the inconvenience of allergen treatment injections was attempted for several years in the early 1900s, but it was abandoned for lack of noticeable efficacy. It has been reinstituted on an experimental basis recently using pollens and house dust mite extracts in capsules or tablets for treatment of allergic rhinitis and asthma.

  1) Much higher doses of allergen are both required and tolerated orally compared to the doses used in treatment by conventional subcutaneous injections.

  2) The results of controlled trials are mixed. A significant clinical effect may be achieved, but only with doses up to 4000 times those tolerated by atopic patients when given subcutaneously.

  3) As with injected allergens, some studies show a rise in allergen-specific IgG antibodies and blunting of the normal seasonal and post-seasonal rise in specific IgE antibodies.

  4) Both clinical and immunologic responses are delayed for more than a year after the treatment is started. Oral immunotherapy is experimental at this time.

e. *Sublingual drop therapy*, presumably because of rapid absorption and avoidance of injections, is used for "neutralization" of symptoms.[35,63,64] It can be performed with or without swallowing after the allergen solution is kept in the mouth in position under the tongue for a few minutes. If the allergen is swallowed, exposure is both sublingual and oral.

  1) Recent double-blind placebo-controlled clinical trials in allergic rhinitis with or without accompanying asthma have yielded

conflicting results for efficacy and evidence of an immune response.[65,66]

  2) Local angioedema of the buccal mucosa or even systemic anaphylaxis is a potential risk and has been documented. A double-blind, double-dummy comparison of sublingual versus subcutaneous treatment for one year showed similar improvement by either method, but there were no untreated control subjects for comparison.[67]

f. *Bronchial inhalation* as a route for immuno-therapy is based on animal studies that suggest that immunologic tolerance with suppression of specific IgE antibodies can be induced by repeated inhalation of allergen. A few controlled trials in human asthma using inhaled house dust mite allergen showed a therapeutic effect, but this requires confirmation.

g. *Local nasal immunotherapy* for allergic rhinitis uses nasal inhalation of allergen to avoid the risk of a systemic reaction. In general, this produces no increased IgG or reduced IgE antibody response in the serum.

  1) One study showed a lessened local inflam-matory response to nasal allergen challenge, and there was some mild clinical efficacy. Improvement may be masked by treatment-induced rhinitis, so the treatment is usually restricted to a preseasonal time frame accom-panied by symptom-reducing medications such as cromolyn.

h. *Injection of food extracts* has not yet been successful in immunizing patients with life-threatening anaphylaxis to specific foods, even though this treatment is highly successful in venom-induced anaphylaxis.

  1) Nevertheless, some practitioners do prescribe food extract injections, often consisting of a combination of foods based on skin test results or patients' reports of intolerance to foods.[68,69]

  2) This form of treatment must be considered unproven as to efficacy and potential danger until appropriate clinical trials have been carried out.

  3) It is most often prescribed for patients with symptoms that are not consistent with allergy, where the relationship of the symptoms to foods is speculative and not proved.

i. *Autogenous urine injections* is a bizarre proce-dure that has surfaced periodically in the past 50 years. It consists of subcutaneous or intramus-cular injections of the patient's urine after it has been chemically treated to extract a substance called "proteose," alleged to be the excreted form of the patient's inhaled or ingested allergens.[70,71]

  1) This is theorized to be more efficacious for immunization than is the allergen extract itself. Uncontrolled anecdotal reports claimed success in treating asthma, rhinitis, anaphylaxis, urticaria, angioedema, and serum sickness. Other reports failed to show efficacy.

  2) The treatment is not only of unproved value but potentially dangerous. This is a critical issue, since small quantities of glomerular basement membrane antigens are found in normal urine.

  3) Chemical treatment of urine during the extraction process could therefore lead to the production of altered renal proteins that might prove to be antigenic, potentially result-ing in autoimmune nephritis.

REFERENCES

1. Speer F: The allergic tension-fatigue syndrome. Pediatr Clin North Am 1954;1:1029.
2. Randolph TG: Sensory aspects of cerebral allergy. J Lab Clin Med 1954;44:910.
3. Feingold B: Why Your Child Is Hyperactive. New York: Random House, 1975.
4. Dohan FC, Grasberger JC: Relapsed schizophrenics: Earlier discharge from the hospital after cereal-free, milk-free diet. Am Psychiatry 1973;130:685.
5. Singh MM, Na SR: Wheat gluten as a pathogenic factor in schizophrenia. Science 1976;191:401.
6. UNEP-ILO-WHO, et al: Conclusions and recommendations of a workshop on multiple chemical sensitivities (MCS). Reg Toxicol Pharmacol 1996;24:S188–S189.
7. Bell IR, Miller CS, Schwartz GE: An olfactory-limbic model of multiple chemical sensitivity syndrome: Possible rela-tionships to kindling and affective spectrum disorders. Biol Psychiatry 1992;32:218–242.
8. McGovern JJ, Lazaroni JA, Saifer P: Clinical evaluation of the major plasma and cellular measures of immunity. Orthomolec Psychiatry 1983;12:60.
9. Randolph TG: The specific adaption syndrome. J Lab Clin Med 1956;48:934.
10. Randolph TG: Human Ecology and Susceptibility to the Chemical Environment. Springfield, IL: Charles C Thomas, 1962.
11. Sparks PJ, Daniell W, Black DW, Kipen HM, Altman LC, Simon GE, Terr AI: Multiple chemical sensitivity syndrome: A clinical perspective. I. Case definition, theories of patho-genesis, and research needs. J Occup Med 1994;36:718–730.
12. Sparks PJ, Daniell W, Black DW, Kipen HM, Altman LC, Simon GE, Terr AI: Multiple chemical sensitivity syndrome: A clinical perspective. II. Evaluation, diagnostic testing, treat-ment, and social considerations. J Occup Med 1994;36:731–737.

13. Simon GE, Daniell W, Stockbridge H, Claypoole K, Rosenstock L: Immunologic, psychological, and neuropsychological factors in multiple chemical sensitivity: A controlled study. Ann Intern Med 1993;119:97–103.
14. Terr AI: Multiple chemical sensitivities: Immunologic critique of clinical ecology theories and practice. Occup Med State Art Rev 1997;2:683–694.
15. Dickey LD (ed): Clinical Ecology. Springfield, IL: Charles C Thomas, 1976.
16. Cullen MR, Pace PE, Redlich CA: The experience of the Yale Occupational and Environmental Medicine Clinics with multiple chemical sensitivities, 1986–1991. Toxicol Ind Health 1996;8:15–19.
17. Levin AS, Byers VS: Environmental illness: A disorder of immune regulation. Occup Med State Art Rev 1987;2:669–682.
18. Levine SA, Reinhart JH: Biochemical pathology initiated by free radicals, oxidant chemicals and therapeutic drugs in the etiology of chemical hypersensitivity disease. J Orthomolec Psychiatry 1983;12:166–183.
19. Miller CS: Possible models for multiple chemical sensitivity: Conceptual issues and role of the limbic system. Toxicol Ind Health 1992;8:181–202.
20. California Medical Association Scientific Task Force on Clinical Ecology: Clinical ecology: A critical appraisal. West J Med 1986;144:239.
21. Staudenmayer H, Selner JC, Buhr MP: Double-blind provocation chamber challenges in 20 patients presenting with multiple chemical sensitivity. Reg Toxicol Pharmacol 1983;18:44–53.
22. Black DW, Rathe A, Goldstein RB: Environmental illness: A controlled study of 26 subjects with "20th century disease." JAMA 1990;264:3166–3170.
23. Brodsky CM: Multiple chemical sensitivities and other "environmental illness": A psychiatrist's view. Occup Med 1987;2:495–704.
24. Haller E: Successful management of patients with "multiple chemical sensitivities" on an inpatient psychiatric unit. J Clin Psychiatry 1993;54:196–199.
25. Selner JC, Staudenmayer H: Neuropsychophysiologic observations in patients presenting with environmental illness. Toxicol Ind Health 1992;8:145–155.
26. Staudenmayer H, Selner ME, Selner J: Adult sequelae of childhood abuse presenting as environmental illness. Ann Allergy 1993;71:538–546.
27. Stewart DE, Raskin J: Psychiatric assessment of patients with "20th-century disease" ("total allergy syndrome"). Can Med Assoc J 1983;133:1001–1006.
28. Crook WG: The Yeast Connection: A Medical Breakthrough. Jackson, TN: Professional Books, 1983.
29. Truss CO: The role of *Candida albicans* in human illness. J Orthomolec Psychiatry 1981;10:228.
30. Bryan WTK, Bryan M: The application of in vitro cytotoxic reactions to clinical diagnosis of food allergy. Laryngoscope 1960;70:810.
31. Bryan MP, Bryan WTK: Cytologic diagnosis of allergic disorders. Otolaryngol Clin North Am 1974;7(4):637.
32. Pasula MJ: The ALCAT test: In vitro procedure for determining food sensitivities. Folia Med Cracov 1993;34:153–157.
33. Lieberman P, Crawford L, Bjelland J, et al: Controlled study of the cytotoxic food test. JAMA 1974;231:728.
34. Benson TE, Arkins JA: Cytotoxic testing for food allergy: Evaluations of reproducibility and correlations. J Allergy Clin Immunol 1976;58:471.
35. Morris DL: Use of sublingual antigen in diagnosis and treatment of food allergy. Ann Allergy 1971;27:289.
36. Willoughby JW: Provocative food test technique. Ann Allergy 1965;23:543.
37. Lee CH, Williams RT, Binkley EL: Provocative testing and treatment for foods. Arch Otolaryngol 1969;90:87.
38. Jewett DL, Fein G, Greenberg MH: A double-blind study of symptom provocation to determine food sensitivity. N Engl J Med 1990;323:429–433.
39. Bock SA, Sampson HA, Atkins FM, et al: Double-blind, placebo-controlled food challenge (DBPCFC) as an office procedure: A manual. J Allergy Clin Immunol 1988:82:986.
40. Voll R: The phenomenon of medicine testing in electroacupuncture according to Voll. Am J Acupunct 1980;8:87.
41. Tsuei JJ, Lehman CW, Lam FMK, Zhu DAH: A food allergy study utilizing the EAV acupuncture technique. Am J Acupunct 1984;12:105.
42. Garrow JS: Kinesiology and food allergy. Br Med J 1988:296:1573.
43. Rinkel HJ, Lee CH, Crown DW Jr, et al: The diagnosis of food allergy. Arch Otolaryngol 1964;79:71.
44. Richardson GS: Titration: Evaluation of an office system of allergy diagnosis and treatment: Its use in otolaryngology. Ann Otol Rhinol Laryngol 70;344:1961.
45. Willoughby JW: Serial dilution titration skin tests in inhalant allergy: A clinical quantitative assessment of biologic skin reactivity to allergenic extracts. Otolaryngol Clin North Am 1974:7:579.
46. Hirsch S, Kalbfleisch JH, Golbert TM, et al: Rinkel method: A controlled study. Second report. J Allergy Clin Immunol 1980;65:192.
47. Van Metre TE, Adkinson NF, Amodio FJ, et al: A comparative study of the effectiveness of the Rinkel method and the current standard method of immunotherapy for ragweed pollen hay fever. J Allergy Clin Immunol 1980;66:500.
48. Coca AF: The Pulse Test. New York: Carol Publishing Group, 1982.
49. Paganelli R, Atherton Di, Levinsky R: The differences between normal and milk allergic subjects in their immune response after milk ingestion. Arch Dis Child 1983;58:201.
50. Husby S, Oxelius V-A, Teisner B, et al: Humoral immunity to dietary antigens in healthy adults: Occurrence, isotype and IgG subclass distribution of serum antibodies to protein antigens. Int Arch Allergy Appl Immunol 1985;77:416.
51. Ammann A: Antibody (B cell) immunodeficiency disorders. In Stites DP, Terr AL (eds): Basic and Clinical Immunology, 7th ed, p 322. Norwalk, CT: Appleton and Lange, 1991.
52. Greenberger PA, Patterson R: Allergic bronchopulmonary aspergillosis and the evaluation of the patient with asthma. J Allergy Clin Immunol 1988;81:646.
53. Inganas M, Johansson SGO, Dannaeus A: A method for estimation of circulating immune complexes after oral challenge with ovalbumin. Clin Allergy 1980;10:293.

54. Haddad ZH, Vetter M, Friedman J, et al: Detection and kinetics of antigen-specific IgE and IgG immune complexes after oral challenge with ovalbumin. Ann Allergy 1983; 51:255.

55. Leary HL, Halsey JF: An assay to measure antigen-specific immune complexes in food allergy patients. J Allergy Clin Immunol 1984;74:190.

56. Cunningham-Rundels C, Brandeis WE, Good RA, Day NK: Bovine proteins and the formation of circulating immune conplexes in selectine IgA deficiency. J Clin Invest 1979;64:272.

57. Root DE, Katzin DB, Schnare DW: Diagnosis and treatment of patients presenting subclinical signs and symptoms of exposure to chemicals which bioaccumulate in human tissue. In Proceedings of the National Conference on Hazardous Wastes and Environmental Emergencies, pp 150–153, 1985.

58. Kailin EW, Collier R: "Relieving" therapy for antigen exposure. JAMA 1971;217:78.

59. Ferguson A: Food sensitivity or self-deception? N Engl J Med 1990;323:476–468.

60. McEwen LM, Nicholson M, Kitchen I, White S: Enzyme potentiated desensitization: III. Control by sugars and diols of the immunological effect of glucuronidase in mice and patients with hay fever. Ann Allergy 1973;31:543.

61. Cantani A, Ragno V, Monteleone MA, Lucenti P, Businco L: Enzyme-potentiated desensitization in children with ashma and mite allergy: A double-blind study. J Invest Allergol Clin Immunol 1996;6:270.

62. Astarita C, Scala G, Sproviero S, Franzese A: Effects of enzyme-potentiated desensitization in the treatment of pollinosis: A double-blind placebo-controlled trial. J Invest Allergol Clin Immunol 1996;6:248.

63. Morris DL: Use of sublingual antigen in diagnosis and treatment of food allergy. Ann Allergy 1969;27:289.

64. Scadding GK, Brostoff J: Low dose sublingual therapy in patients with allergic rhinitis due to house dust mite. Clin Allergy 1986;16:483.

65. Nelson HS, Oppenheimer J, Vatsia GA, Buchmeier A: A double-blind, placebo-controlled evaluation of sublingual immunotherapy with standardized cat extract. J Allergy Clin Immunol 1993;92:229.

66. Malling H-J: Sublingual immunotherapy (editorial). Clin Exp Allergy 1996;26:1228.

67. Quirino T, Iemoli E, Siciliani E, Parmiani S, Milazzo F: Sublingual versus injective immunotherapy in grass pollen allergic patients: A double blind (double dummy) study. Clin Exp Allergy 1996;26:1253.

68. Miller JB: A double-blind study of food extract injection therapy: A preliminary report. Ann Allergy 1977;38:185.

69. Rea WJ, Podell RN, Williams M, et al: Elimination of oral food challenge reaction by injection of food extract. Arch Otolaryngol 1984;110:248.

70. Liberman J, Bigland AD: Autogenous urinary proteose in asthma and other allergic conditions. Br Med J 1937;1:62.

71. Plesch S: Urine therapy. Med Press 1947;218:128.

APPENDIX
Useful Reference Material

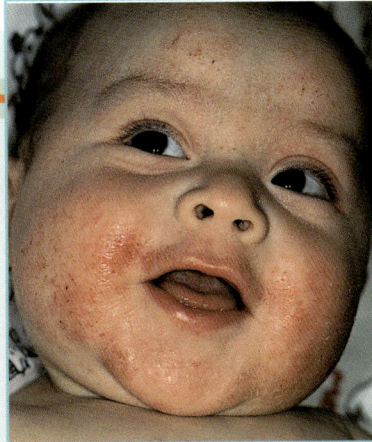

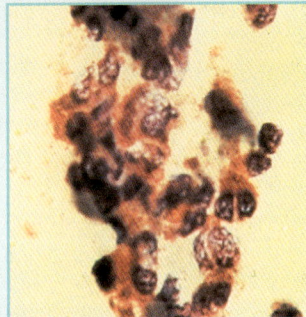

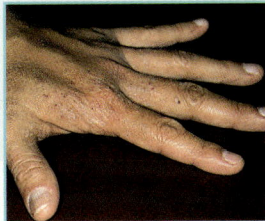

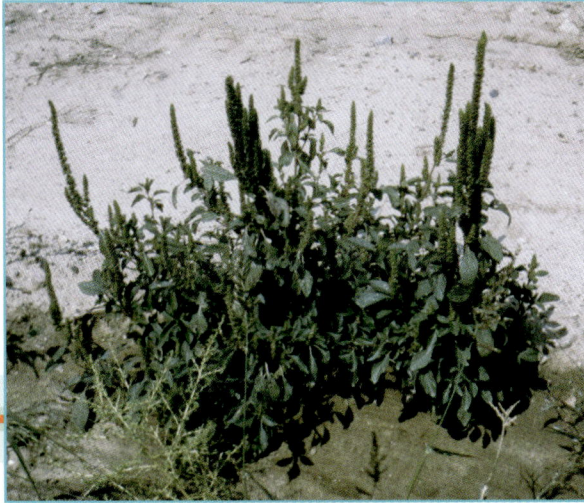

Redroot Pigweed *Courtesy of Hollister-Stier Laboratory*

APPENDIX 1
Basic Materials for an Immunotherapy Program

I. Consent for Immunotherapy

A. Original Consent Form from Prescribing Physician's Office

If immunotherapy is indicated and patients state they desire immunotherapy, oral or written consent must be obtained and noted in the chart of the prescribing physician. It is also included on a consent form from the office if the immunotherapy is to be administered outside the prescribing physician's office. The form may include the following:

1. Patient's name and date of birth
2. Procedure—immunotherapy
3. Risks
4. Benefits
5. Review of office schedule and procedures
6. Costs and method of payment
7. Duration of therapy
8. Patient's responsibilities
   a. Comply with treatment schedule.
   b. Wait in office 20–30 minutes after each shot.
   c. Have EpiPen with self at time of each visit (if appropriate).
   d. Notify staff of any new medications; recognize and notify staff of any immediate or delayed symptoms from previous dose of vaccine. If delayed symptoms occur, patient must call the office or 911 as appropriate.
9. Signature of patient (parent and minor as appropriate) and person doing procedure and date

B. Consent Form for Administration to a Minor with Other Responsible Caregiver

If immunotherapy is to be given to a child without the parent present, a special consent form is necessary. This form includes the name of the authorized adult who will be present at the time of treatment. The treatment form must be signed, witnessed, and dated.

C. Consent Form for "Outside" Physician's Office

A second consent form may be considered for an "outside" physician administering a vaccine. This form may include the name of the patient plus an identification number or birth date.

1. Name of physician administering the vaccine
2. Patient's responsibilities as listed previously
3. Patient's responsibility for cost of service

4. Consent form example. This is presented not as a legal document but to share points that can be emphasized in the final office document (Box A1-1).

II. Treatment Protocols Outline

A. Staffing

Antigen immunotherapy must be delivered by trained staff familiar with the protocols and materials. Supporting staff and a physician must be available.

B. Materials

Vaccine with appropriate dilutions to be available.

1. Cool trays are recommended if antigens are to be out of the refrigerator, because it is necessary to maintain proper storage temperature and conditions at all times.
2. Establish whether the patient is latex sensitive, so that latex-free materials can be made available and latex exposure in the room be limited. Patients can react to the powder from latex gloves.

BOX A1-1

Form Letter

(This example highlights some of the key points of a partial consent form. This is not a legal document.)

I _____ (date of birth _____) authorize specific allergen immunotherapy to be provided for me (or my child _____ —date of birth _____) in the office of Dr X. I understand that this treatment is being provided because of the diagnosis of _____ (allergic rhinitis, asthma). I understand that many patients with allergic rhinitis and asthma can benefit from this procedure with improved control of symptoms. I understand that symptom control may not be noted until after 1 year of treatment.

I understand that antigen (pollen, house dust mite, animal, mold protein) will be administered on a regular schedule for 3 to 5 years with reevaluation at _____ month(s) after starting the program and every _____ month(s) thereafter. I understand I must bring my EpiPen (if necessary) to every visit or the antigen/vaccine will not be administered.

I will wait in the office for 30 minutes after each injection. I will notify the office of any local or systemic symptoms, such as increased nasal congestion, eye irritation, skin itching or flushing, cough, wheeze, or breathing difficulty, or throat swelling or tightness. Any symptoms will be reported so that treatment can begin as soon as possible. I will call 911 or go to the nearest emergency room as appropriate. I will notify the office of any delayed symptoms and seek treatment as appropriate.

I know that if I am sick and have respiratory difficulty, including a decrease in peak flow, I may not be able to obtain the allergen/vaccine. If I miss a shot or have a reaction to the previous vaccine dose, the dose and schedule may be adjusted.

I will maintain a regular schedule. I know the duration of the program is 3 years or longer depending on symptom control.

I know I am responsible for payment if my insurance does not cover the costs. I understand the cost of the immunotherapy program includes the antigen and injection costs.

I know that if I receive immunotherapy in another physician's office the preceding rules equally apply. I will wait in that office 20–30 minutes after the shot. I will carry an EpiPen (if appropriate). If symptoms occur after I have left the office, I will notify the staff of any reactions and will obtain help as soon as possible (call 911 or go to the nearest emergency department).

Signed _____ date _____ Phone Number _____

Print Name _____ Emergency Number _____

Witness _____ date _____

Release for "underage" patients/children who will be coming to the office for their shot without a parent or legal guardian:

My child _____ (date of birth _____) will be with _____ (friend, relative, caregiver), who is the adult who is responsible for his/her care at this time and can authorize treatment as appropriate. I also give permission to have my child treated by your office and the paramedics in case of an emergency.

Signed _____ date _____

Print Name _____

Witness _____ date _____

3. Emergency medications must be available and clearly marked (e.g., epinephrine, oxygen, antihistamines, bronchodilators, corticosteroids).

C. Treatment Protocol

Prior to antigen dosing it is essential to do the following:

1. ***Identify the patient and the appropriate patient record.***
2. ***Question the patient concerning:***
   a. Any reactions to the last dose of antigen
   b. General health at this time—ask whether patient has a cough or a wheeze
   c. Any new medications (e.g., β-blockers)
   d. Peak flow measurement before shot (especially if patient is asthmatic); record this answer
   e. Latex sensitivity or allergy (glove precautions)
3. ***Check the antigen label.***
   a. Identify the antigen by name (e.g., grass).
   b. Identify the antigen by dilution, bottle number, and lid color.
   c. Check the expiration date.
   d. In some offices the patient does a "meds check" with the nursing staff and the patient initials daily treatment sheets, confirming that the proper antigen has been administered.
4. ***Check dose and administer antigen.***
5. ***Record:***
   a. Site of antigen injections (right or left arm)
   b. Any local reactions to that specific injection
6. ***Monitor patient during waiting period and recheck patient after 20–30 minutes (or longer) before discharge.***
7. ***Treat and record any reaction:***
   a. Local reactions—treat with ice pack, steroid cream, and or anti-itch cream.
   b. Systemic reactions (see later discussion).
   c. After treatment, provide an action plan for the patient plus a record of any medications given. Be in contact with the patient within 4–6 hours of the original reaction.
   d. Patients must call and report any delayed symptoms and seek care as appropriate.

D. Documentation and Record Keeping

The patient record should include:

1. Patient consent form.
2. Patient information—name, record number, birth date, picture, emergency and contact phone numbers.
3. Vaccine schedule with contents of extract/vaccine, dilution from the concentrate in vol/vol, vial number, and cap color.
4. Date and time of administration, dose, and site (arm injected).
5. Peak flow as appropriate with asthmatic patients.

6. Clinical notes regarding any reaction, dose adjustments, and clinical status prior to injection (document questions asked concerning acute illness, new medications, reaction to last shot).
7. Initials or signature of person administering the shot.

E. Dosing Schedules

The basic dosing schedule is outlined in Chapter 11. The antigen is prepared initially in four or five vials of usually 10-fold (vol/vol) dilutions of the concentrate provided by the company. Doses are advanced at each treatment interval based on the schedule selected—weekly, biweekly, cluster, or rush schedule. These schedules are reviewed in Chapter 11.

When Schedules May Need to Be Adjusted

a. Large local reaction: Repeat at the same dose or drop back a level, depending on the patient. Prominent local reactions do not predict systemic reactions.
b. Patient is late for a scheduled visit: May require a drop in dose (<3 weeks late—proceed according to schedule; 3–6 weeks late—repeat previous dose; 7–12 weeks late—drop one step per week missed; >12 weeks late—re-evaluate and start over).
c. During heavy pollen season: Patient and physician may decide not to advance the doses of some antigens.
d. New vial: Drop back one or more doses.
e. Systemic reaction from previous shot. Drop back the dose. All systemic reactions must be reported to the prescribing specialist, and consultation will be scheduled.
f. After a patient has reached maintenance (optimal dose for a given patient), the patient may receive shots less frequently, depending on the season and the symptom control. For example, an off-season maintenance schedule may entail an injection once every 4–6 weeks. During the "season," the patient may come in more often (e.g., weekly) to facilitate symptom control. Some patients will remain on the same dose and injection schedule year round.

III. Reactions to Immunotherapy

A. Local Reactions

Local reactions include swelling and itching at the site of the injection. These reactions are not associated with the risk of anaphylaxis; however, it may be necessary to reduce the dose (or dilute with saline) for patient comfort.

B. Systemic Reactions

Systemic reactions are defined as generalized symptoms or signs such as hives, wheezing, or shock.

C. Safety Monitoring

Patients need to be responsible for their own safety monitoring (as well as having the staff monitor the patient). Patients need to:

1. Know the antigens they are receiving and the importance of regular scheduled dosing.
2. Notify staff of any new medications (e.g., β-blockers), any side effects of previous dose, and any intercurrent infection or asthma exacerbation prior to being given an injection.
3. Know the importance of having an adequate peak flow at the time of antigen injection if they have asthma.
4. Know the early signs of an allergic reaction, initial treatment (e.g., with an antihistamine), and the use of an EpiPen if needed; be prepared to call physician's office or 911 as appropriate.
5. Understand the reason for any necessary dose reduction.
6. Understand the importance of waiting in the office 20–30 minutes or longer after each injection.

D. Emergency Equipment (see Chapter 6)

Emergency equipment must always be available and the staff well trained in its use.[1] Epinephrine is first-line treatment for anaphylaxis. Corticosteroids decrease the delayed response but provide little if any support for the immediate reaction. Examples of equipment and medications include the following:

1. Stethoscope
2. Sphygmomanometer
3. Tourniquets
4. Syringes
5. Hypodermic needles
6. Large-bore (14-gauge) needles
7. Epinephrine 1:1000, antihistamines for injection, corticosteroid for injection, bronchodilators
8. Oxygen
9. Oral airway
10. Equipment for administering IV fluids or vasopressors as appropriate

E. Treatment of Anaphylaxis[2,3]

Anaphylaxis to vaccine is rare (life-threatening reactions are estimated to occur in 1 out of 2 million injections). However, minor reactions to injections are more frequently noted and must be treated appropriately. Treat all reactions early and aggressively, because anaphylaxis can proceed rapidly (see Chapter 6).

Acute Care

Monitor the patient continually and record at regular intervals the patient's clinical status and vital signs, including blood pressure, heart rate, oxygen saturation, and peak flow (position the patient in the Trendelenburg position as necessary). Call 911 if necessary.

a. Epinephrine 1:1000 SC or IM (1:10,000 IV)
b. Oxygen (mouthpiece, bag available)
c. Benadryl or other antihistamine
d. Cimetidine or ranitidine
e. Bronchodilators: albuterol, levalbuterol, (Xopenex), atropine (by nebulizer or metered-dose inhaler)
f. Corticosteroids
g. Data are not presently available on the use of antileukotrienes in anaphylaxis.
h. IV fluids if necessary.

F. Monitoring

Monitor over an extended period, because delayed reactions (4–6 hours post reaction) can be equally severe.

G. Discharge

Discharge patient with:

1. A detailed treatment plan (written and verbal) with all medications available.
2. A record of the office treatment received for this reaction, in case the patient is seen later in the ER.
3. Emergency numbers for the physician on call. Needless to say, if delayed symptoms occur after discharge, it may be necessary to call 911. Patients with a generalized anaphylactic reaction are often held overnight in an ER or admitted to the hospital.

H. Dosage Adjustment

If patients continue with immunotherapy, the dose is adjusted and dropped back significantly.

IV. Patient Follow-up—Clinical Questionnaire

Patients need to be seen within the first couple of months after the initiation of therapy and at regular 6- to 12-month intervals while on therapy. Key questions include the following:

A. How long has the patient been receiving immunotherapy (i.e., number of months)?

B. Any local reactions to immunotherapy (date, symptoms, treatment)?

C. Any systemic reactions to immunotherapy (date, symptoms, treatment)?

D. Any change in symptoms
since starting shots?　　　　__Yes　　　__No

1. Nasal congestion
2. Drainage
3. Snoring
4. Sleep pattern
5. Fatigue
6. Sinusitis
7. Wheezing
8. Coughing
9. Bronchitis
10. Missed work/school
11. Other

E. Medications needed for symptom control (e.g., antihistamines, nasal steroids, nasal antihistamines, nasal cromolyn, nasal ipratropium bromide,decongestants, bronchodilators, inhaled steroids, leukotriene receptor antagonists)?

V. Patient Education: Terminology for Allergen Immunotherapy[4,5]

For patients and staff the terms used in the immunotherapy program may be confusing. The following is a list of commonly used terms.

A. Antigen/Allergen

An *antigen* or *allergen* is generally a high-molecular-weight molecule (such as a protein, glycoprotein, or lipoprotein) of foreign animal or vegetable origin[4,6] that has been determined to be a possible cause of a patient's sensitivity reaction. The immunologic response to the antigen is influenced by the duration and amount of exposure, as well as by other environmental factors. Common triggers for allergic reactions include pollen, house dust mite, cockroach, fungi, molds, animal dander, and insect venom. Exposure can be related to natural lifestyle (e.g., household exposure) or to occupational exposure.

Allergens are used for testing as well as for the treatment of the allergic individual.

B. Dilution

An extract or vaccine is usually diluted in series of four to five 10-fold (vol/vol) dilutions.[6] The patient's treatment schedule is based on a stepwise increase in dose to a maintenance level.

Bottles need to be clearly labeled with the patient's name, antigen (name), dilution of concentrate (vol/vol), bottle number (1–4), lid color corresponding to the dilution (red, yellow . . .), expiration date, and name of prescribing physician.

C. Desensitization

During a desensitization procedure, a substance, usually a medication, is given in gradually increasing, small doses to a patient with a history of allergic reactions to that specific antigen. Such treatment allows the immune system to tolerate exposure to the antigen.

D. Immediate Reaction versus Delayed Reaction

Signs or symptoms occurring within a couple of hours of treatment or exposure can be considered an immediate reaction. Delayed reactions typically occur within 4–6 hours of the initial exposure and may occur with or without immediate symptoms. Symptoms can include nasal or pulmonary congestion, hives, or generalized anaphylaxis.

E. Local Reaction versus Systemic Reaction

Local reactions are characterized by symptoms at the site of contact, such as redness, swelling, or itching at the site of the injection. Systemic signs or symptoms can include generalized pruritus, hives, redness, angioedema, laryngeal edema, asthma, hypotension, and anaphylaxis. Patients and staff must be aware of and prepared for such reactions to immunotherapy.

F. Maintenance Concentration

This refers to the individual patient's maximum dose used for ongoing immunotherapy. Once this dose is attained, the patient can often extend the interval between treatments. Efficacy is related to dose. It is important to reach the maintenance dose as quickly as possible and continue at regular intervals.

G. Rush versus Traditional Schedules for Advancing Allergen/Vaccine Doses

"Rush" programs are designed to advance a patient to maintenance therapy in a stepwise manner in 1 or 2 days.[7] "Cluster" schedules allow the patient to receive approximately three shots or dose increases per visit (with an appropriate waiting time between each step). Traditional programs are characterized by a single increase in dose weekly or biweekly. The goal of all schedules is to bring the patient to a maximum or maintenance concentration dose quickly and safely.

H. Standardized Antigen

The FDA has established a standard "strength" for a given antigen based on skin test results or single antigen determination (e.g., Der P 1 antigen). The standardized units are reported as allergy units (AU) or bioequivalent allergy units (BAU). Prior to availability of this standardization, antigens were labeled by wt/vol or PNU (protein nitrogen unit), neither of which provides an index of immunologic activity.

I. Test Dose of Allergen/Vaccine

This is a term that is often used to describe the first dose of antigen or vaccine. This dose is given intradermally. If a significant reaction occurs, it may be necessary to drop back to a lower dilution for the starting dose.

J. Stock Antigen versus Individual Treatment Mixes

The term *stock antigen* usually refers to a single antigen or mix of specific antigens that is prescribed frequently for patients (e.g., cat antigen, house dust mite mix, or special grass mix). The antigen is often packaged in a multidose vial.

Individual mixes include those antigens noted to be reactive on skin or RAST testing. The antigen or formulation may include only one or two specific grasses rather than a "grass mix" because of recognized antigen cross-reactivity.

REFERENCES

1. American Academy of Allergy and Immunology: Personnel and equipment to treat systematic reactions caused by immunotherapy with allergenic extracts (position statement). J Allergy Clin Immunol 1986;77:271–273.

2. American Academy of Allergy and Immunology: Guidelines to minimize the risk from systemic reactions caused by immunotherapy with allergic extracts (position statement). J Allergy Clin Immunol 1994;93:811–812.

3. American Academy of Allergy and Immunology: The use of epinephrine in the treatment of anyphylaxis (position statement). J Allergy Clin Immunol 1994;94:666–648.

4. Kao N: Terminology for allergen immunotherapy (guest editorial). Ann Allergy Asthma Immunol 2000;84:273–274.

5. Blumenthal MN, Rosenberg A: Definition of an allergen. In: Lockey RF, Bukantz SC, eds. Allergens and Allergin Immunotherapy, 2nd ed. New York: Marcel Dekker, 1999, pp 39–51.

6. Nelson HS: Preparing and mixing allergen vaccines. In: Lockey RF, Bukantz SC, eds. Allergens and Allergen Immunotherapy, 2nd ed. New York: Marcel Dekker, 1999, pp 401–422.

7. Grammer LC, Shaughnessy MA, Patterson R (eds.): Administration of Inhalant Allergen Vaccines, pp 423–434.

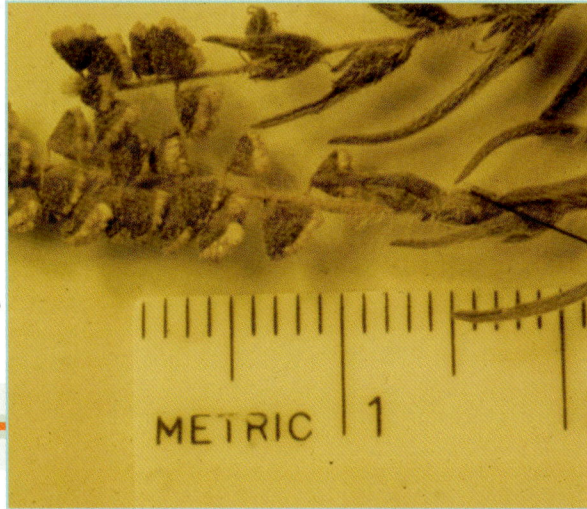

APPENDIX 2
Pollen Distribution in the United States

The following list includes only the most common pollen and mold varieties in each zone. For the most current and comprehensive prevalence reports, readers should refer to the Annual Pollen and Spore Report, published by the American Academy of Allergy, Asthma and Immunology (www.aaaai.org).

Pollen Prevalence in North American Floristic Zones

N (north), S (south), E (east), W (west), and L (local) indicate occurrence limited to these areas within a zone.

I. Northern Forest (Northern New England, Michigan, Minnesota, the Appalachian Peaks)

Trees

Pine, spruce, fir, hemlock, arborvitae	May–July
Birch, hazelnut, poplar, aspen	May–early July

Grasses (relatively low in summer)

Weeds (traditionally low levels, "refuge" for ragweed-sensitive)

II. Eastern Agricultural Region

Trees

Red cedar, hazelnut	Feb–April
Elm	Mar–April
Alder, maple (amphiphilous), poplar, aspen, ash	Mar–May
Birch, paper mulberry (S)	Mar–May
Willow	Mar–July
Box elder (W), sycamore, hackberry (L)	April–May
Beech (N)	April–May
Oak, mulberry, walnut, hickory	April–June

Grasses

Bluegrass, orchard, timothy, red top, bermuda	May–July
Perennial ryegrass, sweet vernal	May–July

Weeds

Sheep (red) sorrel	May–June
Plantain	May–Oct
Nettles, hemp (NW), western water hemp (W)	July–Sept
Russian thistle (W), kochia, pigweed, amaranth	July–Sept
Sages and mugworts	July–Oct
Southern (SW) and perennial (W) ragweed	Aug–Oct
Short and giant ragweed	Aug–Oct
Burweed marsh elder (W)	Aug–Oct
Rough marsh elder (S, W)	Aug–Oct

III. Southeastern Coastal Plain

Trees

Red cedar	Jan–April
Hackberry	Jan–May
Elm, pecan, hickory	Feb–April
Willow	Feb–May
Poplar	Mar–April
Ash, birch, sweet gum, maple	Mar–May
Sycamore, mulberry	Mar–June
Oak, walnut	Mar–May

Grasses

Bermuda (predominant)	Mar–Sept
Eastern agricultural region species	

Weeds

Sheep (red) sorrel	April–June
Plantain	May–Oct
Nettle, sagewort-mugwort (L)	July–Sept
Western water hemp (W), Russian thistle (NW)	July–Sept
Pigweeds, amaranths	July–Sept
Kochia, short and giant ragweed	Aug–Oct
Southern ragweed (W)	Aug–Oct
Rough and burweed marsh elders (W)	Aug–Oct

IV. Florida Subtropical Region

Trees

Bald cypress	Jan–Mar
Oak	Jan–April
Palm	Jan–Dec
Australian Pine	Oct–April (often with early and late peaks)

Grasses

Bermuda	Jan–Dec
Johnson	Jan–Dec
Bahia	Jan–Dec

Weeds

Short ragweed	July–Sept
Baccharis (groundsel)	July–Sept
Chenopod, amaranth	Jan–Dec (peak in late summer)

V. Central Plains

Trees

Mountain cedar (SW)	Dec–Mar
Elm	Jan–April, Aug–Sept (S)
Ash, oak	Jan–May
Poplar, box elder	Feb–April

Willow, hackberry (S)	Feb–May
Sycamore, walnut	Mar–May
Hickory, pecan, mulberry	Mar–May
Osage orange (SE)	April–May

Grasses

Eastern agricultural region species	June–July
Bermuda	
Smooth brome	
Fescue	
Johnson	

Weeds

Sheep (red) sorrel	May–July
Atriplex species	June–Aug
Hemp (NE), Russian thistle, kochia	July–Sept
Greasewood (W), smotherweed (NW)	July–Sept
Burweed & rough marsh elder (S)	July–Oct
Sagebrushes, sages	July–Oct
Western water hemp	July–Oct
Western and burr ragweed	Aug–Oct

VI. Rocky Mountain Region

Trees

Mountain cedar, junipers (SE)	Jan–Mar
Elm	Feb–April
Alder	Mar–April
Ash	Mar–May
Willow	Mar–June
Poplar, aspen	April–May
Birch	April–June
Oak	May–June

Grasses (decrease with elevation)

Central Plains species	May–July

Weeds

Species from adjacent Central Plains,
Great Basin or Arid Southwestern regions (Ragweed, chenopods,
amaranths diminish above 5000 feet)

VII. Arid Southwestern Region

Trees

Mountain cedar (E)	Dec–Mar
Elm	Feb–Mar, Aug–Oct
Arizona cypress (W)	Feb–Mar
Ash, poplar, mulberry	Feb–April
Mesquite	Feb–June
Olive (Sycamore, eucalyptus, pecan, hackberry, acacia present in irrigated areas)	Mar–May

Grasses

Bermuda	All warm months
Great Plains species	All warm months
Salt grass	All warm months
Canary grass	All warm months

Weeds

Burroweed	Feb–June
Sagebrush, sages	Feb–May, July–Oct
Rabbit bush	Mar–May
Shadscale	May–Aug
Greasewood	May–Sept
Kochia, sugar beet (L)	July–Oct
Short and slender ragweed	July–Oct

Pollen Prevalence in North American Floristic Zones (continued)

VIII. Great Basin

Trees

Juniper	Feb–May
Elm, poplar	Mar–April
Willow	Mar–May
Sycamore, box elder (L)	April–May

Grasses (levels generally low)
Central Plains species (N)
Arid Southwest species (S)

Weeds

Sagebrush, sages	June–Nov
Russian thistle	July–Sept
Kochia, greasewood	July–Oct
Short and bur ragweeds	Aug–Oct
Poverty weed	Aug–Nov

IX. California Lowland

Trees

Mulberry, alder, ash, willow	Jan–April
Walnut	Jan–May
Poplar	Feb–April
Elm	Feb–April, Aug–Oct
Sycamore	Feb–April
Oak, birch	Feb–May
Olive	Mar–May

Grasses

Bermuda, brome, ryegrass, wild oats	Mar–Nov

Weeds

Nettle	May–Aug
Bur ragweeds	June–Sept
Western ragweeds	July–Oct
Sagebrush, sages	July–Oct
Chenopods and amaranths	Summer–fall

X. Northwest Coastal Regions

Trees

Hazelnut	Jan–Mar
Alders, willow, ash	Feb–April
Box elder	Mar–April
Birch	Mar–May
Poplar, aspen, elm	Mar–June
Coast maple, oak, walnut (L)	April–June

Grasses

Eastern agricultural species	May–Aug
Sweet vernal, velvet, ryegrass	May–Aug

Weeds (levels relatively low)
(Much of Pacific Northwest remains ragweed-free)

Plantain	May–Sept
Sheep (red) sorrel	June–Aug
Poverty weed (L), nettle	June–Aug
Russian thistle, sagebrush, sages	July–Sept
Short ragweed (L)	Aug–Sept

Adapted from Solomon WR, Platts-Mills TAE: Aerobiology and inhalant allergens. In Middleton E Jr, et al (eds): Allergy: Principles and Practice, 5th ed. St. Louis: Mosby, 1998.

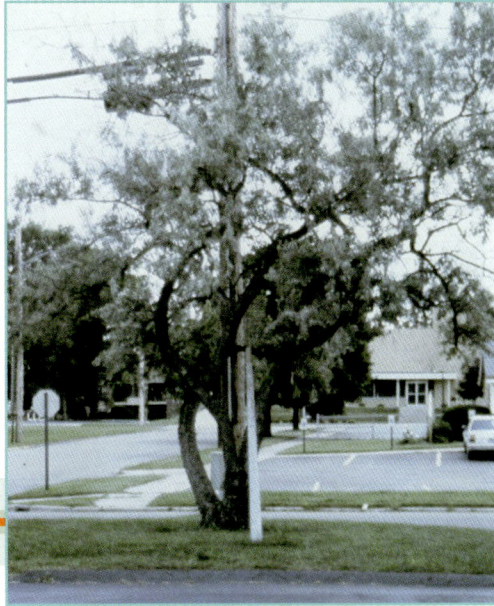

Russian Olive *Courtesy of Hollister-Stier Laboratory*

APPENDIX 3
Allergic Extract Manufacturers

ALK-Abelló, Inc.
1700 Royston Lane
Round Rock, TX 78664
512-251-0037
Fax: 512-251-8450
www.alk-abello.com

Allergy Laboratories, Inc.
1005 SW 2nd St.
Oklahoma City, OK 73109
800-654-3971
Fax: 800-811-3389
www.allergylabs.com

Allergy Laboratories of Ohio, Inc.
623 E. 11th Ave.
Columbus, OH 43211
614-291-7414
Fax: 614-291-2329

Allermed Laboratories, Inc.
7203 Convoy Ct.
San Diego, CA 92111
858-292-1060
Fax: 800-221-2748
www.allermed.com

Antigen Laboratories
3034 S. Main St.
Liberty, MO 64068
816-781-5222
Fax: 816-781-5189

Center Laboratories
35 Channel Dr.
Port Washington, NY 11050
516-767-1800
Fax: 516-767-4229

Greer Laboratories
Box 800
Lenoir, NC 28645
828-754-5327
Fax: 828-754-5320
www.greerlabs.com

Hollister-Stier Laboratories LLC
3525 N. Regal St.
Spokane, WA 99207-5788
509-482-0567
800-992-1120
Fax: 800-752-6258
www.hollister-stier.com

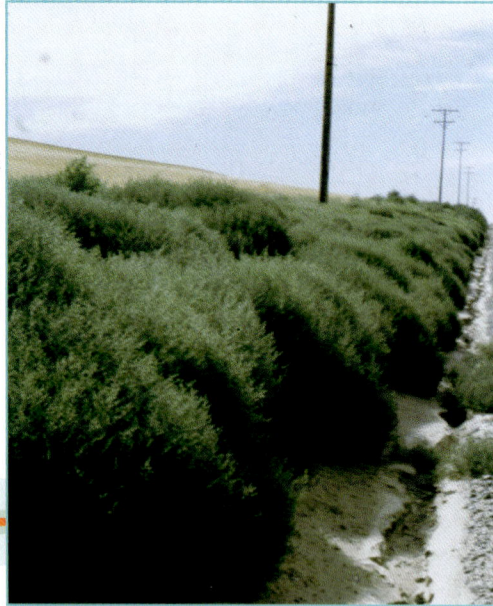

Russian Thistle *Courtesy of Hollister-Stier Laboratory*

APPENDIX 4
Total Serum IgE by Age

Serum IgE Levels in Infants and Younger Children

Age	No.	Geometric Mean (ng/mL)	95th Percentile Limits (ng/mL)
Cord blood	24	0.53	0.1–3.1
6 wk	17	1.67	0.2–15
3 mo	15	1.98	0.4–9.1
6 mo	15	6.49	1.0–39
9 mo	16	5.71	1.8–18
1 yr	12	8.45	1.9–37
2 yr	18	7.33	0.8–71
3 yr	6	4.36	0.5–41
4 yr	7	20.8	2.6–167
7 yr	18	31.2	2.5–390

From Kjellman NIM, Johansson SGO, Roth A: Serum IgE levels in healthy children quantified by a sandwich technique (PRIST). Clin Allergy 1976;6:51. Reproduced with permission.

Total Serum IgE Levels in Skin Test–Negative Older Children and Adults

Age (yr)	No.	Sex	Geometric Mean (IU/mL)	Geometric Mean ± 2 SD (IU/mL)
6–14	69	M	40.9	2.0–824.1
	71	F	40.7	3.4–452.9
15–34	213	M	23.3	0.9–635.3
	201	F	16.5	0.8–349.1
35–54	145	M	20.4	0.9–443.6
	154	F	14.6	0.7–286.4
55–74	224	M	19.8	0.8–484.2
	348	F	10.7	0.6–198.6
75+	61	M	17.8	0.8–387.3
	83	F	8.9	0.4–208.9

From Klink M, Cline MG, Halonen M, et al: Problems in defining normal limits for serum IgE. J Allergy Clin Immunol 1990;85:440. Reproduced with permission.

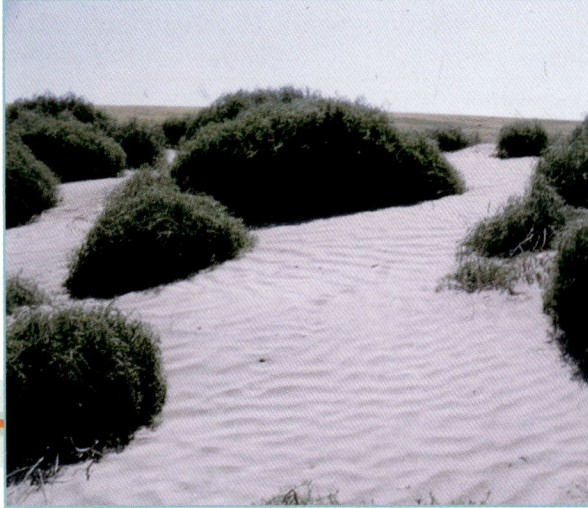

Russian Thistle 2 Courtesy of Hollister-Stier Laboratory

APPENDIX 5
Dermatology Reference Tables

TABLE A5-1

Descriptions of Primary and Secondary Skin Lesions

Lesion	Description
Primary (basic) lesions	
Macule	Circumscribed flat discoloration
Papule	Elevated solid lesion (≤5 mm)
Plaque	circumscribed superficially elevated solid lesion (>5 mm); often a confluence of papules
Nodule	Palpable solid (round) lesion, deeper than a papule
Wheal (hive)	Pale red edematous plaque, round or flat-topped and transient
Pustule	Elevated collection of purulence
Vesicle	Circumscribed elevated collection of fluid (≤5 mm in diameter)
Bulla	Circumscribed elevated collection of fluid (>5 mm in diameter)
Secondary (sequential) lesions	
Scale (desquamation)	Excess dead epidermal cells
Crusts	A collection of dried serum, blood, or purulence
Erosion	Superficial loss of epidermis
Ulcer	Focal loss of epidermis and dermis
Fissure	Linear loss of epidermis and dermis
Atrophy	Depression in the skin from thinning of epidermis or dermis
Excoriation	Erosion caused by scratching
Lichenification	Thickened epidermis with prominent skin lines (induced by scratching)

From Usatine R: Skin problems. In Sloane P, Slatt L, Ebell M (eds): The Essentials of Family Medicine, 3rd ed. Baltimore: Williams and Wilkins, 1999. Reproduced with permission.

TABLE A5-2

Commonly Used Vehicles for Steroids and Other Dermatologic Preparations

Creams
- Mixture of oil and water; may contain alcohol
- White color; may be somewhat greasy
- May cause stinging and irritation to broken skin
- May be drying; best for moist or exudative lesions
- Cosmetically most acceptable
- Better in skin folds than ointments

Ointments
- Base is frequently petroleum jelly (petrolatum)
- Translucent and very greasy
- Best for dry lesions; lubricating
- Greasy feeling persists after application
- May get on clothes and be transferred from hands to surfaces at work
- Cosmetically less acceptable in daytime (may be used at night and apply cream during the day)
- Increased absorption of steroid and therefore enhances potency of the steroid
- Too occlusive for exudative lesions and areas of skin folds (groin)
- Too messy for hair-covered areas.

Gels
- Greaseless mixtures of propylene glycol and water; may contain alcohol
- Clear and jelly-like
- Useful for exudative lesions; may be drying

Solutions and lotions
- Water and alcohol base
- Solutions usually clear; lotions have a milky appearance
- Best for scalp and other hair-covered areas: penetrates easily and doesn't make hair greasy
- May cause stinging and irritation to broken skin

Modified from Habif T: Clinical Dermatology: A Color Guide to Diagnosis and Therapy, 3rd ed. St. Louis: Mosby, 1996.

TABLE A5-3

Topical Glucocorticoid Potency Ranking

Group I (Super high potency)

- Betamethasone dipropionate 0.05% (cream and ointment)
- Clobetasol propionate 0.05% (cream and ointment)
- Diflorasone diacetate 0.05% (ointment)
- Halobetasol propionate 0.05% (cream and ointment)

Group II (High potency)

- Amcinonide 0.1% (ointment)
- Betamethasone dipropionate 0.05% (cream and ointment)
- Desoximetasone 0.25% (cream)
- Desoximetasone 0.05% (gel)
- Diflorasone diacetate 0.05% (ointment)
- Fluocinonide 0.05% (cream, gel, ointment, and solution)
- Halcinonide 0.1% (cream)
- Mometasone furoate 0.1% (ointment)

Group III (Intermediate high potency)

- Amcinonide 0.1% (cream and lotion)
- Betamethasone dipropionate 0.05% (cream)
- Betamethasone valerate 0.1% (ointment)
- Desoximetasone 0.05% (cream)
- Diflorasone diacetate 0.05% (cream)
- Fluocinonide 0.05% (cream)
- Halcinonide 0.1% (ointment and solution)
- Triamcinolone acetonide 0.1% (ointment)

Group IV (Intermediate potency)

- Hydrocortisone valerate 0.2% (ointment)
- Flurandrenolide 0.05% (ointment)
- Fluocinolone acetonide 0.025% (ointment)
- Mometasone furoate 0.1% (cream)

Group V (Intermediate low potency)

- Betamethasone dipropionate 0.05% (lotion)
- Betamethasone valerate 0.1% (cream)
- Fluticasone acetonide 0.025% (cream)
- Fluticasone propionate 0.05% (cream)
- Flurandrenolide 0.05% (cream)
- Hydrocortisone valerate 0.2% (cream)
- Prednicarbate 0.1% (cream)

Group VI (Low potency)

- Alclometasone dipropionate 0.05% (cream and ointment)
- Betamethasone valerate 0.05% (lotion)
- Desonide 0.05% (cream)
- Fluocinolone acetonide 0.01% (cream and solution)
- Triamcinolone acetonide 0.1% (cream)

Group VII (Lowest potency)

- Hydrocortisone hydrochloride 1% (cream and ointment)
- Hydrocortisone hydrochloride 2.5% (cream, lotion and ointment)
- Hydrocortisone acetate 1% (cream and ointment)
- Hydrocortisone acetate 2.5% (cream, lotion, and ointment)
- Pramoxine hydrochloride 1.0% (cream, lotion, and ointment)
- Pramoxine hydrochloride 2.5% (cream, lotion, and ointment)

From Leung D, Hanifin JM, Charlesworth EN: disease management of atopic dermatitis: a practice parameter, 1997, with permission.

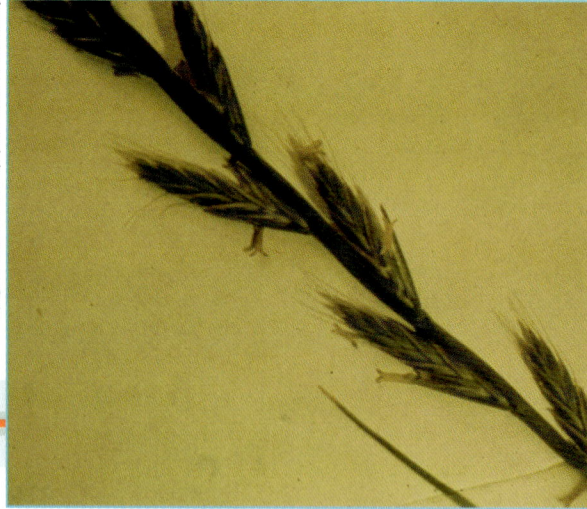

APPENDIX 6
Tips for Managing Food Allergies*

I. Tips for Managing a Milk Allergy

A. Baking

Fortunately, milk is one of the easiest ingredients to substitute in baking and cooking. It can be substituted, in equal amounts, with water or fruit juice. (For example, substitute 1 cup milk with 1 cup water.)

Some hidden sources of milk

a. Deli meat slicers are frequently used for both meat and cheese products.

b. Some brands of canned tuna fish contain casein, a milk protein.

c. Many nondairy products contain casein (a milk derivative), listed on the ingredient labels. The FAAN is currently working with the FDA to have this term eliminated on products that contain milk derivatives.

d. Some meats may contain casein as a binder. Check all labels carefully.

e. Many restaurants put butter on steaks after they have been grilled to add extra flavor. The butter is not visible after it melts.

B. Commonly Asked Questions

1. **Is goat's milk a safe alternative to cow's milk?**
Goat's milk protein is similar to cow's milk protein and may, therefore, cause a reaction in milk-allergic individuals. It is not a safe alternative.

2. **Can I rely on kosher symbols to determine if a product is milk-free?**
The Jewish community uses a system of product markings to indicate whether a food is kosher, or prepared in accordance with Jewish dietary rules. There are two Kosher symbols that can be of help for those with a milk allergy: a "D," or the word *dairy*, on a label next to "K" or "U" (usually found near the product name) indicates the presence of milk protein, and a "DE" on a label indicates the food has been produced on equipment shared with dairy.

   If the product contains neither meat nor dairy products, it is *pareve*. Pareve-labeled products indicate that the products are considered milk-free according to religious specifications. Be aware that under Jewish law, a food product containing a small amount

*Source: Food Allergy and Anaphylaxis Network (FAAN). Available at www.foodallergy.org.

252

of milk may be considered pareve. Therefore, a product labeled as pareve could potentially have enough milk protein in it to cause a reaction in a milk-allergic individual.

3. ***Do these ingredients contain milk?***
These ingredients do not contain milk protein and need not be restricted by someone avoiding milk:

- Calcium lactate
- Calcium stearoyl lactylate
- Cocoa butter
- Lactic acid
- Oleoresin
- Sodium lactate
- Sodium stearoyl lactylate

II. Tips for Managing an Egg Allergy

A. Baking

For each egg, substitute one of the following in recipes:

- 1 tsp baking powder, 1 T liquid, 1 T vinegar
- 1 tsp yeast dissolved in 1/4 cup warm water
- 1 1/2 T water, 1 1/2 T oil, 1 tsp baking powder
- 1 packet gelatin, 2 T warm water. Do not mix until ready to use.
These substitutes work well when baking from scratch and substituting 1 to 3 eggs.

B. Some Hidden Sources of Egg

1. Eggs have been used to create the foam or milk topping on specialty coffee drinks and are used in some bar drinks.
2. Some commercial brands of egg substitutes contain egg whites.

    Most commercially processed cooked pastas (including those used in prepared foods such as soup) contain egg or are processed on equipment shared with egg-containing pastas. Boxed, dry pastas are usually egg-free. Fresh pasta is usually egg-free, too. Read the label or ask about ingredients before eating pasta.

III. Tips for Managing a Peanut Allergy

A. Some Hidden Sources of Peanuts

1. Artificial nuts can be peanuts that have been deflavored and reflavored with a nut, such as pecan or walnut. Mandelonas are peanuts soaked in almond flavoring.
2. Arachis oil is peanut oil.
3. It is advised that peanut-allergic patients avoid chocolate candies unless they are absolutely certain there

is no risk of cross-contact during manufacturing procedures.

4. African, Chinese, Indonesian, Mexican, Thai, and Vietnamese dishes often contain peanuts or are contaminated with peanuts during preparation of these types of meals. Additionally, foods sold in bakeries and ice cream shops are often in contact with peanuts. It is recommended that peanut-allergic individuals avoid these types of foods and restaurants.
5. Many brands of sunflower seeds are produced on equipment shared with peanuts.

B. Keep in Mind

1. Studies show that most allergic individuals can safely eat peanut oil (not cold pressed, expelled, or extruded peanut oil—sometimes represented as gourmet oils).
2. Most experts recommend peanut-allergic patients avoid tree nuts as well.
3. Peanuts can be found in many foods. Check all labels carefully. Contact the manufacturer if you have questions.

C. Commonly Asked Questions

1. ***Can a peanut allergy be outgrown?***
Although once considered to be a lifelong allergy, recent studies indicate that up to 20% of children diagnosed with peanut allergy outgrow it.
2. ***Can alternative nut butters (e.g., cashew nut butter) be substituted for peanut butter?***
Many nut butters are produced on equipment used to process peanut butter, therefore making it somewhat of a risky alternative. Additionally, most experts recommend that peanut-allergic patients avoid tree nuts as well.

IV. Tips for Managing a Tree Nut Allergy

A. Some Hidden Sources of Tree Nuts

1. Artificial nuts can be peanuts that have been deflavored and reflavored with a nut, such as pecan or walnut. Mandelonas are peanuts soaked in almond flavoring.
2. Mortadella may contain pistachios.
3. Natural and artificial flavoring may contain tree nuts.
4. Tree nuts have been used in many foods including barbecue sauce, cereals, crackers, and ice cream.
5. Kick sacks (or hacky sacks), beanbags, and draft dodgers are sometimes filled with crushed nut shells.

B. Commonly Asked Questions

1. ***Should coconut be avoided by someone with a tree nut allergy?***
A coconut is the seed of a drupaceous fruit. Coconuts are not typically restricted in the diet of an

individual allergic to tree nuts. Some people have reacted to coconut; therefore, discuss this with a doctor before introducing coconut to your diet.

2. *Is nutmeg safe?*

Nutmeg is obtained from the seeds of the tropical tree species *Myristica fragrans*. It is safe for an individual with a tree nut allergy.

C. Keep in Mind

1. Most experts advise tree nut-allergic patients to avoid peanuts as well.
2. Most experts advise patients who have been diagnosed with an allergy to specific tree nuts to avoid all tree nuts.

V. Tips for Managing a Fish and/or Shellfish Allergy

A. Keep in Mind

1. Fish-allergic individuals should be cautious when eating away from home. They should avoid fish and seafood restaurants because of the risk of contamination in the food-preparation area of their "nonfish" meal from a counter, spatula, cooking oil, fryer, or grill exposed to fish. In addition, fish protein can become airborne during cooking and cause an allergic reaction. Some individuals have had reactions from walking through a fish market.
2. Allergic reactions to fish and shellfish can be severe and are often a cause of anaphylaxis.

B. Some Hidden Sources of Fish

1. Caponata, a traditional sweet-and-sour Sicilian relish, can contain anchovies.
2. Caesar salad dressings, steak sauce, and Worcestershire sauce often contain anchovies.
3. Surimi (imitation crabmeat) often contains fish.

C. Commonly Asked Questions

1. *Should carrageenan be avoided by a fish- or shellfish-allergic individual?*

Carrageenan is not fish. Carrageenan, or Irish moss, is a red marine alga. This food product is used in a wide variety of foods, particularly dairy foods, as an emulsifier, stabilizer, and thickener. It appears safe for most individuals with food allergies. Carrageenan is not related to fish or shellfish and does not need to be avoided by those with food allergies.

2. *Should iodine be avoided by a fish- or shellfish-allergic individual?*

Allergy to iodine, allergy to radiocontrast material (used in some lab procedures), and allergy to fish or shellfish are not related. If you have an allergy to fish or shellfish, you do not need to worry about cross-reactions with radiocontrast material or iodine.

VI. Tips for Managing a Soy Allergy

A. Soybeans have become a major part of processed food products in the United States. Avoiding products made with soybeans can be difficult.

B. Soybeans alone are not a major food in the diet, but because they are in so many products, eliminating all those foods can result in an unbalanced diet. Consult a dietitian to help you plan for proper nutrition.

C. Keep in Mind

1. Soybeans and soy products are found in baked goods, canned tuna, cereals, crackers, infant formulas, sauces, and soups. At least one brand of peanut butter lists soy on the label.
2. Studies show soy lecithin and soybean oil can be tolerated by most soy-allergic individuals.

D. Soy-Free Stir-Fry Recipe

Stir-Fried Orange Beef

- 1 tsp cornstarch
- 1 cup orange juice
- 1 to 1 1/2 lb trimmed beef, thinly sliced
- 1 to 2 T of oil
- 1/4 to 1/2 tsp crushed red pepper flakes
- 1 clove minced garlic
- 1 T grated fresh ginger root
- 1/4 cup green onion, thin-sliced
- 1/4 cup bell pepper, thin-sliced

Directions: In small bowl, combine cornstarch and orange juice. Set aside. In a wok, add beef, oil, and red pepper flakes. Stir-fry over high heat until beef is browned. Remove beef with slotted spoon. Set aside. Add garlic, ginger root, onion, and bell pepper to oil remaining in the wok. Stir-fry 2 minutes. Add cornstarch/orange juice mixture. Simmer until thickened. Add beef and toss with sauce. Can be served over noodles or rice.

VII. Tips for Managing a Wheat Allergy

A. Baking

1. When baking with wheat-free flours, a combination of flours usually works best. Experiment with different blends to find one that will give you the texture you are trying to achieve.
2. Try substituting 1 cup wheat flour with one of the following:

- 7/8 cup rice flour
- 5/8 cup potato starch flour
- 1 cup soy flour plus 1/4 cup potato starch flour
- 1 cup corn flour

B. Keep in Mind

1. Read labels carefully. At least one brand of hot dogs and one brand of ice cream contain wheat. It is listed on the label.
2. Many country-style wreaths are decorated with wheat products.
3. Some types of imitation crabmeat contain wheat.
4. Wheat flour is sometimes flavored and shaped to look like beef, pork, and shrimp, especially in Asian dishes.

C. Commonly Asked Questions

1. ***What is the difference between celiac disease and wheat allergy?***
   Celiac disease and wheat allergy are two distinct conditions. Celiac disease, or celiac sprue, is a permanent adverse reaction to gluten. Those with celiac disease will not lose their sensitivity to this substance. This disease requires a lifelong restriction of gluten.

   The major grains that contain gluten are wheat, rye, oats, and barley. These grains and their by-products must be strictly avoided by people with celiac disease.

   Wheat-allergic people have an IgE-mediated response to wheat protein. These individuals must only avoid wheat. Most wheat-allergic children outgrow the allergy.

2. ***Are kamut and spelt safe alternatives to wheat?***
   No. Kamut is a cereal grain that is related to wheat. Spelt is an ancient wheat that has recently been marketed as safe for wheat-allergic individuals. This claim is untrue, however. Wheat-allergic patients can react as readily to spelt as they do to common wheat.

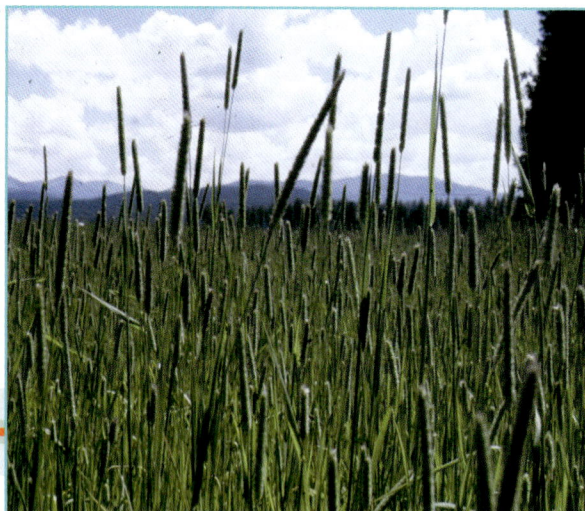
Timothy Courtesy of Hollister-Stier Laboratory

APPENDIX 7
Guide to Sources for Allergy Avoidance Products

Allerderm Laboratories, Inc.
1330 Redwood Way, Ste. C
Petaluma, CA 94954
707-664-8777
800-365-6868
Fax: 800-926-4568
www.allerderm.com

Aller/Guard Corp.
40 Cindy Lane
Ocean, NJ 07712
732-988-6868
800-234-0816
Fax: 732-988-6777
www.allergyhelp.com/allerguard

Allergy & Asthma Technology
8224 Lehigh Ave.
Morton Grove, IL 60053
800-621-5545
Fax: 847-966-3068
www.allergyasthmatech.com

Allergy Clean Environments, Inc.
3641 Garner Blvd.
Arlington, TX 76013
800-882-4110
Fax: 800-561-1077
www.allergyclean.com

Allergy Control Products
96 Danbury Rd.
Ridgefield, CT 06877
203-438-9580
Fax: 203-431-8963
www.allergycontrol.com

Allergy-Free LP
905 Gemini
Houston, TX 77058
281-486-4141 ext. 254
Fax: 281-486-9312
www.allergy-free.com

Allersearch Laboratories
Division of Alkaline Corp.
Box 306
Oakhurst, NJ 07755
908-531-7830
800-686-6483
Fax: 732-531-7160
www.allergyhelp.com/allersearch

ALO Laboratories, Inc.
623 E. 11th Ave.
Columbus, OH 43211
614-291-7414
800-654-5439
Fax: 614-291-2329

Cloud 9 Division
Mason Engineering and Design Corp.
777 Edgewood Ave.
Wood Dale, IL 60191
630-595-5000
Fax: 630-595-5902
www.4cloud9.com

The Easy Breathin' Group, Inc.
21804 Belshire Ave.
Hawaiian Gardens, CA 90716
562-421-5234
Fax: 562-421-5236
www.aller-rx.com

Euroclean
1151 Bryn Mawr Ave.
Itasca, IL 60143
630-773-2111
Fax: 630-773-2859
www.eurocleanusa.com

E.L. Foust Co., Inc.
Box 105
Elmhurst, IL 60126

Gazoontite Stores: www.gazoontite.com
New York:
2151 Broadway
New York, NY 10023
San Francisco:
2157 Union St.
San Francisco, CA 94123
Costa Mesa:
South Coast Plaza
3333 Bear Street
Costa Mesa, CA 92626

Hi-Tech Filter Corp. of America
80 Myrtle St.
North Quincy, MA 02171
617-328-7756
www.hitechfilter.com

Home Diagnostics
12910 Oak Bend Dr.
Austin, TX 78727
512-255-8188
Fax: 512-255-8188
www.homediagnostics.net

MDS Pharma Services
9 Medical Parkway, Plaza 4, Ste. 202
Dallas, TX 75324
972-241-1222
Fax: 972-241-0459
www.mdsps.com

Mycotech Biological
2482 FM 39 N.
Jewett, TX 75846
800-272-3716
Fax: 903-626-4429
www.iaqconsultants.com

National Allergy Supply, Inc.
1620 Satellite Blvd., Ste. D
Duluth, GA 30097
770-623-3237
800-522-1448
Fax: 770-623-5568
www.nationalallergy.com

Nilfisk-Advance America, Inc.
300 Technology Dr.
Malvern, PA 19355
610-647-6420
800-645-3475
Fax: 610-647-6427
www.pa.nilfisk-advance.com

Ogallala Down Co.
Box 830
Ogallala, NE 69153
308-284-8403
Fax: 308-284-8405
www.ogallaladown.com

Vitaire Corp.
Box 88
Elmhurst Annex, NY 11380
973-473-2244
800-552-5533
Fax: 201-592-6612

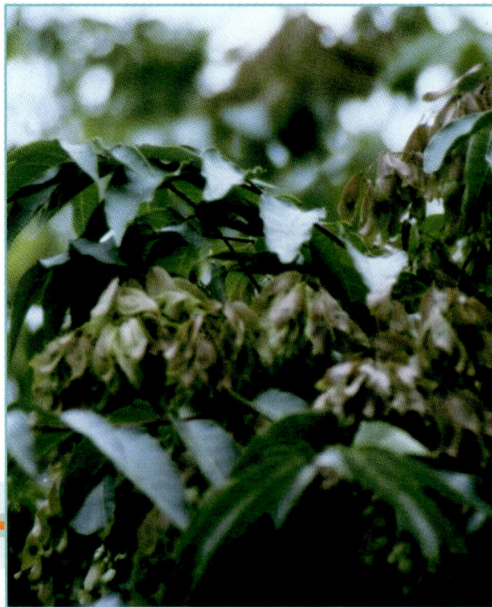

Tree of Heaven FR *Courtesy of Hollister-Stier Laboratory*

APPENDIX 8
Professional and Lay Organizations and Resources

Note: Specific information may be subject to change.

I. Professional Organizations

American Academy of Allergy, Asthma and Immunology
611 East Wells St.
Milwaukee, WI 53202
414-272-6071
Physician referral and information line: 1-800-822-2762
Fax: 414-272-6070
www.aaaai.org

American College of Allergy, Asthma and Immunology
85 West Algonquin Rd., Ste. 550
Arlington Heights, IL 60005
847-427-1200
Fax: 847-427-1294
www.acaai.org

Allergy, Asthma and Immunology Online
For the public: www.allergy.mcg.edu

Nationwide Asthma Screening Program
(Sponsored by the ACAAI)
www.allergy.mcg.edu/lifeQuality/nasp.html

Joint Council of Allergy, Asthma and Immunology
(Sponsored by the AAAAI and ACAAI)
50 N. Brockway, Ste. 3.3
Palatine, IL 60067
847-934-1918
Fax: 847-934-1820
www.jcaai.org

American Academy of Dermatology
930 N. Meacham Rd.
P.O. Box 4014
Schaumburg, IL 60168-4014
847-330-0230
Fax: 847-330-0050
www.aad.org

American College of Chest Physicians
3300 Dundee Rd.
Northbrook, IL 60062-2348
847-498-1400
Fax: 847-498-5460
www.chestnet.org

American Lung Association
1740 Broadway
New York, NY 10019
212-315-8700
Fax: 212-315-8872
1-800-LUNG-USA
www.lungusa.org

American Thoracic Society
1740 Broadway
New York, NY 10019
212-315-8700
Fax: 212-315-6498
www.thoracic.org

National Jewish Medical and Research Center
1400 Jackson St.
Denver, CO 80206
303-388-4461
Lung Line: 800-222-LUNG
www.njc.org

European Academy of Allergology and Immunology
www.eaaci.org

World Allergy Organization
611 East Wells St.
Milwaukee, WI 53202
414-276-1791
Fax: 414-276-3349
www.worldallergy.org

II. Government Agencies

National Heart, Lung and Blood Institute
NHLBI Information Center
P.O. Box 30105
Bethesda, MD 20824-0105
301-592-8573
Fax: 301-592-8563
www.nhlbi.nih.gov

National Institute of Allergy and Infectious Diseases
Bldg. 31, Rm. 7A-50
31 Center Dr., MSC 2520
Bethesda, MD 20892-2520
301-496-5717
www.niaid.nih.gov

National Library of Medicine
8600 Rockville Pike
Bethesda, MD 20894
888-FIND-NLM
888-346-3656
301-594-5983 (local and international calls)
www.nlm.nih.gov

III. Support Groups and Lay Organizations

A. Allergy & Asthma Network/Mothers of Asthmatics

This network facilitates communication of accurate allergy and asthma information among patients, parents, physicians, schools, and industry in an effort to help families create a management program for children who have allergies and asthma. It provides emotional support to individuals and their families with allergies and asthma and promotes the Bill of Rights for Children with Allergies and Asthma.

2751 Prosperity Avenue, Ste. 150
Fairfax, VA 22031
Phone: 800-878-4403 or 703-385-4403
Fax: 703-573-7794
www.aanma.org

B. Asthma and Allergy Foundation of America

The Asthma and Allergy Foundation of America is a not-for-profit, voluntary health organization dedicated to improving the quality of life for people with asthma and allergies and their caregivers through education, research, and advocacy.

1233 20th St., NW, Suite 402
Washington, DC 20036
Phone: 800-7-ASTHMA (800-727-8462) or 202-466-7643
Fax: 202-466-8940
www.aafa.org
Alabama chapter: www.asthmaandallergy.org
Florida chapter: www.aafaflorida.org
Maryland/Washington, DC chapter: www.aafa-md.org
North Texas chapter: www.aafa-ntx.org
Southern California chapter: www.aafasocal.org
Washington chapter: www.aafawa.org

C. Food Allergy and Anaphylaxis Network (FAAN)

FAAN's mission is to increase public awareness about food allergies and anaphylaxis, and to provide education, emotional support, and coping strategies to individuals with food allergies.

10400 Eaton Place, Ste. 107
Fairfax, VA 22030-2208
Phone: 800-929-4040 or 703-691-3179
Fax: 703-691-2713
www.foodallergy.org

D. Immune Deficiency Foundation (IDF)

This foundation is devoted to research and education in primary immune deficiency diseases, IDF has established chapters across the country. On behalf of those with primary immune deficiency diseases, IDF promotes and supports scientific research in the causes, prevention, and treatments; promotes and supports training in medical research and clinical treatment; coordinates and disseminates information; and conducts educational campaigns to increase public awareness.

25 West Chesapeake Ave., Ste. 206
Towson, MD 21204
Phone: 800-296-4433 or 410-321-6647
Fax: 410-321-9165
www.primaryimmune.org

E. International Food Information Council (IFIC)

IFIC's mission is to serve as the critical link between the scientific community, food manufacturers, health professionals, government officials and the news media. With clear, factual information as the cornerstone, these groups have the tools to build better understanding of nutrition and food safety issues for the benefit of the consuming public.

1100 Connecticut Ave., N.W., Ste. 430
Washington, DC 20036
Phone: 800-296-4433
www.ificinfo.health.org/

F. Consortium on Childrens' Asthma Camps

This consortium was established in 1988 to coordinate the camp activities of national organizations involved in the care of children with asthma. Their purpose is to promote and foster camps for children with asthma. The Camp Directory is a comprehensive list of asthma camps across the United States.

490 Concordia Ave.
St. Paul, MN 55103-2441
651-227-8014
Fax: 651-227-5459
www.lungusa.org/asthmacamps/

G. National Allergy Bureau (NAB)

NAB is the section of the American Academy of Allergy, Asthma, and Immunology's (AAAAI) Aeroallergen Network that is responsible for reporting current pollen and mold spore levels to the media. NAB works in cooperation with the American College of Allergy, Asthma and Immunology (ACAAI).

Year-round indoor allergies: 1-877-9-ACHOOO
Pollen and mold report: 1-800-9-POLLEN
www.aaaai.org/nab

H. MedicAlert

This company makes emergency information bracelets for patients.

2323 Colorado Ave.
Turlock, CO 95382
1-888-633-4298
Fax: 209-669-2495
www.medicalert.org

IV. Prescription Assistance Programs

The following programs are sponsored by pharmaceutical companies:

Aventis, Inc.
Indigent Patient Program
10236 Marion Park Dr.
P.O. Box 9950
Kansas City, MO 64134-9950
800-552-3656

Bayer Corporation
Indigent Patient Program
P.O. Box 29209
Phoenix, AZ 85038-9209
800-998-9180

Boehringer Ingelheim Pharmaceuticals
Partners in Health Prescription Assistance
900 Ridgebury Rd.
P.O. Box 368
Ridgefield, CT 06877-0368
800-556-8317

Forest Pharmaceuticals, Inc.
Indigent Care Program
13622 Lakefront Dr.
St. Louis, MO 63045
800-678-1605 x207

GlaxoSmithKline
Patient Assistance Program
P.O. Box 52185
Phoenix, AZ 85072-9711
800-722-9294

Merck & Co., Inc.
Patient Assistance Program
P.O. Box 4 (WP35-258)
West Point, PA 19486-0004
800-999-1796
800-994-2111 (health providers only)

Pfizer Pharmaceuticals
Prescription Assistance
P.O. Box 25457
Alexandria, VA 22313-5457
800-646-4455

Schering Laboratories
Patient Assistance Program
P.O. Box 52122
Phoenix, AZ 85072
800-656-9485

Astra-Zeneca Pharmaceuticals
Foundation Patient Assistance Program
P.O. Box 15197
Wilmington, DE 19850-5197
800-424-3727

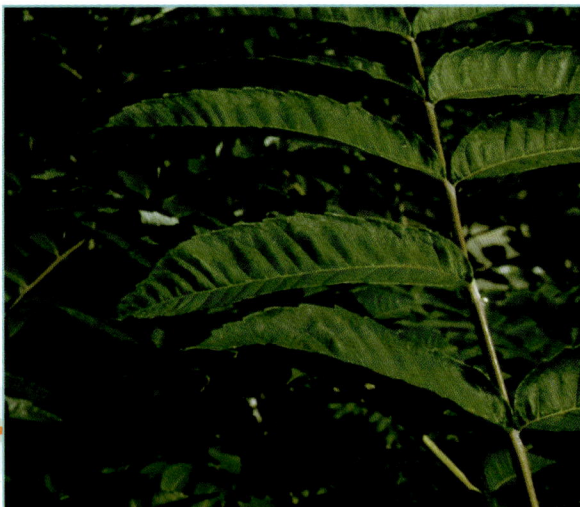

Tree of Heaven 2 Courtesy of Hollister-Stier Laboratory

APPENDIX 9
Internet Resources

Note: The web sites of professional organizations, government agencies, support groups and lay organizations devoted to allergy and immunology (see Chapter 29, Professional and Lay Organizations and Resources) are the most reliable sources of information and should be consulted first in any Internet search.

The following list of additional web sites is by no means comprehensive and may be subject to change.

I. Consumer Web Sites

A. Allergy, Asthma and Immunology Online

www.allergy.mcg.edu
Web site targeted to the public by the American College of Allergy, Asthma and Immunology

B. National Allergy Bureau

www.aaaai.org/nab
The National Allergy Bureau (NAB) is the section of the American Academy of Allergy, Asthma, and Immunology's (AAAAI) Aeroallergen Network that is responsible for reporting current pollen and mold spore levels to the media. The NAB works in cooperation with the American College of Allergy, Asthma and Immunology (ACAAI).

C. Asthma All-Stars

www.asthmaallstars.com
Olympic swimmer, Amy Van Dyken, NFL star, Jerome Bettis, and Olympic runner, Jackie Joyner-Kersee—three world-class athletes with one important message: People with asthma can live without limits.

D. MEDEM

www.medem.com
Health care information site founded by the nation's leading medical societies.

E. MSNBC Health News Page

www.msnbc.com/news/health_front.asp
Current news and interesting information about asthma and other allergic diseases for patients, parents, and physicians.

F. PDR's Getting Well Network

www.pdr.net
Current news and interesting information about asthma and other allergic diseases for patients, parents, and physicians.

G. Pedianet: Allergies

www.pedianet.com/news/allergies
General information on allergies.

H. Asthma Management Model System

www.nhlbisupport.com/asthma/index.html
Interactive web site developed by the National Asthma Education and Prevention Program (NAEPP). Sponsored by the National Heart, Lung, and Blood Institute.

I. National Committee on Quality Assurance

www.ncqa.org
Find out how your health plan measures up.

J. Bravekids

www.bravekids.org/
Information on children's diseases; chat rooms and message boards for parents of children with chronic illnesses.

K. Centros Para el Control y la Prevención de Enfermedades

www.cdc.gov/spanish/
Information on children's diseases; chat rooms and message boards for parents of children with chronic illnesses.

L. Asma: Como Controlar esta Enfermedad

www.nhlbi.nih.gov/health/public/lung/asthma/
Sponsored by the National Heart, Lung, and Blood Institute.

M. Clinical Trials Database

www.apps.nhlbi.nih.gov/clinicaltrials/
Sponsored by the National Heart, Lung, and Blood Institute.

N. Clinical Trials: Asthma Sponsored by CenterWatch, Inc.

www.centerwatch.com/studies/

O. MayoClinic.com

www.mayoclinic.com
General health information including allergies and asthma from the Mayo Clinic.

II. Publications Available On-Line

A. Asthma and Allergy Statistics (National Institute of Allergy and Infectious Diseases)

www.niaid.nih.gov/factsheets/allergystat.htm

B. Allergy-Immunology Glossary (American College of Allergy, Asthma and Immunology)

www.allergy.mcg.edu/glossary/index.html

C. AAAAI Public Education Materials: Tips to Remember (American Academy of Allergy, Asthma and Immunology)

www.aaaai.org/patients/publicedmat/tips/default.stm

D. Asthma and Allergy Prevention (National Institute of Environmental Health Sciences)

www.niehs.nih.gov/airborne/prevent/intro.html

E. Allergy Shots: Could They Help Your Allergies? (American Academy of Family Physicians)

www.familydoctor.org/handouts/232.html

F. Treating People with Allergic Diseases (National Institute of Allergy and Infectious Diseases)

www.niaid.nih.gov/publications/allergens/treating.htm

G. Living with Allergies (National Institute of Allergy and Infectious Diseases)

www.niaid.nih.gov/factsheets/allergyr.html

H. Environmental Control Measures (Nemours Foundation)

www.kidshealth.org/parent/general/body/environ_control.html

I. Something in the Air: Airborne Allergens (National Institute of Allergy and Infectious Diseases)

www.niaid.nih.gov/publications/allergens/title.htm

J. Antihistamines (American Academy of Family Physicians)

www.familydoctor.org/handouts/262.html

K. How to Create a Dust-Free Bedroom (National Institute of Allergy and Infectious Diseases)

www.niaid.nih.gov/factsheets/dustfree.html

L. Dust Mites in the Home (American Academy of Family Physicians)

www.familydoctor.org/handouts/683.html

M. Treating Allergic Conjunctivitis (American Academy of Family Physicians)

www.familydoctor.org/handouts/678.html

N. Managing Your Asthma Flare-ups (American Academy of Family Physicians)

www.familydoctor.org/handouts/681.html

O. Getting Your Asthma Under Control: A Self Evaluation (American College of Chest Physicians)

www.chestnet.org/health.science.policy/asthmacontrol.html

P. Your Asthma Can Be Controlled: Expect Nothing Less (National Heart, Lung, and Blood Institute)

www.nhlbi.nih.gov/health/public/lung/asthma/asthma.htm

Q. 8 Questions to Ask When Your Asthma Doesn't Get Better (American Academy of Family Physicians)

www.familydoctor.org/handouts/682.html

R. AMA Physician Select Reference Library: Asthma (American Medical Association)

www.ama-assn.org/aps/asthma/asthma.htm

S. Learn How to Clear Your Home of Asthma Triggers (Environmental Protection Agency)

www.epa.gov/iaq/asthma.index.html

T. Asthma & Physical Activity in School (National Heart, Lung, and Blood Institute)—Links to a PDF Document

www.nhlbi.nih.gov/health/public/lung/asthma/phy_asth.pdf

U. Asthma, Air Quality, and Environmental Justice: EPA's Role in Asthma Education and Prevention (Environmental Protection Agency)

www.epa.gov/iaq/asthma/index.html

V. National Asthma Education Prevention Program

www.nhlbi.nih.gov/about/naepp/index.htm

W. Environmental Tobacco Smoke: A Hazard to Children (RE9716) (American Academy of Pediatrics)

www.aap.org/policy/re9716.html

X. Living with Asthma: Special Concerns for Older Adults (National Heart, Lung, and Blood Institute)

www.nhlbi.nih.gov/health/public/lung/asthma/asth_ap.htm

Y. FASTATS: Asthma (National Center for Health Statistics)

www.cdc.gov/nchswww/fastats/asthma.htm

Z. Sulfites: Safe for Most, Dangerous for Some (Food and Drug Administration)

www.cfsan.fda.gov/~dms/fdsulfit.html

AA. Food Allergies: Rare but Risky (Food and Drug Administration)

www.cfsan.fda.gov/~dms/wh-alrg1.html

BB. Food Allergy and Intolerances (National Institute of Allergy and Infectious Diseases)

www.niaid.nih.gov/factsheets/food.htm

CC. Latex Allergy (American Academy of Family Physicians)

www.familydoctor.org/handouts/254.html

DD. Preventing Allergic Reactions to Natural Rubber Latex in the Workplace (Centers for Disease Control and Prevention)

www.cdc.gov/niosh/latexalt.html

III. Pharmaceutical Company–Sponsored Web Sites

Note: The authors do not endorse these companies' products but include these web sites as a source of useful general information.

A. Allerdays

www.allerdays.com
Sponsored by Hoechst Marion Roussel

B. IBreathe.com

www.ibreathe.com
Sponsored by GlaxoSmithKline

C. Schoolasthmaallergy.com

www.schoolasthma.com
Sponsored by Schering/Key

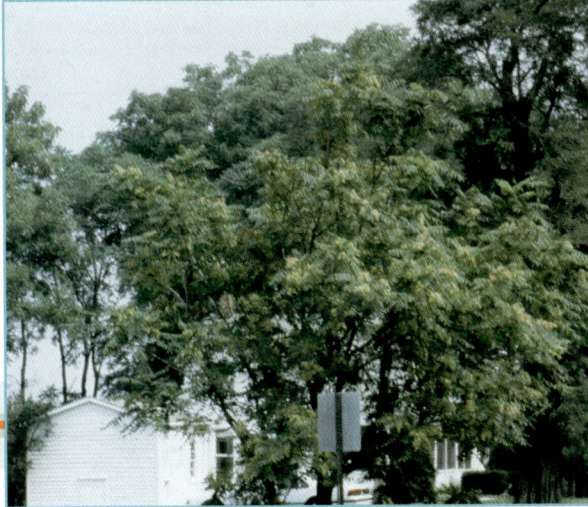

Tree of Heaven *Courtesy of Hollister-Stier Laboratory*

Antihistamines for Allergic Disorders

TABLE A10-1

Antihistamines for Use in Allergic Disorders

Generic Name	Trade Name	Dosage Adults	Children (<12 years of age)
Sedating			
Ethanolamine			
Diphenhydramine HCl	Benadryl	25–50 mg 3 or 4 times daily	5 mg/kg in 3 or 4 divided doses
Ethylenediamines			
Tripelennarmine	PBZ	25–50 mg 3 or 4 times daily	5 mg/kg in 3 or 4 divided doses
Alkylamines			
Chlorpheniramine maleate	Chlor-Trimeton	4 mg 3 or 4 times daily	0.4 mg/kg in 3 or 4 divided doses (<2 years: 1.25 mg 2 or 3 times daily)
Brompheniramine maleate	Dimetane	4 mg 3 or 4 times daily	0.4 mg/kg in 3 or 4 divided doses
Piperazines			
Hydroxyzine HCl	Atarax Vistaril	10–50 mg 3 or 4 times daily	2 mg/kg in 4 divided doses
Phenothiazines			
Promethazine HCl	Phenergan	12.5–25.0 mg 2 or 3 times daily	1 mg/kg divided into one-half dose before bedtime and 2 one-fourth doses during the day
Piperidines			
Azatadine maleate	Optimine	1–2 mg 2 times daily	
Miscellaneous			
Cyproheptadine HCl	Periactin	4 mg 3 or 4 times daily	0.25 mg/kg in 3 or 4 divided doses
Clemastine fumarate	Tavist	2.68 mg 2 times daily	
Nonsedating			
Fexofenadine	Allegra	60 mg 2 times daily or 180 mg once daily	
Loratadine	Claritin (Alavert, available OTC)	10 mg once daily	2–5 yrs: 5 mg once daily ≥6 yrs: 10 mg once daily
Desloratadine	Clarinex	5 mg once daily	
Certirizine	Zyrtec	5 or 10 mg tablets once daily	

Modified and updated with permission from Milgrom EC: Allergic rhinitis, part 2: Meeting the challenges of patient management. Fam Pract Recertification 1993;15:45–46.

INDEX

Note: Page numbers followed by "f" refer to figures; those followed by "t" refer to tables; and those followed by "b" refer to boxes.

A

Acne, steroid, 57, 58f
Acupuncture, 228
Adenoidal pad, 216f
β-Adrenergic agonists, in asthma, 29, 30t, 31
β-Adrenergic antagonists
  asthma and, 23
  epinephrine interactions with, 104, 106
Adverse drug reaction. *See* Drug allergy.
Adverse food reaction, 110, 111b. *See also* Food allergy.
Aerochamber, 185, 185f
African Americans
  atopic dermatitis in, 41f, 47f, 61
  urticaria in, 82, 84f
Africanized honeybee, 131, 131f, 132f. *See also* Insect
    hypersensitivity.
Air pollution, asthma and, 23
Alamast, in conjunctivitis, 126
Albuterol
  in anaphylaxis, 106
  in asthma, 29, 30t, 31
  in food allergy, 115
Allergen immunotherapy, 155–167
  alternative routes for, 166
  anaphylaxis with, 162–163, 240
  antigen for, 159–162
    classification of, 159
    dilutions of, 160–161, 161t
    dosages of, 160, 162
    manufacturers of, 247
    potency of, 162
    preparation of, 159–160, 159b, 160b
    selection of, 159
    terminology for, 241–242
  at home, 166
  away from home, 165–166

consent for, 237–238, 238b
controversial forms of, 230–232
documentation for, 239
duration of, 163–164
efficacy of, 156–157, 157b, 163, 229–230
emergency equipment for, 240
evaluation of, 163
food allergy and, 115
guidelines for, 157
ICD-9 codes for, 166–167
in allergic rhinitis, 156, 165
in asthma, 33, 156–157
in autoimmune disease, 165
in children, 164–165, 165b
in conjunctivitis, 126
in immunodeficiency disease, 165
in insect hypersensitivity, 134
in older adults, 164
in pregnant women, 164
in rhinitis, 10–11
indications for, 158
internet resources on, 166
local reactions to, 239
mechanism of action of, 155–156
negative studies of, 157
patient compliance with, 158
patient education on, 16
patient follow-up for, 240–241
patient selection for, 157–158, 158b
protocol for, 239
reactions to, 239–240
safety for, 162–163, 162t, 240
schedules for, 160, 161–162, 161t, 239
staffing for, 238–239
systemic reactions to, 240
terminology for, 241–242

Hormonal rhinitis, 6
Hornet, 130f. *See also* Insect hypersensitivity.
House dust mites, 5, 5f
    in asthma, 22
    in rhinitis, 8
    in skin test screening panel, 172t
Hydralazine, allergic reaction to, 140
Hydration, in atopic dermatitis, 57
Hydroxychloroquine, in asthma, 33
Hydroxyzine HCl (Atarax, Vistaril)
    in atopic dermatitis, 59–60
    in rhinitis, 9t, 266t
Hypersensitivity pneumonitis, vs. asthma, 20
Hypertension, ocular, steroids and, 32
Hypotension, in anaphylaxis, 105–106
Hypothyroidism, rhinitis and, 6

I
ICD-9 codes
    for allergen immunotherapy, 166–167
    for anaphylaxis, 107
    for asthma, 34
    for atopic dermatitis, 62
    for chronic hoarseness, 214b
    for chronic postnasal drip, 214b
    for chronic rhinitis, 214b
    for chronic sinusitis, 214b
    for conjunctivitis, 127
    for contact dermatitis, 76
    for drug allergy, 150
    for food allergy, 116
    for foreign body, possible, 214b
    for insect hypersensitivity, 135
    for nasal bleeding, 214b
    for nasal polyp(s), 214b
    for ocular allergy, 127
    for rhinitis, 13
    for urticaria, 93
Ichthyosis, 53, 53f
Idiopathic environmental intolerances, 223–224
Immediate IgE contact reaction, vs. contact dermatitis, 69
Immune complexes, 227
Immune globulin, intravenous, in asthma, 33
Immunoglobulin E (IgE), serum, 227
    by age, 248t
    in asthma, 21, 22
    in atopic dermatitis, 52
    in conjunctivitis, 123
    in rhinitis, 8
Immunoglobulin G (IgG), 226–227
Immunotherapy. *See* Allergen immunotherapy.
Infants, atopic dermatitis in, 41–42, 42f, 43f, 52, 61
Infectious rhinitis, 5
Inhalers, 183–185, 184f, 185f
    spacers with, 185–187, 186f
Insect hypersensitivity, 129–135
    age and, 134
    clinical manifestations of, 131
    consultation for, 134

death from, 132
diagnosis of, 133, 135f
differential diagnosis of, 131–132
drug effects in, 134
epidemiology of, 129, 130f, 131f
etiology of, 129, 131
ICD-9 codes for, 135
internet resources for, 135
laboratory evaluation of, 132–133
large local reaction in, 131, 134
lifestyle and, 134
patient education on, 135, 135b
physical examination in, 132
practice guidelines for, 134–135
sting reaction in, 131
systemic allergic reaction in, 131
toxic reaction in, 131
treatment of, 133–134, 133t, 135f
vs. urticaria, 85, 85f
InspirEase device, 185, 186f
Interferon, in atopic dermatitis, 61
Internet resources, 262–264
    for consumers, 262–263
    for journals, 263–264
    on anaphylaxis, 107
    on asthma, 35–36
    on atopic dermatitis, 62
    on conjunctivitis, 127
    on contact dermatitis, 76
    on drug allergy, 149
    on food allergy, 115–116
    on insect hypersensitivity, 135
    on ocular allergy, 127
    on rhinitis, 13
    on urticaria, 93
    pharmaceutical company–sponsored, 264
Interstitial nephritis, in drug allergy, 141
Interstitial pneumonitis, in drug allergy, 141
Iodoxamide tromethamine (Alomide), in conjunctivitis, 125t
Ioteprednol (Alrex), in conjunctivitis, 125t
Ipratropium
    in asthma, 30t, 31
    in rhinitis, 10, 11t
    patient education on, 16
Irrigation, in conjunctivitis, 123, 124t
Itching
    in anaphylaxis, 99
    in atopic dermatitis, 46
    in urticaria, 82

J
Jewelry, dermatitis with, 75, 75f

K
Kamut, 255
Keratoconjunctivitis
    atopic, 120t, 121f, 122, 122b
    vernal, 120t, 121f, 122
Keratosis pilaris, 53, 53f